# PARKINSON'S DISEASE
Neurophysiological, Clinical, and Related Aspects

# ADVANCES IN EXPERIMENTAL MEDICINE AND BIOLOGY

## Recent Volumes in this Series

# PARKINSON'S DISEASE
Neurophysiological, Clinical,
and Related Aspects

Edited by
## Fathy S. Messiha
## and Alexander D. Kenny
Texas Tech University School of Medicine
Lubbock, Texas

PLENUM PRESS • NEW YORK AND LONDON

Library of Congress Cataloging in Publication Data

Tarbox Parkinson's Disease Symposium, 1st, Lubbock, Tex., 1976.
  Parkinson's disease.

  (Advances in experimental medicine and biology; v. 90)
  Includes index.
  1. Parkinsonism—Congresses. I. Messiha, Fathy S. II. Kenny, Alexander D. III.
Texas Tech University. Dept. of Pharmacology and Therapeutics. IV. Tarbox
Parkinson's Disease Institute. V. Title. VI. Series. [DNLM: 1. Parkinsonism—Con-
gresses. W1 AD559 v. 90 1976/WL359 T179 1976p]
RC382.T37 1976                    616.8'33                    77-21498
ISBN 978-1-4684-2513-0     ISBN 978-1-4684-2511-6 (eBook)
DOI 10.1007/978-1-4684-2511-6

Proceedings of the First Tarbox Parkinson's Disease Symposium held
at Lubbock, Texas, October 14–16, 1976, and sponsored by

Texas Tech University School of Medicine
  Department of Pharmacology and Therapeutics
  Tarbox Parkinson's Disease Institute
  Office of Continuing Education and Faculty Development

and
American Association of Neurological Surgeons

© 1977 Plenum Press, New York
Softcover reprint of the hardcover 1st edition 1977
A Division of Plenum Publishing Corporation
227 West 17th Street, New York, N.Y. 10011

## SYMPOSIUM CHAIRMAN

Alexander D. Kenny, Ph.D., Professor and Chairman
Department of Pharmacology and Therapeutics, and
Acting Director, Tarbox Parkinson's Disease Institute
Texas Tech University School of Medicine, Lubbock.

## COMMITTEE MEMBERS

Roy C. Allen, Ed.D., Office of Continuing Education and
Faculty Development, Texas Tech University School of
Medicine (TTUSM).

Charles D. Barnes, Ph.D., Professor and Chairman,
Department of Physiology, TTUSM.

James E. Dyson, Ph.D., Director, Continuing Education
and Faculty Development, TTUSM.

Tamas L. Frigyesi, M.D., Professor, Department of
Physiology, TTUSM.

William H. Gordon, Jr., J.D., M.D., Clinical Professor
and Chairman, Department of Neurology, TTUSM.

J. Barry Lombardini, Ph.D., Associate Professor, Department of Pharmacology and Therapeutics, TTUSM.

Fathy S. Messiha, Ph.D., Associate Professor, Departments of Pharmacology and Therapeutics and Psychiatry,
TTUSM; Chairman, Program Committee.

Peter K. T. Pang, Ph.D., Associate Professor, Department of Pharmacology and Therapeutics, TTUSM.

James H. Pirch, Ph.D., Associate Professor, Department
of Pharmacology and Therapeutics, TTUSM.

David E. Potter, Ph.D., Associate Professor, Department
of Pharmacology and Therapeutics, TTUSM.

Lou A. Roberts, Ph.D., Instructor, Department of
Physiology, TTUSM.

Donald L. Wilbur, Ph.D., Assistant Professor, Department of Anatomy, TTUSM.

v

# INVITED SPEAKERS

DONALD B. CALNE, M.D., F.R.C.P.

Clinical Director, National Institute of Neurological and
Communicative Disorders and Stroke, National Institutes
of Health, Bethesda, Maryland, U.S.A.

JACK C. DE LA TORRE, Sc.D.

Associate Professor of Neurosurgery and Psychiatry,
Division of Neurosurgery, Pritzker School of Medicine,
University of Chicago, Chicago, Illinois, U.S.A.

ROGER C. DUVOISIN, M.D.

Professor of Neurology, Mount Sinai School of Medicine,
The City University of New York, New York, New York, U.S.A.

STANLEY FAHN, M.D.

Professor of Neurology, Department of Neurology and
Neurological Institute of New York, College of Physicians
and Surgeons, Columbia University, New York, New York,
U.S.A.

TAMAS L. FRIGYESI, M.D.

Professor of Physiology, Texas Tech University School of
Medicine, Lubbock, Texas, U.S.A.

OLEH HORNYKIEWICZ, M.D.

Director, Biochemical Pharmacology Institute, University
of Vienna School of Medicine, Vienna, Austria; Professor
of Pharmacology and Head, Department of Psychopharmacology,
Clarke Institute of Psychiatry, Toronto, Canada.

HAROLD L. KLAWANS, M.D.

Professor of Neurology and Director, Division of Neurology,
Department of Medicine, Pritzker School of Medicine,
University of Chicago, and Michael Reese Hospital and
Medical Center, Chicago, Illinois, U.S.A.

# OTHER SPEAKERS AND DISCUSSANTS

C. D. Barnes, Department of Physiology, Texas Tech University School of Medicine, Lubbock, Texas.

R. W. Bell, Department of Psychology, Texas Tech University, Lubbock, Texas.

E. C. Clark, Department of Neurosciences, Mount Zion Medical Center, San Francisco, California.

Y. D. Clement-Cormier, Deparment of Pharmacology, University of Texas Medical School at Houston, Houston, Texas.

C. P. De Francisco, National Institute of Neurology, Mexico City, Mexico.

H. M. Erickson, Departments of Psychiatry and Pediatrics, Texas Tech University School of Medicine, Lubbock, Texas.

A. Flemenbaum, Department of Psychiatry, Texas Tech School of Medicine, Lubbock, Texas.

W. Flores, Lovington, New Mexico.

D. N. Franz, Department of Pharmacology, University of Utah School of Medicine, Salt Lake City, Utah.

S. J. Fung, Department of Physiology, Texas Tech University School of Medicine, Lubbock, Texas.

M. M. Hoehn, Department of Neurology, University of Colorado School of Medicine, Denver, Colorado.

G. M. Hunt, Loma Linda University Medical Center, Loma Linda, California.

D. Lake, Department of Physiology, Texas Tech University School of Medicine, Lubbock, Texas.

K. A. Lloyd, Department of Psychopharmacology, and Clarke Institute of Psychiatry, University of Toronto, Toronto, Canada.

H. Mars, Department of Neurology, Case-Western Reserve Medical School, Cleveland, Ohio.

F. A. Messiha, Departments of Pharmacology and Therapeutics and
    Psychiatry, Texas Tech University School of Medicine,
    Lubbock, Texas.

J. H. Pirch, Department of Pharmacology and Therapeutics, Texas
    Tech University School of Medicine, Lubbock, Texas.

D. E. Potter, Department of Pharmacology and Therapeutics, Texas
    Tech University School of Medicine, Lubbock, Texas.

U. K. Rinne, Department of Neurology, University of Turku, Turku,
    Finland.

A. Rix, Oklahoma City, Oklahoma.

C. N. Still, Department of Neuropsychiatry and Behavioal Sciences
    and the William S. Hall Psychiatric Institute, University of
    South Carolina School of Medicine, Columbia, South Carolina.

P. Volkman, Department of Pharmacology, University of Chicago
    Pritzker School of Medicine, Chicago, Illinois.

D. D. Webster, Department of Neurology, University of Minnesota
    School of Medicine and Veterans Administration Hospital,
    Minneapolis, Minnesota.

R. L. Weddige, Department of Psychiatry, Texas Tech University
    School of Medicine, Lubbock, Texas.

# PREFACE

These Proceedings are the outcome of the First Tarbox Parkinson's Disease Symposium held October 14-16, 1976, at the South Park Inn in Lubbock, Texas. The Symposium was sponsored by the Department of Pharmacology and Therapeutics and the Tarbox Parkinson's Disease Institute of the Texas Tech University School of Medicine at Lubbock.

The Tarbox Parkinson's Disease Institute was established in 1973 with funds appropriated by the State of Texas and is dedicated to research, patient care, and educational activities related to Parkinson's disease. The Institute is named after Mr. Elmer L. Tarbox, who recently served the Lubbock area as a Representative to the Texas Legislature, and is himself a parkinsonian patient. Mr. and Mrs. Tarbox attended the Symposium as honored guests.

The First Tarbox Parkinson's Disease Symposium was devoted to both basic and clinical aspects of Parkinson's disease, with an emphasis on discussion of drug therapy. This discussion focused not only on readily available drugs such as levodopa, but also on new investigational drugs such as bromocriptine.

Thanks are especially due to Thelma Saunders and the office staff of the Department of Pharmacology and Therapeutics, Texas Tech University School of Medicine, for their excellent service in producing camera-ready copy for the Publisher. Thanks are also due to Fathy S. Messiha, Program Chairman, to the other committee members, and to the staff of the Office of Continuing Education and Faculty Development. The Symposium could not have succeeded without their help.

Alexander D. Kenny

# CONTENTS

Invited Speakers

# HISTORICAL ASPECTS AND FRONTIERS OF PARKINSON'S DISEASE RESEARCH

OLEH HORNYKIEWICZ

Institute of Biochemical Pharmacology
University of Vienna
Vienna, Austria

## I HISTORICAL ASPECTS

From the historical point of view it would appear that right from the beginning of the era that we call modern medicine, drugs have been regarded as important tools in elucidating the biochemical pathology of disease.  In the history of Parkinson's disease there has been hardly a drug that has not been tried as a potential remedy.  The long list includes such oddities as ferrisulfate, barium chloride, strychnine, metrazol, thyroid and parathyroid hormones, and - surprizingly - striaphorin, an extract of the striatum.  Of all the older antiparkinson drugs, anticholinergics attained special significance because of their unquestionable (though low) therapeutic efficacy.  However, these drugs also led the thinking of researchers astray because for a long time the effectiveness of the anticholinergic agents was taken as evidence that Parkinson's disease may be primarily a disorder of cholinergic brain mechanisms.

The new era of the neurochemistry of Parkinson's disease began in the early fifties with the drug reserpine, one of the pharmacologically active ingredients of the Indian plant Rauwolfia serpentina.  The reserpine story has been often recounted.  After the introduction of reserpine in the western hemisphere as an anti-hypertensive and antipsychotic medication, it soon became evident that apart from its therapeutic properties, this drug produced

highly interesting and unusual side effects. Among reserpine's
manyfold side effects, catalepsy in laboratory animals and a reversible Parkinsonism-like condition in the human were most intriguing.
Therefore, when in the late fifties, Carlsson and his collaborators
showed that reserpine, in addition to its already known effects on
brain noradrenaline (NA) and serotonin (5-HT), also depleted the
brain of its dopamine (DA) (whose preferential localization in the
corpus striatum of laboratory animals had also been established at
about the same time by this research group) and that L-dopa, the
precursor of DA and NA in the body, antagonized the reserpine-in-
duced catalepsy, the stage was set for the story of brain DA to
begin *(Bertler and Rosengren, 1959; Carlsson, 1959; Carlsson et al.
1957, 1958)*.

However, the brain DA story had an intriguing prelude - a prelude that potentially could have significantly accelerated progress
in the field of neurochemistry of Parkinson's disease.  Starting in
the late forties, Wilhelm Raab described the occurrence of a new
catechol compound in the mammalian brain, including human brain
*(Raab and Gigee, 1951)*.  Raab named this compound encephalin.  After
establishing its occurence, Raab determined the regional distribution of encephalin in the human brain, and found that its highest
concentrations could be measured in the caudate nucleus.  Not content
with this observation Raab went on studying the effect of drugs on
the concentration of this new "adrenaline-like" substance in the
rat brain.  He discovered that out of a host of diverse drugs, only
L-dopa affected significantly the concentration of encephalin.  It
is quite exiting to read Raab's report on the time course of the
L-dopa induced increase in the encephalin level in the rat brain;
this account reads like a recent description of the typical L-dopa
effect on brain DA.  There can be little doubt that - albeit unknow-
ingly - Raab had discovered most of the relevant facts about brain
DA.  Had Raab included in his study, in addition to human control
brains, also brains of patients with Parkinson's disease, he probably would have discovered the characteristic deficiency of his
"encephalin" in this disorder.  This short prelude to the DA story
properly demonstrates how close one can come to making an important
discovery - and how easily one can miss it.

Ten years after Raab's observations, the discoveries of the
Swedish workers provided the first useful basis for the beginning
of the new era in neurochemistry of Parkinson's disease.  The story
of DA in Parkinson's disease began in 1959 in the basement of the
Department of Pharmacology of the University of Vienna where, at
that time, I had my laboratory.  Putting aside all at that time
justifiable doubts regarding the usefulness of postmortem material
for biochemical studies, we began to examine the behaviour of DA
and NA in the brain of patients with Parkinson's disease, comparing
the results with those obtained in the brain of non-neurological
controls of comparable pre- and postmortem history.  Already the

very first results showed that in Parkinson's disease there was a
characteristic deficiency of DA in the nuclei of the basal ganglia,
notably the caudate nucleus, putamen, substantia nigra and globus
pallidus *(Bernheimer et al. 1963; Ehringer and Hornykiewicz, 1960;
Hornykiewicz, 1963).* Subsequently, it was shown in a series of
systematic studies, that a similar decrease was present in the DA
metabolite homovanillic acid, and in the synthesizing enzymes
tyrosine hydroxylase and L-dopa decarboxylase *(Bernheimer and
Hornykiewicz, 1965; Lloyd and Hornykiewicz, 1970; Lloyd et al.,
1975).* All of these biochemical alterations are apparently due
to the degeneration of the pars compacta of the substantia nigra;
the latter change represents a characteristic morphological feature
of Parkinson's disease. This conclusion is supported by the observation that the degree of DA deficiency in the striatum was directly
proportional to the degree of cell loss in this part of the substantia nigra *(Bernheimer et al., 1973).* Since striatal DA deficiency proved to be a constant finding in the Parkinsonian syndrome
regardless of etiology *(Ehringer and Hornykiewicz, 1960; Bernheimer
et al., 1973),* a replacement therapy with L-dopa (DA's immediate
metabolic precurosr which passes the blood-brain barrier) was a
logical and, as it turned out, important clinical consequence of
this line of neurochemical research *(Birkmayer and Hornykiewicz,
1961; Barbeau et al., 1962; Cotzias et al., 1967).* The possibility
that L-dopa was a specific (though mainly symptomatic) drug for
Parkinson's disease, was indirectly supported by findings that
seemed to establish a link between the striatal DA deficiency and
the main extrapyramidal symptomatology of this disorder, namely:
(a) in hemiparkinsonism, the degree of DA deficiency was shown to
be more pronounced in the striatum contralateral to the side of
the symptoms *(Barolin et al., 1964);* and (b) the degree of extrapyramidal symptoms (especially akinesia) was found to correlate
significantly with the degree of DA changes in the nuclei of the
basal ganglia *(Bernheimer et al., 1973).* More recently, direct
evidence has been furnished for L-dopa's potential to replace the
missing DA by showing that in patients treated with L-dopa, the
striatal DA levels were greatly increased as compared with untreated cases, approaching control values in some individuals
*(Lloyd et al., 1975).*

All of the above observations permit the conclusion that deficiency of striatal DA represents a neurochemical alteration characteristic for Parkinson's disease. Although most of this work is of
recent date, already it can be regarded as representing part of the
historical aspects of the development of our concepts on Parkinson's
disease.

II FRONTIERS

Turning to the frontiers of Parkinson's disease research, I

want to focus especially on two aspects, namely the behaviour of
the recently much discussed mesolimbic DA, and secondly, the possible neurohumoral interactions in the striatum.

A. *The mesolimbic DA*.  It has been known for some time that in
addition to the large nigro-striatal DA system, there are other
dopaminergic pathways in the mammalian brain (*cf. Fuxe et al.,
1970*).  Among these, the mesolimbic DA system has attracted particular attention.  In the human brain (*Farley et al., 1977*) most of
the areas of the classical limbic lobe as defined by Broca, are poor
in DA; an exception is the parolfactory gyrus (area 25 in Brodmann's
classification) with DA concentrations ranging between 0.3 - 0.4
ug/g fresh tissue.  In contrast, the distribution of DA in the subcortical areas of the limbic forebrain is more widespread.  Similar
as in laboratory animals, the highest DA concentration is found in
the nucleus accumbens.  The next highest levels are found in the
nucleus of the stria terminalis and the medial olfactory area, the
ventral septum, the lateral hypothalamic area, and the mammillary
bodies.  In the brain of patients with Parkinson's disease, the DA
concentration in these limbic structures was found to be affected
in an uneven manner (*Farley et al., 1977*).  In the parolfactory
gyrus, the DA concentration was less than 10 per cent of the normal
value.  In the nucleus accumbens, the level was 40 per cent of the
control value.  In contrast, DA in the medial and lateral olfactory
areas did not show significant changes from normal.  These recent
observations seem to indicate that in respect to limbic DA, Parkinson's disease apparently has a characteristic effect predominantly
on the parolfactory gyrus and the nucleus accumbens.  In this
respect it is interesting to note that in these areas DA is depleted to the same extent as in the putamen and caudate nucleus,
respectively.  Although in laboratory animals the main source of
the dopaminergic innervation of the limbic forebrain seems to be
the A10 cell group of the mesencephalic tegmentum (*cf. Fuxe et al.,
1970*), there is evidence to show that the substantia nigra also may
contribute to this limbic DA (*Nauta, 1977*).  It is thus possible
that the parallel depletion of DA in the parolfactory area and the
putamen, as observed in patients with Parkinson's disease, may be
the result of cell loss in those subdivisions of the compact layer
of the substantia nigra (namely the posterior and lateral parts)
which are known to project to the putamen (*cf. Bernheimer et al.,
1973*).  In analogy, the fact that the DA decrease in the nucleus
accumbens was quite similar to that seen in the caudate nucleus,
may also indicate a common origin of dopaminergic innervation of
these two regions.  This possibility seems to be supported by
recent observations showing that there is a considerable overlap
between the nigral and A10 innervations of the basal ganglia
(*Nauta, 1977*).

The decrease of DA in the nucleus accumbens and the parolfactory
gyrus in patients with Parkinson's disease can be expected to have

functional implications.  At present nothing is known about the significance of the DA in the parolfactory region.  However, the nucleus
accumbens has recently been implicated in several aspects of motor
behaviour *(Pijnenburg et al., 1976)*.  It is therefore possible that
certain aspects of motor deficits in Parkinson's disease (such as for
instance akinesia) may not be solely striatal in origin but may, in
addition, involve the dopaminergic innervation of the nucleus accumbens.

   *B. Neurohumoral Interactions in the Striatum*.  In addition to
DA, the basal ganglia contain high concentrations of other neuro-
humors, e.g. gamma-aminobutyric acid (GABA), 5-HT, acetylcholine
(ACh), and NA (the latter preferentially in the nucleus accumbens).
In the regulation of normal movement the striatal cells must somehow
integrate multiple inputs involving many neurochemically distinct
transmitter substances *(cf. Hornykiewicz, 1976)*.  Although we are
just at the very beginning of our understanding of these complex
neurochemical relationships, some of the patterns of interactions
are becoming known.  Thus, there is evidence showing that the GABA
system inhibits the DA system *(Andén, 1974; Lahti and Losey, 1974;
Tarsy et al., 1975)*.  Similarly, the 5-HT system seems to be
inhibitory in respect to the DA and NA systems *(Grabowska and
Michaluk, 1974; Hollister et al., 1975; Maj et al., 1974)*.  Both of
these effects may involve the recently demonstrated GABAergic and
the serotonergic innervations respectively, of the substantia nigra.
With the nigro-striatal and limbic DA systems deranged in Parkinson's
disease, it is perhaps not surprizing that these other neurohumoral
systems in the basal ganglia also show abnormalities.  For example,
in Parkinson's disease the level of glutamic acid decarboxylase (GAD),
the enzyme that synthesizes GABA from glutamate, is also reduced,
especially in the caudate nucleus, putamen, globus pallidus and the
substantia nigra *(Bernheimer and Hornykiewicz, 1962; Lloyd and
Hornykiewicz, 1973)*.  Similarly, the concentration of 5-HT and its
metabolite 5-hydroxyindoleacetic acid is subnormal in Parkinson's
disease in many forebrain areas, including the basal ganglia regions
*(Bernheimer et al., 1961; Lloyd, Farley and Hornykiewicz, manuscript
in preparation)*.  Finally, the NA forebrain system, which is
especially well represented in the nucleus accumbens and the
hypothalamus, is also affected in Parkinson's disease; particularly
pronounced decreases are seen in the nucleus accumbens, the hypothalamus and the olfactory areas, with other forebrain regions,
such as the septum, showing smaller or no NA changes *(Farley and
Hornykiewicz, 1977)*.

   At present, it is difficult to assess the functional significance
of these changes in neurotransmitter systems other than DA.  Thus, it
is possible that the deficiencies seen in GAD and 5-HT do not have an
antomical substrate at all; rather, they may represent only functional
changes so as to compensate for the loss of the dopaminergic influence
upon the striatum.  There is reason to believe that the decrease of

striatal DA is primarily related to akinesia (and possibly rigidity) *(Bernheimer et al., 1973)*; the foremost effect of L-dopa is to counteract this symptom by restoring striatal DA to functionally critical levels *(Lloyd et al., 1975)*. However, the decrease in NA in the nucleus accumbens (and elsewhere) may significantly contribute to the Parkinsonian akinesia. Pharmacological evidence suggests that brain NA plays an important auxiliary role for the DA-controlled locomotor activity *(for ref. cf. Lloyd and Hornykiewicz, 1975)*. L-dopa's strong anti-akinesia effect may have something to do with this, since the drug can be expected to have an effect on brain NA levels as well as DA levels. Since according to recent evidence the 5-HT system in the brain is inhibitory to the DA and NA systems (see above) the lowered levels of brain 5-HT in Parkinson's disease simply may represent an attempt of the affected brain regions to prevent (compensate for) excessive inhibition of an already underactive (DA and NA) system. This would perhaps act to lessen symptoms such as akinesia which result from the striatal DA deficiency. An analogous situation may pertain with regards to the (possibly) lowered activity of the GABA system in the basal ganglia of patients with Parkinson's disease. As mentioned above, the GABA system also seems to inhibit the nigro-striatal DA system (at the level of the substantia nigra). In contradistinction, the cholinergic striatal systems are normally inhibited by the DA system *(cf. Bartholini et al., 1975)*. In Parkinson's disease the cholinergic systems may become overactive due to disinhibition (because of the striatal DA deficiency) and thus contribute to the symptoms of Parkinsonism. L-dopa may normalize the cholinergic hyperactivity in the basal ganglia by reinstating the dopaminergic inhibition. Although the above conclusions regarding neurohumoral interactions in Parkinson's disease are at present rather hypothetical, future research on diseases of the basal ganglia should pay close attention to these possibilities. For some of the as yet neurochemically poorly defined basal ganglia disorders these possibilities may turn out to be of primary importance.

## REFERENCES

Andén, N.-E. (1974). Inhibition of the turnover of the brain dopamine after treatment with the gamma-aminobutyrate:2-oxyglutarate transaminase inhibitor aminooxyacetic acid. *Arch Pharmacol.* *283*, 419-424.

Barbeau, A., Sourkes, T.L. and Murphy, G. (1962). Les catecholamines dans la maladie de Parkinson. *In Monoamines et System Nerveux Central* (Ajuriaguerra, J.de, Ed.) pp. 247-262. Georg, Geneva and Masson, Paris.

Barolin, G.S., Bernheimer, H. and Hornykiewicz, O. (1964). Seitenverschiedenes Verhalten des Dopamins (3-Hydroxytyramin) im Gehirn eines Falles von Hemiparkinsonismus. *Schweiz. Arch. Neurol. Psychiat. 94*, 241-248.

Bartholini, G., Stadler, H. and Lloyd, K.G. (1975). Cholinergic-dopaminergic interregulations within the extrapyramidal system. *In Cholinergic Mechanisms* (Waser, P.G., Ed.) pp. 411-418. Raven Press, New York.

Bernheimer, H. and Hornykiewicz, O. (1962). Das Verhalten einiger Enzyme im Gehirn normaler und Parkinsonkranker Menschen. *Arch. exp. Path. Pharmak. 243,* 295.

Bernheimer, H. and Hornykiewicz, O. (1965). Herabgesetzte Konzentration der homovanillinsäure im Gehirn von Parkinsonkranken Menschen als Ausdruck der Störung des zentralen Dopaminstoffwechsels. *Klin.Wschr. 43,* 711-715.

Bernheimer, H., Birkmayer, W. and Hornykiewicz, O. (1961). Verteilung des 5-Hydroxytryptamins (Serotonin) im Gehirn des Menschen und sein Verhalten bei Patienten mit Parkinson-Syndrom. *Klin.Wschr. 39,* 1056-1059.

Bernheimer, H., Birkmayer, W. and Hornykiewicz, O. (1963). Zur Biochemie des Parkinson-Syndroms des Menschen. *Klin. Wschr. 41,* 465-469.

Bernheimer, H., Birkmayer, W., Hornykiewicz, O., Jellinger, K. and Seitelberger, F. (1973). Brain dopamine and the syndromes of Parkinson and Huntington. *J. Neurol. Sci. 20,* 415-455.

Bertler, A. and Rosengren, E. (1959). Occurrence and distribution of dopamine in brain and other tissues. *Experientia 15,* 10-11.

Birkmayer, W. and Hornykiewicz, O. (1961). Der L-Dioxyphenylalanin (= L-DOPA)-Effekt bei der Parkinson-Akinese. *Wien.Klin.Wschr. 73,* 787-788.

Carlsson, A. (1959). The occurrence, distribution and physiological role of catecholamines in the nervous system. *Pharmacol. Rev. 11,* 490-493.

Carlsson, A., Lindqvist, M. and Magnusson, T. (1957). 3,4-Dihydroxyphenylalanine and 5-hydroxytryptophan as reserpine antagonists. *Nature 180,* 1200.

Carlsson, A., Lindqvist, M., Magnusson, T. and Waldeck, B. (1958). On the presence of 3-hydroxytyramine in brain. *Science 127,* 471.

Cotzias, G.C., Van Woert, M.H. and Schiffer, L.M. (1967). Aromatic amino acids and modification of parkinsonism. *New Engl. J. Med. 276,* 374-379.

Ehringer, H. and Hornykiewicz, O. (1960). Verteilung von Noradrenalin und Dopamin (3-Hydroxytyramin) im Gehirn des Menschen und ihr Verhalten bei Erkrankungen des extrapyramidalen Systems. *Klin.Wschr. 38,* 1236-1239.

Farley, I.J. and Hornykiewicz, O. (1977). Noradrenaline in subcortical brain regions of patients with Parkinson's disease and control subjects. *In Advances in Parkinsonism, Biochemistry, Physiology, Treatment* (Birkmayer, W. and Hornykiewicz, O., Eds.) Editiones Roche, Basel (in press).

Farley, I.J., Price, K.S. and Hornykiewicz, O. (1977). Dopamine in
    the limbic regions of the human brain: normal and abnormal.
    *In Advances in Biochem. Psychopharmacol. vol. 16* (Costa, E.
    and Gessa, G.L., Eds.) pp. 57-64. Raven Press, New York.
Fuxe, K., Hökfelt, T. and Ungerstedt, U. (1970). Morphological and
    functional aspects of central monoamine neurons. *Int. Rev.
    Neurobiol. 13*, 93-126.
Grabowska, M. and Michaluk, J. (1974). On the role of serotonin in
    apomorphine-induced locomotor stimulation in rats. *Pharmacol-
    ogy, Biochemistry and Behavior 2*, 263-266.
Hollister, A.S., Breese, G.R., Kuhn, C.M., Cooper, B.R. and Shanberg,
    S.M. (1975). Evidence for an inhibitory function of brain
    serotonin systems in the locomotor stimulant effects of
    D-amphetamine. *Neurosci. Abstr. 1*, 297.
Hornykiewicz, O. (1963). Die topische Lokalisation und Verhalten
    von Noradrenalin und Dopamin (3-Hydroxytyramin) in der Sub-
    stantia nigra des normalen und Parkinsonkranken Menschen.
    *Wien.Klin.Wschr. 75*, 309-312.
Hornykiewicz, O. (1976). Neurohumoral interactions and basal ganglia
    function and dysfunction. *In The Basal Ganglia* (Yahr, M.D.,
    Ed.) pp. 269-278. Raven Press, New York.
Lahti, R.A. and Losey, E.G. (1974). Antagonism of the effects of
    chlorpromazine and morphine on dopamine metabolism by GABA.
    *Res. Commun. Chem. Pathol. Pharmacol. 7*, 31-40.
Lloyd, K.G. and Hornykiewicz, O. (1970). Parkinson's disease:
    activity of L-DOPA decarboxylase in discrete brain regions.
    *Science 170*, 1212-1213.
Lloyd, K.G. and Hornykiewicz, O. (1973). L-Glutamic acid decarboxy-
    lase in Parkinson's disease: effect of L-dopa therapy.
    *Nature 243*, 521-523.
Lloyd, K.G. and Hornykiewicz, O. (1975). Catecholamines in regulation
    of motor function. *In Catecholamines and Behavior, vol. 1*
    (Friedhoff, A.J., Ed.) pp. 41-57. Plenum Publ. Comp., New York.
Lloyd, K.G., Davidson, L. and Hornykiewicz, O. (1975). The neuro-
    chemistry of Parkinson's disease: effect of L-dopa therapy.
    *J. Pharmacol. 195*, 453-464.
Maj, J., Pawlowski, L. and Sarnek, J. (1974). The role of brain
    5-hydroxytryptamine in the central action of L-DOPA. *In
    Advances in Biochem. Psychopharmacol. vol. 10* (Costa, E.,
    Gessa, G.L. and Sandler, M., Eds.) pp. 253-256. Raven Press,
    New York.
Nauta, W.J.H. (1977). Some cross-roads of limbic and striatal
    circuitry. *In The Continuing Evolution of the Limbic System
    Concept* (Livingston, K. and Hornykiewicz, O., Eds.). Plenum
    Press, New York (in press).
Pijnenburg. A.J.J., Honig, W.M.M., Van der Heyden, J.A.M. and Van
    Rossum, J.M. (1976). Effects of chemical stimulation of the
    mesolimbic dopamine system upon locomotor activity. *Europ.
    J. Pharmacol. 35*, 45-58.

Raab, W. and Gigee, W. (1951). Concentration and distribution of "encephalin" in the brain of humans and animals. *Proc. Soc. exp. Bio. 76,* 97-100.

Tarsy, D., Pycock, C., Meldrum, B. and Marsden, C.D. (1975). Rotational behaviour induced in rats by intranigral picrotoxin. *Brain Res. 89,* 160-165.

## *DISCUSSION*

### *Dr. Flemenbaum*

Dr. Frigyesi, could you summarize the question so that some of us that are not so knowledgeable can understand what your question is?

### *Dr. Frigyesi*

Electrophysiological data seem to indicate that the substantia nigra is connected by a large fiber system to the nucleus accumbens and by a small fiber system to the rest of the caudate nucleus. Biochemical, histochemical, other studies indicate that only the large cells contain dopamine in the substantia nigra. My question: are there dopamine containing cells in the nigra?

### *Dr. Hornykiewicz*

I cannot answer the question from my own experience, but I find this a very interesting point; I must admit that I was not really familiar with these details like the latencies which you studied in your work, which is as such known to me. Now, one could say the following. Firstly, the flourescence histochemical work suggests that the dopamine is in the nucleus accumbens, in the rat at least, is contained in neurons originating not in the substantia nigra proper, but in the area A-10 which is just dorsal and lateral to the inter-peduncular nucleus. This pathway belongs to the so-called mesolimbic dopamine system. Now, it cannot be excluded that these neurons might actually have electrophysiological characteristics which are different from those of the nigra striatal neurons. I cannot remember the exact stimulation parameters in your studies. Possibly the electrical current also involved the stimulation of the mesolimbic system which passes very close to the nigro-striatal pathway. Now, for the human brain, the situation is not so simple. We have new data to support the idea that at least part of the dopamine in the nucleus accumbens derives from the substantia nigra and not from the area A-10. This, by the way, may also be the case in the cat. Moore, Bhatnagar and Heller have shown that clearcut destruction of the substantia nigra which, according to the anatomical pictures which they show in their work certainly does not involve the area A-10, does decrease the dopamine in the nucleus accumbens. The second point is that in your work you did not stimulate exclusively the dopaminergic neurons. The accumbens receives a substantial input

from the noradrenergic system, expecially in the human brain, but
also in the animal brain; you may have stimulated the noradrenergic
neurons terminating in the accumbens.  The noradrenergic neurons
may well possess neurophysiological characteristics quite different
from those of the nigro-striatal dopamine neurons.  So there are
several different possibilities; you were correct in mentioning the
Zona reticulata of the substantia nigra whose projection system may
contain acetylcholine and might also have a higher conduction velocity than the dopaminergic neurons.

## Dr. de la Torre

I think we should make a distinction when we talk about the
nucleus accumbens between the rat and the human.  When we talk about
the nucleus accumbens in the human, we are talking about the nucleus
accumbens septi, which correlates more neuroanatomically to the rat
septal region while the nucleus accumbens in the rat is functionally
another area that does not correlate with any neuroanatomical structure in the human brain.  I also had a question regarding your work
with GAD and the decreasing turnover in GABA; in view of the fact
that there has been some reports showing a decrease in the amounts
of GABA in Huntington's chorea, I wonder if you would comment as to
the relationship between Huntington's chorea and Parkinson's
disease, as far as the fact that L-dopa appears to exacerbate the
syndrome of Huntington's chorea and appears to increase GAD in
parkinsonian patients?

## Dr. Hornykiewicz

I do not think that L-dopa's aggravating effect in Huntington's
chorea is related to the "increase" in GAD activity as observed in our
Parkinsonian patients.  One has to keep in mind that the effect on
GAD in Parkinsonian patients only becomes apparent after very prolonged administration of L-dopa (one year or longer) whereas L-dopa
aggravates the Huntington's chorea symtomatology acutely after a
single dose.  On the contrary, it is known that acute L-dopa administration decreases brain GAD activity by binding vitamin $B_6$, GAD's
co-factor.  This effect may very well be involved in worsening of the
choreatic condition produced acutely by L-dopa.  On the other hand,
it is of course quite interesting that Huntington's chorea, which
clinically is the mirror image of Parkinson's disease, qualitatively
has the same alteration in striatal GAD activity as in Parkinson's
disease.  What that means functionally, I simply don't know.  In a
way, it is a disquieting situation even casting some doubt as to the
specificity of the derangement of the striatal GABA system in Huntington's chorea.

## Dr. Fahn

Just a followup on the previous question about the origin of
the dopamine fibers to the accumbens.  I would like to ask if you

have any information about the possible existence of an equivalent
to the A-10 nucleus in the human compared to the rat; the substantia
nigra increases phylogenetically and it reaches its maximum dimen-
sion in total neurons in humans.  I wondered if perhaps in humans
it incorporates what in a rat might be the A-10 nucleus.  I don't
know the answer and I wonder if you possibly have that information?

*Dr. Hornykiewicz*

I have studied quite extensively the available literature on
the human substantia nigra.  There seem to exist only a few studies
on this subject.  From these studies, it becomes apparent that in
the human brain the anatomical correlate of the area A-10 as described in the animal brain may be the nucleus paranigralis as described in the Atlas of the Human Brain Stem by Olszewski and Baxter.
Hausler describes under this area under a completely different name.
Hausler also studied the behavior of the paranigral region in Parkinson's disease, and observed that it does degenerate in postencephalitic cases but not in idiopathic cases.  Neurochemically in the
human brain, the paranigral nucleus is predominantly noradrenergic
in nature; it contains high amounts of noradrenalin and less dopamine than in the rat brain or cat brain.  This seems to represent
an important species difference.  As a matter of fact, it is possible that in contradistinction to e.g. the rat brain, in the human
brain, the paranigral region gives rise to a noradrenergic projection to the forebrain, especially to the nucleus accumbens, and to
some other limbic areas which possess noradrenergic connections.

*Dr. Flores*

I wish to ask you a question about the use of reserpine that
has been given for a long time in patients with hypertension.  Do
you think that this drug causes a chronic deficiency in the dopamine
in the nucleus of the base of the brain and thereby induces the
parkinsonism syndrome?

*Dr. Hornykiewicz*

Well, the reserpine treatment of hypertension does occassionally
give rise to a drug-induced parkinsonism, especially in some sub-
ceptible cases.

*Dr. Volkman*

The data you presented showed decreased serotonin in the brain
of some of the Parkinson patients.  It has been suggested by Cools
and Janssen *(European Journal of Pharmacology 28: 266-275, 1974)*
that lesions in the median raphe area, which would effect brain
serotonin, may produce symptoms similar to lesions in the caudate
nucleus.  Do you think it is possible that there exists a subgroup
of Parkinsonian patients whose symptoms result from lesions in the

median raphe?  These patients might benefit from 5-hydroxytryptophan
therapy but not respond to L-dopa.

*Dr. Hornykiewicz*

It is not an effect of chronic L-dopa therapy, because you
can see the changes in patients not treated with L-dopa.  There
have been a few studies on the effects of 5-hydroxytryptophan and
parachlorophenylalanine on the parkinsonian symptomatology.  In
general, the results were disappointing.  5-HTP has been, I think,
reported to worsen, but not at all dramatically, the symptomatology
of Parkinson's disease.  This would not be surprising because
5-hydroxytryptophan competes with L-dopa for the decarboxylating
enzyme.  Parachlorophenylalanine, in a study by Chase, did not
produce any effects as far as I can remember.  But of course, with
human patients, one is never sure that the doses of such experimental drugs are high enough to produce large changes in the brain
amines; it is only such large changes that can be expected to produce clinical symptoms.

*Dr. Fahn*

There is another aspect in regards to these other neurotransmitter substances in parkinsonism, which I would like to discuss.
Instead of just looking only at the motor system in parkinsonism,
the akinesia or rigidity, there are other changes that take place
in parkinsonism such as mood changes, memory impairment, sensory
symptoms even.  It is possible that some of these other neurotransmitters may be involved in these other symptoms, which are generally overlooked when the akinesia is so severe and which is what
you are trying to treat.  But as the akinesia is treated with
levodopa therapy and that symptom comes under control, the other
symptoms may become more significant to the patient.  It is in
this context that perhaps these other neurotransmitters should be
looked at further.  As you know, there are reports that L-tryptophan,
given in the presence of levodopa therapy, can overcome some of the
toxic effects, that is some of the hallucinatory effects of levodopa.
We have also seen it overcome some of the hypokinesias.  Now, part of
its mechanism may well be that it competes with the absorption of
levodopa across the intestine or into the brain and it may not
actually have anything to do with brain mechanisms of serotonin *per
se*.  It just may be a way of reducing the amount of available levodopa into the brain.  But nevertheless, we must keep an open mind
that increasing serotonin in the brain, by giving L-tryptophan, may
really be of primary importance in overcoming some of the symptoms.
Perhaps some of the people in the audience have experiences they
would like to share with us.  In regard to serotonin, I would like
to ask another question.  You showed the reduction of serotonin in
Parkinson brains.  Do you have any data on what levodopa therapy
does to serotonin in the parkinsonian brain?  We know in animal

brains that levodopa decreases serotonin levels, but is it always
depleted in parkinsonian brain?

*Dr. Hornykiewicz*
    Yes, we do. According to our unpublished observations the
serotonin concentrations in the brain do not change in patients on
levodopa; in such patients, the brain serotonin is still about as
low as in untreated patients. However, if I remember correctly,
the 5-hydroxyindoleacetic acid concentration is slightly higher
than in non-dopa treated patients. This suggests that there is a
slight effect of L-dopa on the serotonin metabolism in Parkinson's
disease. But the changes are by no means as large as in animals
receiving L-dopa in acute experiments. This difference is due,
I think, to a very simple fact: the doses of L-dopa given to
parkinsonian patients are comparatively low on a per kilogram basis,
especially if the plasma levels attained are considered. In contrast, in the animal experiments which demonstrated the effect of
L-dopa on brain serotonin, something like 200 mg/kg of L-dopa were
injected intraperitoneally. With the usual oral L-dopa regimen,
such high levels are never reached in human brain. As to the
possible involvement of these non-dopaminergic systems, in Parkinson's disease I quite agree with you. The mood changes could be
related both to noradrenaline changes in the limbic system as well
as to the changes of brain serotonin.

*Dr. Frigyesi*
    Could the biochemical deficiency you described in the nucleus
account for some of the symptoms in Parkinson's disease?

*Dr. Hornykiewicz*
    Well, I think that the human nucleus accumbens is a very
curious area. It is my working hypothesis that the nucleus accumbens is both limbic and striatal. I would like to regard the dopaminergic innervation of the accumbens as being more or less functionally the same as that of the rest of the striatum. As you know,
anatomically, the nucleus accumbens looks very much like the striatum,
which makes it morphologically pretty hard to distinguish the
accumbens in the human brain. Also in respect to the dopamine, the
human nucleus accumbens looks just like the caudate nucleus. Furthermore, in Parkinson's disease the accumbens dopamine behaves exactly
like the caudate nucleus dopamine. It is from this point of view
as if the nucleus accumbens were part of the caudate nucleus. On
the other hand, the human nucleus accumbens receives a very dense
noradrenergic innervation and this noradrenergic innervation possibly
is the true limbic component of the nucleus accumbens. It is temp-
ting to speculate that the decrease of noradrenalin in the nucleus
accumbens in Parkinson's disease, may be related to some of the
limbic symptoms of Parkinson's disease. In contrast, the decrease in

dopamine in the nucleus accumbens might be actually related to
the striatal symptomatology of Parkinsonism which might be, as far
as we know, more in the area of the motor deficit, seen in Parkinson's disease.  Clearly the nucleus accumbens is quite a unique
area in the human brain.  It seems to be the only brain area that
contains high amounts of nearly everything that you find in the
human brain: dopamine, noradrenaline, serotonin, acetylcholine, and
I think GABA, too.

*Dr. Mars*
     We have been C.T. scanning patients with Parkinson's disease,
and become aware of just how much significant cerebral atrophy is
present in many people with this disorder. Can we link the cerebral
atrophy to what is happening biochemically?

*Dr. Hornykiewicz*
     We have recently studied the behavior of noradrenaline and
dopamine in the cortex of parkinsonian patients.  In many cortical
areas noradrenaline concentrations are decreased in Parkinson's
disease.  However, the atrophy does not have much in common with
any possible degeneration of the noradrenergic inputs to the cortex,
since this would not show up as an atrophy; from what you say there
must be a genuine atrophy of the cell bodies in the cortex in Parkinson's disease.

*Dr. Mars*
     One always hates to bring up the question, but it always
arises.  A few years ago, in some of the very earlier symposiums
we had on Parkinson's disease, it was brought to our attention that
a very definite percentage of 6-hydroxydopamine is present in the
synthesized levodopa preparations.  Do we know that still to be so;
and if so, could this perhaps represent an effective chronic treatment
to all of the natural history of the disease?

*Dr. Hornykiewicz*
     Well, all I can say is that we have to assume that the L-dopa
preparations on the market are subject to strict quality controls
and do not contain toxic contaminants.

*Dr. Klawans*
     I would like to comment a little bit upon that.  I don't think
there is much evidence that there is really 6-hydroxydopa present in
presently available synthesized levodopa.  But the more general question that Harold Mars asked, does the chronic exposure to the medicine
alter the natural history of the disease?  I think that can be answered and I think the answer is yes.  Chronic exposure of brains to high
doses of dopamine agonists clearly changes the response of that brain
to subsequent dopaminergic innervation.  It occurs in chronic levodopa

in man and can be shown with other dopamine agonists in man and in the animals, including amphetamine, cocaine, bromocriptine, lergotrile, and methylphenidate. I think that chronic exposure to these dopamine agonists does change the subsequent brain response to dopamine agonism, and probably does contribute to the psychiatric side effects of levodopa, the hallucinations, the paranoid psychosis and to the pathophysiology and pathogenesis of L-dopa induced dyskinesias.

*Dr. Hornykiewicz*

Yes, I assume everybody would agree on that.

*Dr. Mars*

Again, one hates to be the devil's advocate, but I think the administration of any drug in large quantity to an organism must result in biochemical adaptations to that drug. We have demonstrated this with respect to how a human will handle pyridoxine and the transformations of pyridoxine to pyridoxal-5-phosphate, when that individual has been chronically treated with levodopa. This is a question that we must address ourselves to, in trying to delineate exactly what biochemical modifications arise from the chronic treatment with the drug and whether there is some adaptation and possibly loss of effect; whether there are perhaps adverse effects in terms of the progression of the disease; and even whether there is any truth to what Dr. Cotzias has reported in the literature recently, we may have tapped the spring of longevity.

*Dr. Duvoisin*

I want to take you back just a little bit to your historical perspective and I would like to ask you to review your rationale for using levodopa in the first place. Was it simply replenishment of dopamine in surviving neurons that were deficient; and if so, why? And what do you think it is now? You know there are some contrary opinions and there are some clinical facts that don't seem to fit with the notion that it is only a question of replenishing dopamine in sick neurons?

*Dr. Hornykiewicz*

I like to think that in principle it is still a simple problem. The situation, in my opinion, is the following: As long as there are still a certain number of functioning neurons remaining in the parkinsonian striatum, you will have a formation, from the exogenous L-dopa, of dopamine in these neurons. Now, there is reason to believe that the neurons that survive in Parkinson's disease are in a state of overactivity. This is made probable by the fact that the ratio of homovanillic acid to dopamine in these neurons is shifted in favor of homovanillic acid as compared with the normal brain. Thus the surviving neurons are turning over the dopamine at a higher

than normal rate.  Therefore, it you supply them with exogenous
L-dopa, they will be in a position to form more dopamine, and release more dopamine, than under normal conditions.  Therefore, the
administration of L-dopa to such a parkinsonian striatum with overactive neurons will actually result in an increased supply of the
intact dopamine receptors with the transmitter.  The other point
that is very important in this respect is the fact that the dopaminergic innervation of the striatum has an extremely high degree
of divergence.  That means that one nigro-striatal dopamine fiber
supplies thousands of striatal cells with synaptic contacts; in
other words there is a large innervation overlap in respect to the
dopaminergic innervation of the striatum.  A partial degeneration
of the substantia nigra will leave a substantial portion of the
striatum basically innervated, although the innervation density
may be reduced.  It is thus not too outlandish to assume that if
supplied with large amounts of the precursor L-dopa, still preserved and functionally overactive, dopamine neurons will produce
and release onto receptors large amounts of the dopamine.  The
released dopamine will reach wide enough areas of the striatum to
have functional consequences.  This is the reason why I think that
as long as there are still functioning dopamine neurons left in
the parkinsonian striatum the dopamine replenishment can be expected to produce functional effects.  That is the main reason why
I don't favor those hypotheses that stress the difficulties, because as long as we can answer the question in a simple way, we
should, I think, try to do so.  Of course, the important point would
be what happens if the parkinsonian striatum loses all of its dopaminergic innervation?  Such cases, of course, may exist.  But again,
there exist cases that do not respond to L-dopa, and these might
be exactly the cases with a complete loss of the nigro-striatal
dopamine innervation.  In addition to the above we have to keep in
mind the noradrenergic and sertoninergic innervations of the
striatum which are not reduced to the same extent as the dopaminergic.  It is well-known that L-dopa will be converted to dopamine
both in the noradrenaline neurons and in the serotonin neurons.
From these neurons, the dopamine may easily diffuse to the sites of
dopamine receptors, and by doing so exert dopaminergic effects,
despite the fact that a large portion of the dopaminergic neurons
are gone.

*Dr. Duvoisin*
        I am glad to hear that, but there are problems, as you know.
First of all, it was suggested that some structural change is involved and that some neurons other than dopaminergic neurons might
be processing the dopa.  I don't know of any satisfactory identification of which ones; but there are possibilities.  Clinically, the
postencephalitic patients who have by far the most severe nigral loss
and the most marked dopamine depletion, as your own work shows, and

as appeared in the slides you showed this morning, responded to very
small doses of levodopa, whereas the most far advanced Parkinson's
disease patients, do not have such severe cell loss and may no longer
respond to levodopa.  There is a paradox here that must have some
explanation.  For clinicians trained in classical anatomy and physiology, it is difficult to accept that dopamine receptors may be
just sitting there waiting for some dopamine to reach them, somehow.
If it's true that nature abhors an empty synapse, what happens to
the synapses that are vacated following the death of a nigral neuron?
Surely there must be some reorganization in the striatum which affects
the response to levodopa therapy.  What are your thoughts?

*Dr. Hornykiewicz*
     Well, the first consequence of a degeneration of the neuronal
supply that we would expect to occur is a supersensitivity of
that receptor to the responding neurotransmitter.  This is exactly
what I think happens in Parkinson's disease.  Your mention of the
postencephalitic cases as being the more severely affected as to
the degeneration of the nigral neurons, and those reacting more
sensitively to L-dopa, quite nicely illustrates that possibility;
actually it can be interpreted as supporting the whole dopamine
concept of L-dopa's effect, and not contradicting it.  What happens,
in my opinion, in the parkinsonian striatum are two events , two
developments which have opposite effects on the functional abilities
of the parkinsonian striatum.  On one hand, the degeneration of the
dopamine neurons will reduce the dopaminergic control of the striatum.
On the other hand, the more the degeneration progresses, the more
there is a development of a receptor supersensitivity in the striatum
to dopamine; counterbalances, make up for, the loss of transmitter.
Thus, ideally, the loss of dopamine neurons can, at a certain point,
be functionally counterbalanced by the development of supersensitivity
to the corresponding transmitter.  In such cases, L-dopa will be, I
think, quite effective in replenishing functionally the missing dopamine.  When degeneration reaches very severe degrees the supersensitivity will not be of much help; there will not be enough dopamine
neurons left, so as to supply the supersensitive dopamine receptors
with the transmitter.  In conclusion, I would like to propose that
there is a very critical balance between supersensitivity, loss of
neurons, and the effectiveness of L-dopa.  With regard to your observation of clinally far advanced Parkinson's disease patients who do
not have such severe cell loss in the substantia nigra and may not
respond any more to L-dopa, there are several possibilities.  Thus,
it could be that these cases are atypical in the sense that other
neuropathological changes are superimposed on the Parkinsonian
neuropathology, e.g. striatonigral degeration, other system degenerations, or supranuclear palsy etc.; or, the predominant parkinsonian
symptoms may be, in such cases, exactly those that are known to be

less sensitive to L-dopa, namely rigidity and especially tremor.
It is not certain at present whether these symptoms, in contrast
to akinesia, are directly related to the degree of cell loss in
the substantia nigra. Finally, the idea that the vacated dopamine receptors in the parkinsonian striatum may become occupied
by other terminals, is quite attractive. Of course, one would
first of all think of the same remaining dopamine terminals as
occupying, by way of sprouting, these empty receptors. This
would be, from a functional point of view, very advantageous in
Parkinson's disease. In addition, non-dopaminergic terminals may
establish synaptic contacts with such empty receptor sites. Of
these, some, e.g. noradrenergic or serotoninergic neurons, may
actually contain dopa decarboxylase, thus being able to form
dopamine from exogenous L-dopa, and release it upon the appropriate
dopamine receptors. This too would be, functionally speaking, a
meaningful event in Parkinson's disease.

*Dr. Frigyesi*

Is it your experience that nigral axons diffusely and randomly
engage caudate neurons in man? The neuroanatomy and neurophysiology
of nigrocaudate relations in subhuman primates and felines seem to
indicate a reasonable topographical arrangement.

*Dr. Hornykiewicz*

Well, as a matter of fact, I was not referring to the human
striatum at all, since I don't think there is any evidence available.
I was referring to the fluorescence histochemical work done mainly in
the rat. By counting the dopamine cell bodies in the nigra and the
monoamine boutons in the striatum, and comparing these figures with
the dopamine content of these two regions, Hökfelt came out with
something like five hundred thousand synaptic boutons for each dopamine neuron in the striatum, which is, or course, a tremendous number. From that, he concluded that there is a large degree of divergence of that innervation, and I simply assumed that it's similar in
the human brain. As to the topographical arrangement of the nigro-
striatal projections, as far as I am aware of, this applies in a
rather general manner; the rostral portions of the substantia nigra
predominantly innervate the caudate nucleus and the caudal and medial
portions, innervate predominantly the putamen. I am not aware of any
further well-established somatotopic distribution of the nigral dopamine neurons within the striatum.

*Dr. Frigyesi*

Carpenter states that the substantia nigra and the striatum are
not only reciprocally but also topographically linked. The recent
work of Nauta shows the caudate to be a mosaic; my data are in full
agreement with this. It also appears that nigral neurons feed into

some of these interneuronal pools. Both Nauta's and my own work
seem to indicate that there is at least one "nucleus" in the head
of the caudate. It appears that nigral stimulation exerts a frequency specific drive on the postsynaptic negatively here. Thus,
it would be curious if the nigral axons would randomly distribute
in the caudate.

*Dr. Hornykiewicz*

Well, I really didn't want to give the impression that I
think that one nigral fiber goes all over the whole caudate and
supplies it with terminal branches. In my opinion, it is, however,
important to realize that, the field of innervation in the striatum
of, let us say two neighboring neurons may overlap. Thus, if one
of these two nigral neurons degenerates, the other will still supply
the same area in the striatum. Since this can be repeated all over
the striatum such an anatomical innervation pattern would favor
preservation of a critical amount of innervation. On the other hand,
the possibility of a monoamine neuron going all over the place,
giving off branches and innervating several brain structures, is not
at all that strange. It is known that for example the noradrenaline
neurons originating in the locus coeruleus, and innervating the cerebral cortex, give branches all over the place on the way to the cerebral cortex; some of the branches going into the reticular formation
and some even turning back to the cerebellum. This is a good example
of one neuron innervating, by way of extensive branching, a wide area
of the central nervous system. This, in principle could also apply
to the nigro-striatal dopamine neurons. However, in my opinion, the
most important point about the nigral dopamine neurons is the overlap
of their fields of innervation in the striatum.

*Dr. Calne*

Since you have traced the historical background right up to
the recent and very complex problems, I wondered whether you might
comment on the receptors which haven't been mentioned so far: the
nigral dopamine receptors and the striatal presynaptic dopamine
receptors. Can you see any way of fitting that added complexity
to all the other problems which you have discussed this morning,
into the functional disturbances of parkinsonism or the complications of anti-parkinsonism therapy?

*Dr. Hornykiewicz*

I would prefer, for the time being, to wait for further clari-
fication of the experimental data on the physiological significance
of the presynaptic dopamine receptors as well as the dopamine receptors in the substantia nigra. I feel it would be somewhat premature
to put forward a hypothesis as to the implications of these receptors

in Parkinson's disease.  However, I think these new discoveries will
turn out to be relevant to clinical problems as well as the pathophysiology of basal ganglia diseases.  This is one of the exciting,
and a little frightening, things about the brain dopamine, that now
it really seems to be everywhere in the brain, doing nearly everything.  One wonders, with a self-critical smile, how neuroscience
could do without dopamine for such a long time!

# RECENT ADVANCES IN THE BIOCHEMICAL PHARMACOLOGY OF EXTRAPYRAMIDAL MOVEMENT DISORDERS

HAROLD L. KLAWANS,[1,2] CHRISTOPHER GOETZ,[1] PAUL A. NAUSIEDA,[1,2] AND WILLIAM J. WEINER, [1,2]

[1]Division of Neurology, Michael Reese Hospital and Medical
   Center, and
[2]Department of Medicine (Neurology), University of Chicago
   Pritzker School of Medicine, Chicago, Illinois.

## ABSTRACT

The biochemical pharmacology of parkinsonism and choreatic disorders has been reviewed in relationship to recent observations in
the synaptic pharmacology of dopaminergic systems. Despite the
fact that parkinsonism is usually due to a failure of presynaptic
dopamine input into the striatum, an identical clinical syndrome can
result from postsynaptic striatal dysfunction. Although clinically
identical, these two states differ both biochemically and pharmacologically. Presynaptic parkinsonism is associated with decreased
dopamine turnover in the brain and responds to levodopa. Neither
of these facts applies to postsynaptic parkinsonism.

Denervation hypersensitivity has been proposed as a mechanism
in the production of levodopa-induced dyskinesias and neuroleptic-
induced tardive dyskinesias. The role of chronic dopamine agonism
in the former suggests that denervation hypersensitivity is not the
only factor and raises the question that the treatment of parkinsonism with such agonists may inevitably be associated with dyskinesias and psychosis.

Recent theories of the biochemical pharmacology of extrapyramidal movement disorders are largely derived from three separate sets
of hypotheses:

   1) Dopamine and acetylcholine have antagonistic effects on

striatal neurons and that the normal function of these neurons depends
upon a balance of the influences of these two neurotransmitters.

2) A shift of this balance such that there is a decrease in
dopamine activity results in the signs and symptoms of parkinsonism.
In most, if not all, of these patients this decrease is felt to come
about as a result of decreased dopamine input (i.e., presynaptic
dysfunction).

3) A shift of this balance such that there is a relative increase in dopaminergic activity results in choreatic movement disorders. This increase in dopaminergic activity is felt to be due to
dysfunction of the striatal neurons (postsynaptic dysfunction). This
is felt to be related to primary neuronal disease in Huntington's
chorea and to denervation hypersensitivity in tardive dyskinesias
and levodopa-induced dyskinesias.

These basic concepts are based on a wide diversity of clinical
and preclinical observations which have been reviewed extensively
(Hornykiewicz, 1966, Klawans, 1968, Klawans et al., 1970, Klawans,
1973). Rather than review these data once again, this review will
focus on selected recent observations which serve to qualify and
redefine these basic premises. We will focus on three particular
issues:

1) The occurrence of parkinsonism as a result of striatal cell
dysfunction, i.e., postsynaptic parkinsonism.

2) The role of chronic dopaminergic agonism in the pathogenesis
of levodopa-induced hypersensitivity, i.e., agonist-induced hypersensitivity.

3) Further observation on the development of denervation hypersensitivity within the central nervous system.

PARKINSONISM AS A POSTSYNAPTIC DISORDER

Viewed from the perspective of the striatal dopamine receptor
sites, parkinsonism in almost all instances is a disorder of presynaptic dopaminergic mechanisms. In both idiopathic and postencephalitic parkinsonism, degeneration of the dopaminergic neurons of the
substantia nigra (Greenfield and Bosanquet, 1953) results in decreased
dopaminergic activity at striatal dopamine receptors (Klawans, 1973).
This decreased dopamine input is felt to be the pathophysiologic
basis of the signs and symptoms of parkinsonism (Klawans, 1973),
Hornykiewicz, 1966, Klawans, 1968). The clinical improvement in
parkinsonism resulting from levodopa is presumed to be due to increased
dopamine activity at relatively normal dopamine receptors. If parkinsonism is a reflection of altered response of striatal dopamine
receptors, parkinsonism could also result from primary dysfunction
of the striatal neurons -- a form of postsynaptic receptor site dysfunction. Although the clinical manifestations of parkinsonism may
be identical in "presynaptic" and "postsynaptic" parkinsonism, the

biochemical basis and pharmacologic responses of the two states may
be quite different.  Decreased dopaminergic input ("presynaptic dopamine deficiency") should be reflected by biochemical evidence of
decreased dopamine turnover as reflected by spinal fluid homovanillac
acid levels (Weiner et al., 1969) and should respond to increased
dopamine turnover as a result of levodopa therapy.  Most patients
with parkinsonism fall into this category.  Most patients with
parkinsonism have decreased spinal fluid homovanillic levels (Wiener
et al., 1969, Bertler et al., 1971, Chase and Ng, 1972, Gumpert et
al., 1973, Weiner and Klawans, 1973, Rinne et al., 1973).  In most
such patients, levodopa results in definite clinical improvement.
     Three early studies consisting of limited numbers of patients
all suggested that patients with higher homovanillic acid levels
prior to levodopa therapy show less clinical improvement when placed
on levodopa, see Table 1 (Godwin-Austen et al., 1971, Jequier and
Dufresne, 1972, Gumpert et al., 1973).  Although larger studies have

TABLE 1.   RELATIONSHIP BETWEEN PRETREATMENT CEREBROSPINAL FLUID
           HOMOVANILLIC ACID AND SUBSEQUENT RESPONSE TO LEVODOPA

| Response | Number | Source |
|---|---|---|
| Four of 5 patients without repsonse had normal pretreatment homovanillic acid levels | 16 | Godwin-Austen et al. (1971) |
| Patients with higher pretreatment homovanillic acid levels tended to be relatively resistant | 26 | Gumpert et al. (1973) |
| The mean homovanillic acid level in cerebrospinal fluid in 11 patients who were most responsive to levodopa was significantly lower than the mean homovanillic acid level in 10 poorly responsive patients* | 21 | Jequier and Dufresne (1972) |
| No correlation | 14 | Weiner and Klawans (1973) |
| No correlation | 151 | Rinne et al. (1973) |

*Cerebrospinal fluid was obtained by suboccipital puncture.

failed to show any correlation at all (Weiner and Klawans, 1973, Rinne
et al., 1973), these studies do raise the possibility that parkinsonism
can occur as a result of postsynaptic dysfunction.  Parkinsonism in
such patients need not be associated with any alteration in cerebro-

spinal fluid homovanillic acid.  If parkinsonism in such patients is
caused by loss of striatal response to dopamine, the efficacy of
levodopa may be quite limited.  This raises the possibility that at
least some of the patients reported by Godwin-Austen *et al. (1971)*,
Gumpert *et al. (1973)*, and Jequier and Defresne *(1972)* may have had
postsynaptic striatal dysfunction which could produce clinical parkinsonism not associated with altered cerebrospinal fluid homovanillic
acid and unresponsive to levodopa.  It has become clear that several
such states do exist.  The first of these is striatonigral degeneration.
This disease is characterized clinically by parkinsonism and pathologically by degeneration of both the substantia nigra and the putamen.
Table 2 shows the results of clinical trials of levodopa in 10 patients *(Andrews et al., 1970, Fahn and Greenberg, 1972, Izumi et al.,*
*1971, Rajput et al., 1972, Sharpe et al., 1973, Trotter, 1973)* with

*TABLE 2.  EFFICACY OF LEVODOPA IN STRIATONIGRAL DEGENERATION (10*
*PATIENTS)*

| Source | Number | Response | |
|---|---|---|---|
| *Andrews et al. (1970)* | 1 | No improvement | 1 |
| *Fahn and Greenberg (1972)* | 3 | No improvement | |
| | | Significant but only | 1 |
| | | transient improvement | 2 |
| *Izumi et al. (1971)* | 2 | No improvement | 2 |
| *Rajput et al. (1972)* | 2 | No improvement | 2 |
| *Sharpe et al. (1973)* | 1 | Transient response | 1 |
| *Trotter (1973)* | 1 | Transient response | 1 |
| TOTAL | 10 | No improvement | 6 |
| | | Transient improvement | 4 |

pathologically proved striatonigral degeneration.  Six of the 10 patients showed no response at all to levodopa, while four improved but
only transiently.  This is clearly inferior to the expected response
in classic parkinsonism.  While there are no studies of cerebrospinal
fluid homovanillic acid in such patients, clearly these patients do not
respond as well to chronic levodopa therapy as patients with parkinsonism per se.
    Postsynaptic striatal dysfunction also results in parkinsonism
in the so-called rigid or akinetic form of Huntington's chorea *(Klawans,*
*1973)*.  Although the akinetic form of Huntington's disease usually occurs before the age of 20, the clinical manifestations include parkin-
sonlike akinesia and rigidity.  The parkinson like manifestations of

the akinetic form of Huntington's disease are felt to be related to
degeneration of striatal neurons and loss of response to dopamine
(Klawans et al., 1971).  If the parkinsonian features of this form
of Huntington's disease are related to a decreased effect of dopamine,
it is reasonable to use levodopa in an attempt to increase the
activity of dopamine within the striatum.  Table 3 summarizes the
results of levodopa trials in such patients.  Barbeau (1969) gave

TABLE 3.   EFFICACY OF LEVODOPA IN THE RIGID FORM OF HUNTINGTON'S
           DISEASE (9 PATIENTS)

| Source | Number | Response | |
|--------|--------|----------|---|
| Barbeau (1969) | 2 | Significant improvement | 1 |
| | | No improvement | 1 |
| Bird and Paulson (1970) | 1 | Transient improvement | 1 |
| Klawans (1975) | 5 | Transient improvement | 2 |
| | | No improvement | 3 |
| Low et al. (1974) | 1 | No improvement | 1 |
| TOTAL | 9 | No improvement | 5 |
| | | Transient improvement | 3 |
| | | Significant improvement | 1 |

levodopa to two such patients, one of whom improved significantly.
Bird and Paulson (1970) reported significant but transient improvement in one patient.  Low et al. (1974) have recently reported another
case unresponsive to levodopa.  We have given levodopa to five such
patients and observed a transient response in two and no improvement
in the other three.  In three of these patients, the cerebrospinal
fluid homovanillic acid was normal.  Akinetic Huntington's disease
apparently is associated with normal cerebrospinal fluid homovanillic
acid and a limited response to levodopa.  We recently studied a
patient with levodopa-resistant parkinsonism due to basal gangliar
calcification related to surgically-induced hypoparathyroidism (Klawans
et al., 1976a).  The parkinsonism in this patient was associated with
normal levels of cerebrospinal fluid homovanillic acid and the patient
showed no clinical response to levodopa.

A fourth state in which parkinsonism is related to postsynaptic
striatal pathology is the Shy-Drager syndrome.  The results of the
few clinical trials of levodopa in this disorder are summarized in
Table 4.  Here again the response to levodopa therapy is poor.  None
of the eight patients showed any significant improvement when treated
with levodopa.

TABLE 4.  *EFFICACY OF LEVODOPA IN SHY-DRAGER SYNDROME (8 PATIENTS)*

| Source | Number | Response | |
|---|---|---|---|
| *Aminoff et al. (1973)* | 5 | No improvement | 5 |
| *Klawans (1975)* | 3 | No improvement | 3 |

These various observations have several possible implications for the study of the biochemistry and pharmacology of parkinsonism and any other neurologic disorder involving decreased activity of any neurotransmitter.
1) Presynaptic deficiency and postsynaptic dysfunction in relation to the same amine system can result in identical clinical pictures.
2) Only the presynaptic deficiency state is associated with detectable alterations in amine metabolites in the cerebrospinal fluid.
3) The two states may well differ in the response to amine precursors.

## THE ROLE OF DOPAMINE AGONISM IN THE PATHOGENESIS OF LEVODOPA-INDUCED DYSKINESIAS

Numerous side effects occur in patients with Parkinson's disease receiving long-term levodopa therapy.  One of the most severe side effects is levodopa-induced abnormal movements or dyskinesias.  The appearance of these movements usually requires a decrease in levodopa, thereby preventing maximal improvement in the parkinsonian disability. Neither the pathophysiology nor the pathogenesis of levodopa-induced dyskinesias is well understood.  It is generally felt that these levodopa-induced dyskinesias and other similar movement disorders are related to increased activity of dopamine at striatal dopamine receptor sites.  The pathogenesis of this increased striatal dopaminergic activity has been suggested by some investigators to involve denervation hypersensitivity *(Anden 1970, Carlsson, 1970, Klawans et al., 1970)*.  As pointed out by Klawans *et al.* (1975a), however, a number of clinical observations regarding levodopa-induced dyskinesias are not compatible with denervation hypersensitivity as the pathogenic mechanism of this disorder.  Recent work in our animal laboratory on the effect of chronic levodopa exposure on amphetamine- and apomorphine-induced stereotyped behavior sheds light on both the pathophysiology and the pathogenesis of these movements in relation to levodopa-induced dyskinesias.

In these experiments the chronic administration of doses of
levodopa known to be subthreshold for acute induction of stereotyped
behavior produced definite stereotyped behavior after daily ingestion
for 7 to 14 days. This alteration was also characterized by a
decrease in the latent period between the ingestion of levodopa and
the onset of stereotyped behavior. This decreased latency and threshold for stereotypy following chronic levodopa pretreatment may be
viewed as a form of chronic agonist or "innervation-induced hypersensitivity." It is of interest that the same phenomenon has been
reported with experimental animals using other means of chronic
dopaminergic agonism. When long-term subthreshold amphetamine, an
indirect dopamine agonist, is administered to animals the threshold
and latency for stereotyped behavior can likewise be decreased (Klawans et al., 1975a, Klawans and Margolin, 1975). In addition,
Nausieda et al. (in press) administered bromocriptine, a dopaminergic
agonist thought to act directly at postsynaptic dopaminergic receptors, and induced a decrease in the threshold needed to induce
stereotypy.

In laboratory animals exposure to long-term levodopa leads to an
increased sensitivity to dopaminergic stimulation. Possible mechanisms
for this increased response include an alteration in presynaptic
metabolism, distribution, storage and release of dopamine, or an alteration of postsynaptic neuronal structure in the striatum. Further experiments with apomorphine and amphetamine threshold for stereotyped
behavior after chronic levodopa pretreatment clarified the exact
pathophysiology of the hypersensitivity phenomenon.

The guinea pigs pretreated with chronic levodopa demonstrated
a decreased threshold for both apomorphine and amphetamine-induced
stereotyped behavior. This response may again be viewed as hypersensitivity induced by chronic dopaminergic agonism. The fact that
the hypersensitivity is demonstrated with amphetamine does not differentiate presynaptic from postsynaptic mechanisms since amphetamine
is an indirect dopamine agonist and acts to increase dopamine release from presynaptic vescicles onto the postsynaptic membrane.
Apomorphine, however, is believed to be a direct dopamine agonist,
exerting its predominant effect directly on the postsynaptic dopamine
receptor site. The fact that levodopa pretreatment produced a supersensitivity to apomorphine stereotypy suggests that a postsynaptic
mechanism is involved in the pathophysiology of this levodopa-induced
supersensitivity.

As mentioned above animals treated chronically with other dopaminergic agents demonstrate similar hypersensitivity. Klawans and
Margolin (1975) pretreated guinea pigs with chronic amphetamine and
noted a decreased threshold and latency for both apomorphine- and
amphetamine-induced stereotyped behavior. Similarly, pretreatment
with a direct dopamine agonist leads to the same phemonenon.
Nausieda et al. (in press) studied the threshold doses of apomorphine
and amphetamine needed to induce stereotyped behavior after chronic

pretreatment with bromocriptine. They reported that chronic bromocriptine administration reduced the threshold of stereotyped behavior
to both apomorphine and amphetamine. Bromocriptine, a direct dopa-
menergic agent, is structurally unrelated to levodopa or amphetamine
and yet was able to alter the striatal sensitivity to dopaminergic
stimulation with both agents. Bromocriptine, like levodopa- and
amphetamine-induced hypersensitivity to both direct and indirect
dopaminergic agonists in the central nervous system. The chronic
bromocriptine, levodopa, and amphetamine data, viewed together,
demonstrate that dopaminergic hypersensitivity can be induced by long-
term pretreatment with agents that affect the dopamine system differently. Amphetamine, an indirect dopamine agonist, bromocriptine,
a direct acting agonist, and levodopa, a dopamine precursor, are all
able to induce hypersensitivity. The characteristic that all three
agents share is that they are dopaminergic agents administered chronically. These data suggest that while the pathophysiology of the
stereotypy relates to dopaminergic hypersensitivity, the pathogenesis
of the hypersensitivity relates to chronic dopaminergic agonism.

These experiments may serve as a model for levodopa-induced
dyskinesias in humans, and help to clarify both the pathophysiology
and pathogenesis of the disorder. Dyskinesias are seen in as high
as 80% of the patients with Parkinson's disease receiving levodopa
and are considered to be the major dose limiting side effect of
levodopa therapy (Barbeau et al., 1971). The appearance of the
abnormal movements usually necessitates a decrease in the medication
or prevents an increase in medication thereby preventing maximum
improvement of the parkinsonian disability.

Several studies suggest that the pathophysiology of levodopa-
induced dyskinesias is related to increased striatal dopaminergic
sensitivity either pre- or postsynaptic. The pathogenesis of this
increased dopamine sensitivity has been suggested by some investigators to involve denervation hypersensitivity (Anden, 1970, Carlsson,
1970, Klawans et al., 1970). There are, however, a number of
observations that are difficult to explain if levodopa-induced
dyskinesias are due entirely to denervation hypersensitivity. These
include:

1) The direct relationship between duration of levodopa therapy
and prevalence of levodopa-induced dyskinesias.

2) The direct relationship between duration of dyskinesias and
the severity of the dyskinesias.

3) The inverse relationship between duration of dyskinesia in
the individual patient and the dosage of levodopa necessary to elicit
dyskinesias (threshold dosage).

4) The change in time relationship between the dyskinesia and
the individual dose of levodopa as the duration of dyskinesia increases.

The concept of chronic agonist-induced hypersensitivity helps to
explain these observations and may play a role in the pathogenesis
of levodopa-induced dyskinesias.

First, there appears to be a direct relationship between the duration of levodopa therapy and the prevalence of levodopa-induced dyskinesias. In our parkinsonian population, comprising greater than 200 patients, the prevalence of levodopa-induced dyskinesias increases from 37% at 6 months to 66% at 18 months to over 70% after 2 years of therapy. Similarly, in the experimental animals the prevalence of stereotypy increased from 40% after 7 days of levodopa ingestion to 74% after 14 days. In the same way that the chronic subthreshold stimulation increased the prevalence of stereotyped behavior in animals, it is possible that chronic dopaminergic stimulation can contribute to the development of dopamine receptor site hypersensitivity in humans.

The concept of chronic agonist-induced hypersensitivity helps further to explain observations about the duration of the dyskinesias and their severity. The dyskinesias are often quite mild at first and increase in severity as they persist. This increase often includes a wider distribution from solely lingual-facial-buccal movements to involvement of the trunk or limbs. There may also be an increase in the degree and severity of isolated, individual movements. The presence of these abnormal movements appears to indicate increased dopaminergic stimulation. While denervation hypersensitivity may play a pathogenic role in the initial excessive stimulation seen in these patients, our experiments suggest that continuation of levodopa stimulation by itself may further increase the sensitivity and account for the pathogenesis of these dyskinesias and their increasing severity with time.

The third observation pertinent to levodopa-induced dyskinesias is that there is often an inverse relationship between the duration of dyskinesias and the dosage of levodopa necessary to elicit the abnormal movements. It is likely that the chronic exposure to levodopa in patients with Parkinson's disease, like the guinea pigs exposed to chronic levodopa, has altered striatal dopaminergic sensitivity and thereby decreased the threshold dose of levodopa needed to elicit dyskinesias.

The final observation clarified by the concept of chronic agonist-induced hypersensitivity is the change in latency between time of levodopa ingestion and the appearance of dyskinesias. We have noted a large number of patients in whom dyskinesias were initially present one to two hours after levodopa ingestion. This time correlated approximately with the maximal levodopa effect on the patient's parkinsonian signs and symptoms. After several months of chronic levodopa therapy, however, dyskinesias begin within minutes after levodopa ingestion and often precede all antiparkinsonian effects. The animal studies demonstrated a similar altered latency after chronic levodopa administration.

The clinical presentation and course of levodopa-induced dyskinesias are compatible with the concept of chronic agonist-induced hypersensitivity. Altered dopaminergic physiology may be induced by chronic levodopa stimulation in humans.

From a therapeutic standpoint, it may be an unfortunate fact that chronic dopamine stimulation in guinea pigs via three different mechanisms all result in hypersensitivity. Chronic presynaptic stimulation, postsynaptic stimulation, and amino acid precursor load all induce a long-term sensitization to low dose dopamine agonism. This suggests that at least these three drugs can induce dopaminergic side effects of dyskinesias after long-term exposure. There is ample evidence that this prediction is correct in the case of levodopa and amphetamine. The frequency and severity of levodopa-induced dyskinesias have already been discussed. Chronic amphetamine exposure can induce dyskinesias in humans similar in appearance to those seen after levodopa exposure. The movements involve the facial and masticatory musculature and consist primarily of licking, teeth grinding, and tongue protrusion (Kramer et al., 1967, Ellinwood, 1967, Rylander, 1972). Our studies would predict that dyskinesias are a possible and perhaps a likely complication of bromocriptine when used in the treatment of parkinsonism.

These observations suggest that chronic high dose dopamine agonism may in some ways be detrimental to striatal function and raises the possibility that such pharmacologic agents may not be the best approach to the treatment of parkinsonism.

## DENERVATION HYPERSENSITIVITY IN THE CENTRAL NERVOUS SYSTEM

Phenomenologically, tardive dyskinesia is a choreiform movement disorder (Klawans, 1973, Tarsy and Baldessarini, 1976). Pharmacologically, it appears that the activity of dopamine at striatal dopamine receptors plays the same primary role in the pathophysiology of the abnormal movements of tardive dyskinesia as it does in other choreatic disorders such as Huntington's disease (Klawans, 1973) and levodopa-induced dyskinesias (Klawans et al., 1970).

In tardive dyskinesias it has been suggested that prolonged pharmacologic blockade of the striatal dopamine receptors by neuroleptic agents produces a state of denervation hypersensitivity (Klawans, 1973, Klawans and Rubovits, 1975). The prolonged pharmacologic denervation of the striatal dopamine receptors by the continuous administration of these dopamine agonists is thought to produce an alteration in the receptor site responsiveness. As a result of this physiological insult, these neurons respond in an abnormal manner to any dopamine which is able to act upon their altered receptors. It is quite possible that tardive dyskinesia may be the overt manifestation of the abnormal response of such neurons.

The concept of neuroleptic-induced denervation hypersensitivity to dopamine raised two significant questions:

1) Is such denervation hypersensitivity solely a property of dopaminergic systems?

2) Is neuroleptic-induced denervation hypersensitivity limited to such dopaminergic systems?

Recent work in our laboratory sheds some light on these two questions. These experiments involved the study of stereotyped behavior and 5-hydroxytryptophan-induced myoclonus. As mentioned above dopaminergic mechanisms are believed to mediate stereotyped behavior in animals. Chronic pretreatment with dopaminergic blocking agents, such as chlorpromazine and haloperidol, has been shown to intensify this behavior *(Klawans and Rubovits, 1972, Tarsy and Baldessarini, 1976)*. Such neuroleptic pretreatment increases the response to the subsequent administration of both amphetamine and apomorphine. Since apomorphine is felt to act primarily as a direct agonist on dopamine receptors *(Ersnt, 1967)*, it has been postulated that the prolonged pharmacologic blockade of dopamine receptors in these experiments resulted in a form of denervation hypersensitivity.

Subcutaneous injections of 300 mg/kg of D,L-5-hydroxytryptophan, the precursor of serotonin, elicit a rhythmic myoclonic behavior in intact guinea pigs *(Klawans et al., 1973a)*. This behavior is maximal at 1 hour post injection, and is not prevented by chlorpromazine (5, 10 mg/kg), scopolamine (0.1, 0.5 mg/kg), phentolamine (1, 5 mg/kg), or propranolol (0.1, 0.2, 0.5 mg/kg) pretreatments *(Klawans et al., 1973b)*. However, methysergide (0.6 mg/kg) blocks all manifestations of the behavior, without preventing the rise in whole brain serotonin following 5-hydroxytryptophan injections *(Klawans et al., 1973b)*.

Klawans *et al.* (1975b) have studied the effect of chronic methysergide pretreatment on 5-hydroxytryptophan-induced myoclonic behavior in guinea pigs. By analogy to amphetamine-induced stereotyped behavior, we felt that chronic pretreatment with a serotonin antagonist would produce denervation hypersensitivity of serotonin receptors if such a phenomenon could occur in a nondopaminergic system.

Our study showed that chronic methysergide pretreatment produced an increased response to the subsequent administration of 5-hydroxytryptophan *(Klawans et al., 1975b)*.

Evidence has accumulated that a wide variety of pharmacologic and surgical maneuvers can produce supersensitivity in the central nervous system analogous to the denervation hypersensitivity seen in the peripheral nervous system. For the nigrostriatal dopaminergic system, chronic receptor site blockade with neuroleptics *(Tarsy and Baldessarini, 1974, Klawans and Rubovits, 1972)*, acute transmitter synthesis inhibition with alpha-methylparatyrosine *(Costall and Naylor, 1973)*, chronic alpha-methylparatyrosine *(Tarsy and Baldessarini, 1974)*, acute reserpine *(Jonas and Scheel-Kruger, 1969, Goetz and Klawans, 1974)*, chronic reserpine *(Tarsy and Baldessarini, 1974)*, 6-hydroxy-dopamine-induced neuronal degeneration *(Ungerstedt, 1971)*, and neurosurgical lesions *(Ohye et al., 1970)* all result in a supersensitive behavior response (stereotypy) to direct and indirect dopaminergic agents such as apomorphine and amphetamine. The mechanisms by which supersensitivity develops in each of the above cases remain

unknown; however, the general principle has emerged that interruption
of dopaminergic synaptic transmission results in subsequent supersensitivity.

In a subsequent study we have found that the chronic administration of neuroleptics (either chlorpromazine or haloperidol) results
in behavioral hypersensitivity to both direct and indirect dopamine
agonists but does not alter the behavioral sensitivity to the serotonin precursor, 5-hydroxytryptophan *(Klawans et al., 1976b)*. At
the same time, the chronic administration of the serotonin antagonist,
methysergide, results in behavioral hypersensitivity to the subsequent
administration of 5-hydroxytryptophan, but does not produce an increased response to either direct (apomorphine) or indirect (d-amphetamine) dopamine agonism (see Tables 5 and 6).

*TABLE 5.  THE EFFECT OF CHRONIC PRETREATMENT ON SUBSEQUENT RESPONSE
           TO d-AMPHETAMINE AND APOMORPHINE*

| Pretreatment | Test Drug | Dosage (mg/kg) | Number | Number Developing Stereotyped Behavior (3+ or 4+) | Significance |
|---|---|---|---|---|---|
| Control | d-Amphetamine | 3 | 12 | 0 | |
| Chlorpromazine | d-Amphetamine | 3 | 12 | 12 | $p < .01$ |
| Haloperidol | d-Amphetamine | 3 | 6 | 6 | $p < .01$ |
| Methysergide | d-Amphetamine | 3 | 6 | 0 | Not significant |
| Control | Apomorphine | 0.2 | 12 | 0 | |
| Chlorpromazine | Apomorphine | 0.2 | 12 | 12 | $p < .01$ |
| Haloperidol | Apomorphine | 0.2 | 6 | 6 | $p < .01$ |
| Methysergide | Apomorphine | 0.2 | 6 | 0 | Not significant |

The development of hypersensitivity to dopamine agonists by dopamine antagonists has been well documented in a variety of animal species *(Klawans and Rubovits, 1972, Tarsy and Baldessarini, 1974, Fjalland
and Moller-Nielsen, 1974; Gianutsos et al., 1974)*. The fact that
animals pretreated with neuroleptics are hypersensitive to both indirect dopamine agonists such as d-amphetamine *(Klawans and Rubovits,
1976)* and methylphenidate *(Fjallard and Moller-Nielsen, 1974)* and
direct dopamine agonists such as apomorphine *(Klawans and Rubovits,
1975, Tarsy and Baldessarini, 1974, Gianutsos et al., 1974)* suggests
that postsynaptic mechanisms underly this hypersensitivity. It has
been suggested, in fact, that specific pharmacologic denervation-
induced hypersensitivity of dopamine receptors is the basis of the

TABLE 6.  *THE EFFECT OF CHRONIC PRETREATMENT ON THE SUBSEQUENT*
*RESPONSE TO 5-HYDROXYTRYPTOPHAN*

| Pretreatment | Dosage of 5-Hydroxytryptophan (mg/kg) | Number | Number Developing Stereotyped Behavior | Significance |
|---|---|---|---|---|
| Control | 200 | 6 | 0 | |
| Chlorpromazine | 200 | 6 | 0 | |
| Haloperidol | 200 | 6 | 0 | |
| Methysergide | 200 | 6 | 6 | $p < .025$ |

behavioral supersensitivity *(Rubovits and Klawans, 1972)* and that this mechanism may play a role in the pathophysiology of neuroleptic-induced tardive dyskinesia in man *(Klawans, 1973)*.

As pointed out by Tarsy and Baldessarini *(1976)* specific pharmacologically-induced dopaminergic receptor site hypersensitivity remains unproven as the mechanism of prolonged neuroleptic-induced hypersensitivity.  This effect could be due to other effects of neuroleptic agents on cell membranes or cellular respiratory mechanisms as suggested by Faurbye *(1970)*.  If this latter were the case, neuroleptic-induced behavioral hypersensitivity might well be nonspecific.  The possibility that neuroleptic-induced behavioral hypersensitivity is not specifically limited to dopaminergic systems had not previously been examined.

Chronic methysergide-induced hypersensitivity to 5-hydroxytryptophan is also felt to be related to postsynaptic events since methysergide pretreatment does not alter the 5-hydroxytryptophan-induced increases in brain serotonin concentration *(Klawans et al., 1975b)*.  It has been suggested that this behavioral hypersensitivity is also related to specific receptor site hypersensitivity induced by chronic pharmacologic denervation.  The specificity of this behavioral hypersensitivity had not previously been investigated.

These observations show that chronic dopaminergic antagonism results in hypersensitivity to dopamine agonism but does not change the response to serotonin agonism as gauged by 5-hydroxytryptophan-induced myoclonus.  Chronic serotonin antagonism is also shown to result in hypersensitivity to serotonin agonism which is not associated with any increase in the behavioral response to either direct or indirect dopamine antagonists.  These findings are consistent with the hypothesis that the chronic administration of dopamine and serotonin antagonists result in behavioral hypersensitivity which is specifically limited to the system antagonized (i.e., dopamine antagonists

induce specific dopamine hypersensitivity while serotonin antagonists
induce specific serotonin hypersensitivity). These observations are
also consistent with the hypothesis that antagonist-induced hypersensitivity involves the transmitter specific receptors blocked by
the antagonist in question.

## ACKNOWLEDGMENTS

This work was supported in part by the United Parkinson Founda-
tion, the Michael Reese Medical Research Institute Council, and the
Boothroyd Foundation, Chicago, Illinois. The authors wish to thank
Ms. Pat Gerdes for her preparation of the manuscript.

## REFERENCES

Aminoff, M.F., Wilcox, C.S., Woakes, M.M. and Kremer, M. (1973).
    Levodopa therapy for parkinsonism in the Shy-Drager syndrome.
    J. Neurol. Neurosurg. Psychiatry 36, 350-353.
Anden, N.E. (1970). Pharmacological and anatomical implications of
    induced abnormal movements with L-dopa. In L-Dopa and Park-
    insonism (Barbeau, A. and McDowell, F.H., Eds). pp. 132-143.
    F.A. Davis, Philadelphia.
Andrews, J.M., Terry R.D. and Spataro, J. (1970). Striatonigral
    degeneration. Arch. Neurol. 23, 319-327.
Barbeau, A. (1969). L-dopa and juvenile Huntington's disease.
    Lancet 2, 1066.
Barbeau, A., Marsh, H. and Gillo-Joffroy, L. (1971). Adverse clinical
    side effects of L-dopa therapy. In Recent Advances in Park-
    inson's Disease (McDowell, F.A. and Markham, C.H., Eds.),
    pp. 204-237. F.A. Davis, Philadelphia.
Bertler, A., Jeppson, P.G., Nordgren, L., et al. (1971). Serial
    determinations of homovanillic acid in the cerebrospinal
    fluid of parkinson patients treated with L-dopa. Acta Neurol.
    Scand. 47, 393-402.
Bird, M.T. and Paulson, G.W. (1970). Early onset rigid Huntington's
    chorea. Neurology (Minneap.) 20, 400.
Carlsson, A. (1970). Biochemical implications of dopa-induced actions
    on the central nervous system, with particular reference to
    abnormal movements. In L-Dopa and Parkinsonism (Barbeau, A.
    and McDowell, F.H., Eds.). pp. 205-213. F.A. Davis, Phila-
    delphia.
Chase, T.N. and Ng, L.K.Y. (1972). Central monoamine metabolism in
    Parkinson's disease. Arch. Neurol. 27, 486-491.
Costall, B. and Naylor, R.J. (1973). On the mode of action of
    apomorphine. Eur. J. Pharmacol. 21, 350-361.
Ellinwood, E.H. (1967). Amphetamine psychosis. I. Description of
    the individuals and process. J. Nerv. Ment. Dis. 144, 273-283.

Ernst, A.M. (1967). Mode of action of apomorphine and dexamphetamine on gnawing compulsion in rats. *Psychopharmacologia (Berl.) 10*, 316-323.

Fahn, S. and Breenberg, J. (1972). Striatonigral degeneration. *Trans. Am. Neurol. Assoc. 97*, 275-277.

Faurbye, A. (1970). The structural and biochemical basis of movement disorders in the treatment with neuroleptic drugs in extrapyramidal diseases. *Comp. Psychiatry 11*, 205-224.

Fjalland, B. and Moller-Nielsen, I. (1974). Enhancement of methylphenidate-induced stereotypies by repeated administration of neuroleptics. *Psychopharmacologia (Berl.) 34*, 105-109.

Gianutsos, G., Drawbaugh, R.B., Hynes, M.D. and Lal, H. (1974). Behavioral evidence for dopamine supersensitivity after chronic haloperidol. *Life Sci. 14*, 887-898.

Godwin-Austen, R.B., Kantamarreni, B.D. and Curzon, G. (1971). Comparison of benefit from L-dopa in parkinsonism with increase of amine metabolites in the CSF. *J. Neurosurg. Psychiatry 34*, 219-223.

Goetz, C. and Klawans, H.L. (1974). Studies on the interaction of reserpine, d-amphetamine, apomorphine, and 5-hydroxytryptophan. *Acta Pharmacol. Toxicol. 34*,119-L30.

Greenfield, J.G. and Bosanquet, F.D. (1953). The brain stem lesion in parkinsonism. *J. Neurol. Neurosurg. Psychiatry 16*, 213-226.

Gumpert, J., Sharpe, D. and Curzon, G. (1973). Amine metabolites in the cerebrospinal fluid in Parkinson's disease and the response to levodopa. *J. Neurol. Sci. 19*, 1-12.

Hornykiewicz, O. (1966). Dopamine (3-hydroxytyramine) and brain function. *Pharmacol. Rev. 18*, 925-964.

Izumi, K., Inoue, N., Shirabe, T., Miyazaki, T. and Kuroiwa, Y. (1971). Failed levodopa therapy in striatonigral degeneration. *Lancet 1*, 1355.

Jequier, E. and Dufresne, J.J. (1972). Biochemical investigations in patients with Parkinson's disease treated with L-dopa. *Neurology (Minneap.) 22*, 15-21.

Jonas, W. and Scheel-Kruger, J. (1969). Amphetamine-induced stereotyped behavior correlates with the accumulation of O-methydopamine. *Arch. Int. Pharmacody. 177*, 379-386.

Klawans, H.L. (1968). The pharmacology of parkinsonism. *Dis. Nerv. Syst. 29*, 805-816.

Klawans, H.L. (1973). The Pharmacology of Extrapyramidal Movement Disorders. S. Karger, Basel.

Klawans, H.L. (1975). Amine precursors in neurologic disorders and the psychoses. *In Biology of Major Psychoses* (Freedman, D.X., Ed.), pp. 259-272. Raven Press, New York.

Klawans, H., Itaki, M.M. and Sheuher, D. (1970). Theoretical of the use L-dopa in parkinsonism. *Acta Neur. Scand. 46*, 409-441.

Klawans, H.L. and Margolin, D.I. (1975). Amphetamine-induced dopaminergic hypersensitivity in guinea pigs. *Arch. Gen. Psychia-*

*try 32*, 725-732.

Klawans, H.L. and Rubovits, R.  (1972).  An experimental model of tardive dyskinesia.  *J. Neural Transm. 33*, 235-246.

Klawans, H.L. and Rubovits, R.  (1975).  The pharmacology of tardive dyskinesia and some animal models.  *In Proceedings of the IX Confress of the Collegium Internationale Neuropsychopharmacologicum* (Boissier, J.R., Hippius, H. and Pichot, P., Eds.), pp. 58-67.  Excerpta Medica, Amsterdam.

Klawans, H.L., Ilahi, M.M. and Ringel, S.P.  (1971).  Toward an understanding of the pathophysiology of Huntington's chorea.  *Confin. Neurol. 33*, 297-303.

Klawans, H.L., Goetz, C., Westheimer, R. and Weiner, W.J.  (1973a).  5-Hydroxytryptophan-induced behavior in intact guinea pigs.  *Res. Commun. Chem, Pathol. Pharmacol. 5*, 555-559.

Klawans, H.L., Goetz, C. and Weiner, W.J.  (1973b).  5-Hydroxytryptophan-induced myoclonus in guinea pigs and the possible role of serotonin in infantile myoclonus.  *Neurology (Minneap.) 23*, 1234-1240).

Klawans, H.L., Crosset, P. and Dana, N.  (1975a).  Effect of chronic amphetamine exposure on stereotyped behavior: Implications for pathogenesis of L-dopa-induced dyskinesias.  *In Advances in Neurology, vol. 9* (Calne, D.B., Chase, T.N. and Barbeau, A., Eds.), pp. 105-112.  Raven Press, New York.

Klawans, H.L., D'Amico, D.J. and Patel, B.C.  (1975b).  Behavioral supersensitivity to 5-hydroxytryptophan induced by chronic methysergide pretreatment.  *Psychopharmacologia (Berl.) 44*, 297-300.

Klawans, H.L., Lupton, M.D. and Simon, L.  (1976a).  Calcification of the basal ganglia as a cause of levodopa resistant parkinsonism.  *Neurology (Minneap.) 26*, 221-225.

Klawans, H.L., D'Amico, D.J., Nausieda, P.A. and Weiner, W.J.  (1976).  The specificity of neuroleptic- and methysergide-induced behavioral hypersensitivity.  Presented at the American Academy of Neurology Annual Meeting, April, 1976, Toronto, Canada.

Kramer, J., Fischman, V.S. and Littlefield, D.S.  (1967).  Amphetamine abuse -- pattern and effects of high doses taken intravenously.  *J.A.M.A. 201*, 305-309.

Low, P.A., Allsop, J.L. and Halmayi, G.M.  (1974).  The rigid form (Westphal variant) treated with levodopa.  *Med. J. Aust. 1*, 393-394.

Nausieda, P.A., Crosset, P. and Klawans, H.L.  (in press): Effect of chronic dopaminergic agonism on subsequent response to amphetamine and apomorphine.  Encephale.

Ohye, C., Bouchard, R., Boucher, R. and Poirier, L.J.  (1970).  Spontaneous activity of the putamen after chronic interruption of the dopaminergic pathway.  *J. Pharmacol. Exp. Ther. 175*, 700-708.

Rajput, A., Kazi, D.A. and Rozdilsky, B.  (1972).  Striatonigral degeneration: Response to levodopa therapy.  *J. Neurol. Sci.*

16, 331-341.

Rinne, U.K., Sonninen, V. and Surtola, T. (1973). Acid monoamine
    metabolites in the cerebrospinal fluid of parkinson patients
    treated with levodopa alone or combined with a decarboxylase
    inhibitor. Eur. Neurol. 9, 349-362.

Rubovits, R. and Klawans, H.L. (1972). Implications of amphetamine-
    induced stereotyped behavior as a model for tardive dyskinesia.
    Arch. Gen. Psychiatry 27, 502-507.

Rylander, G. (1972). Psychoses and the punding and choreiform
    syndromes in addiction to central stimulant drugs. Psychiatr.
    Neurol. Neurochir. 75, 203-212.

Sharpe, J.A., Newcastle, N.B., Lloyd, K.G., et al. (1973). Stria-
    tonigral degeneration. J. Neurol. Sci. 20, 275-286.

Tarsy, D. and Baldessarini, R.J. (1974). Behavioral supersensitivity
    to apomorphine following chronic treatment with drugs which
    interfere with the synaptic function of catecholamines.
    Neuropharmacology 13, 927-940.

Tarsy, D. and Baldessarini, R.J. (1976). The tardive dyskinesia
    syndrome. In Clinical Neuropharmacology (Klawans, H.L., Ed.),
    pp. 29-61. Raven Press, New York.

Trotter, J.L. (1973). Striatonigral degeneration, Alzheimer's
    disease, and inflammatory changes. Neurolofy (Minneap.) 23,
    1211-1216.

Ungerstedt, U. (1971). Postsynaptic supersensitivity after 6-hydroxy-
    dopamine induced degeneration of the nigrostriatal dopamine
    system. Acta Physiol. Scand. (Suppl.) 367, 69-93.

Weiner, W.J. and Klawans, H.L. (1973). Failure of cerebrospinal
    fluid homovanillic acid to predict levodopa response in Parkin-
    son's disease. J. Neurol. Neurosurg. Psychiatry 36, 747-752.

Weiner, W.J., Harrison, W.H. and Klawans, H.L. (1969). L-dopa and
    cerebrospinal fluid homovanillic acid in parkinsonism. Life
    Sci. 8, 971-976.

## DISCUSSION

Dr. Frigyesi

In your presentation, you convincingly demonstrated the paradox, namely the difference between biochemical phenomena and the behavior of patients following a single dose or a repeated dose of L-dopa.
It may be that the biochemistry is only one of the parameters; there
are several others. In this regard, I would like to recall a series
of experiments we did in cats and monkeys in which we injected L-dopa
in much the same way as you did, and then we observed the electrophysiological relations and to our amazement, we found that following single effective doses of L-dopa, in a vast majority of the
animals, we did not observe the recovery of the control potentials.
L-dopa produced the changes, and I don't want to go into details.
We observed certain changes within minutes or half an hour, and these

changes gradually subsided, but before they were actually recovered, a second type of abnormality was observed on these electrophysiolog-ical conditions; and a third one and so forth. After a period of about eighteen hours, which was the longest observation period, these later effects are clearly not L-dopa effects; what kind of effects they are, I don't know. Whether they are various metabo-lites or they are initiating some kind of "reverberating activity" within the neuron mechanisms within the basal ganglion, I really don't know at the present time. The point which I want to indicate is that the electrophysiology clearly shows a much closer correla-tion to the behavior than to the biochemical picture.

*Dr. Klawans*
     Right.  I think the biochemical correlates just merely go to show that it's not due to purely biochemical phenomena; that's fur-ther correlated not only by the variety of drugs which assure differ-ent metabolisms and different mechanisms of action to which this crosses over, but the fact that you can put your animal on this pretreatment schedule for two weeks, and then come back with these other different drugs a month later, and they are still hypersensi-tive.  One can always hypothesize that other metabolites that may be around that we haven't looked for yet, but it's hard to imagine that they are going to be around a month later from bromocriptine or from levodopa or from apomorphine or from many of the other things, and still have an effect a month later.

*Dr. Flemenbaum*
     To pursue your answer a little bit further, I think it would be worthwhile to look into related subjects; Snyder's paper on agonist-antagonist states of the dopamine receptor may help to explain some.  But that is not my question.  My question refers to your mention of the word kindling.  I would like you to expound a little bit more in the sense that the phenomenon for electrical kindling is present in cases in which the stimulation is intermit-tent.  I found in your papers and in most of the other literature, that the pharmacological stimulation utilized is a continuous (non-intermittent) stimulation; the phenomena of electrical kindling, as summarized beautifully by Post *et al.* recently in the *American Journal of Psychiatry*, is present after intermittent and noncontin-uous stimulation.  Continuous stimulation actually retards the phenomena of hypersensitivity.  I would like you to expound a little bit more on that, and what are your theories in that respect?

*Dr. Klawans*
     Yes, the original kindling, all of the Goddard work and Frank Morrell's work has been intermittent subliminal stimulation.  I

am not sure, by the way, that my models are not that; after all, I give levodopa to an animal once a day. I don't think he is getting constant dopaminergic input for the 24 hours, until I give him his next dose. Clearly, if I give him the amphetamine, he is not; the amphetamine effects are all worn off within four to six hours, and at eighteen hours, we can't find any amphetamine in his brain, much less at 24 hours when we are going to start again. So it's not a constant stimulus. In our experiments all medications have been given once a day at the same time. Bromocriptine, I am not so sure that it's all gone in 24 hours. Methylphenidate is; the amphetamine is; the apomorphine is gone long before that; levodopa is gone long before that. I am not sure that we really have a big difference between intermittent electrical and chemical kindling.

*Dr. Duvoisin*

It seems to me that in cases of supranigral parkinsonism, where there is a loss of the dopamine receptors in the striatum, such as striatonigral degeneration, cerebellar atrophy, even in those in which we have pushed the dose of levodopa to astronomical levels, as high as eight grams of levodopa plus carbidopa daily, which would be close to thirty grams of levodopa a day, do not get dyskinesias. They get no response and no dyskinesia; they get psychotic to other toxicities, but not dyskinesia.

*Dr. Klawans*

Right. The interesting thing about the patients we have seen with that is that other than the original Huntington's, who have a propensity to choreic movements anyway, as they often have a little bit of chorea at the time; a lot of the patients with primarily post-synaptic disease do not seem to be susceptible to dyskinesia; they just may not have receptors. You know, it's whipping a dead horse. They can either get better or get worse from giving dopamine agonists.

*Dr. Fahn*

I wonder if part of our problem with inducing on-off effects in Parkinson patients is because most of these patients have been treated with really toxic levels; I think everyone of them that have on-off effects have had choreic movements at one time in the treatment. Now, by definition that implies a toxic level; it's true that the toxic level may still not have a good clinical efficacy. Yet, it's in these patients that we see on-off effects developing. And I just wonder if Parkinson patients wouldn't be better off if we under-treated them to avoid choreic movements, rather than push them to choreic movements? And in a way, you can say what happens in neuroleptic treatment is that the schizophrenic goes into tardive dyskinesia; maybe the doses that they have been having for so long have changed the receptors.

*Dr. Klawans*

Birkmayer at the World Congress of Neurology in '69 in New York
made a profound observation.  He reminded people that the therapeutic efficacy of levodopa was first demonstrated independently in
Canada and Vienna; and the side effects were first described in the
United States.  And one of the big differences between the Vienna
and Canadian experience and the American experience, of course, is
the massive doses used chronically.  I think you are right, Stan.
I think that I am now much less aggressive; I don't know if Roger
is or not; I am much less aggressive.  If I am starting a patient
on levodopa now, I get them up to an average of three grams levodopa per day.  Now, whether the patient is going to be better off
in the long run, I don't know.  But I clearly have the feeling that
when I pushed them more, they were worse off.

*Dr. Fahn*

Well, I agree with you.  That's why I raised it.

*Dr. Mars*

Harold, a year or two ago there was a paper in *Experientia*
which suggests that the co-administration of a monoamine oxidase
inhibitor, together with haloperidol or other agents of the phenothiazine group might prevent the onset of tardive dyskinesia, and
they presented some evidence to suggest this was so.  Now of course
I am not recommending the use of such drugs in a combination with
levodopa, but I wonder whether there is anything in the work that you
have done that might suggest that MAOI's might inhibit the formation
of receptor hypersensitivity?

*Dr. Klawans*

There is nothing I have done that even addresses that issue.
I would remind you that Birkmayer has also suggested that depranil,
which is an MAO inhibitor, with small doses of levodopa, (a hundred
milligrams a day of levodopa) is, he feels, the single best therapy
for Parkinson's disease, at least this one paper.  Now, nobody else
has used MAO inhibitors; they are not available anywhere else that
I know of.  I don't know.  I would have you look at that paper.

*Dr. Calne*

Could I ask you another question about the agonist induced
supersensitivity?  Do you have any explanation for why some receptors seem to respond with continuing administration to an agonist
by developing tolerance, say those receptors involved in producing
hypotension, or emesis, while others in the striatum apparently are
responding in a different way, by increasing that sensitivity?

*Dr. Klawans*

The answer really is no. I have given a great deal of thought to it; after all, we worked on that when you were in Chicago and demonstrated that the same animals who were hypersensitive in chronic amphetamine administration in relation to stereotypy behavior, were tolerant to the anorexic effect of amphetamine. As the work you and I did showed, they became tolerant to the hypothermic effect. So the same animals, at the same time are becoming tolerant to some receptors and hypersensitive at others. I don't really know an explanation for that. My own feeling is that it probably has to do with other things than just the postsynaptic membrane itself. I use the term denervation hypersensitivity, agonist induced hypersensitivity, and we talk about it as a membrane phenomena in the postsynaptic cell; but really all we know is that something in the millieu of the systems in which the postsynaptic cell acts is altered. Now, whether it is really that single cell that is changed or the total sum of influences on the systems to which that cell relates, which have adapted or learned; after all, all this is basically learning, and we do think the central nervous system is capable of learning. My own feeling is that this may well relate to the type of system involved beyond the postsynaptic membrane; that's just a thought. I don't know how to test it, but it is a thought.

*Dr. Pirch*

Could you comment on the possibility that activation of the receptors might lead to increased activity of feedback pathways, which might change tyrosine hydroxylase activity or release mechanisms, resulting in decreased transmitter output in those periods where you don't have the exposure of the receptor to the agonist. This could lead to a long term denervation and a change in receptor activity.

*Dr. Klawans*

Although in answer to a previous question, I have said that the stimulation is intermittent. We can demonstrate this when the stimulation is not intermittent, also; so I don't think you of necessity have to have denervation. I do not think that periods of denervation explain it, because the degree of denervation one needs in order to do this is relatively severe. You know, just partially decreasing dopamine levels doesn't do it. And so I don't think that denervation plays a role in this, in the mechanism that produces this.

*Dr. Fahn*

That is a point well taken. I do not want to discuss that right now, but I want to make a comment about the changing patterns of dyskinesia with chronic therapy with levodopa. The following is a clinical observation which is very striking to me. I have just returned from a year's sabbatical leave and had not seen the patient for over a year and just recently saw her again. This is a woman who has very severe clinical fluctuations on levodopa, but when she was on her "on" phase she would be so choreic that she would fall, and lose her balance, It was very distressing and disabling. But now when I see her, chorea no longer exists; it is mainly dystonic, sustained posture and sustained contractions. She had a little dystonia even before I left a year ago; but it was mainly chorea. Now she has almost no chorea and mainly only toxic dystonia. So there is a changing pattern, even to this type of dyskinesia, perhaps.

*Dr. Klawans*
    Yes. The change from a very very mobile kind of movement in some patients to mostly posturing dystonia.

*Dr. Duvoisin*
    Harold, I think the original suggestion for striatal dopamine receptor supersensitivity came from Ungerstedt's work with the rat, with the unilateral nigral lesion to account for the counter-rotation in levodopa.

*Dr. Duvoisin*
    The interesting thing about it is that in these rats, as Ungerstedt noted the counter-rotational behavior to apomorphine and L-dopa, is not present initially; it builds up slowly and it takes about three months to reach its peak; it then reaches its plateau, and remains that way thereafter for up to two to three years. It's a somewhat different story than the sheer agonist-induced supersensitivity that you have been describing occurring within one week. And I would like to make a second comment, if I may. I think the clinical experience that you described somewhat overstates the delay with which the dyskinesias develop. The table you showed with the percentage of patients developing dyskinesia on levodopa therapy, gradually increasing and ultimately reaching around 70 to 80 percent after six months, reflects the fact that in those days we were starting with low doses and building up gradually. But when sinemet became available, this delay became much less.

*Dr. Klawans*
    I think so; and it shifts the dose response curves way over.

*Dr. Duvoisin*
    Although we have -- I don't have numbers with me -- seen the dyskinesia appear after the first dose of sinemet, requiring no sustained chronic administration. Part of the delay, even if there

is a short delay, may reflect the so-called long duration effect;
it's not only that the patients develop dyskinesia, but they get
further benefit over those months during which they were developing
the dyskinesia, their parkinsonism was also getting better without
further increases in the dose.

*Dr. Klawans*
     Actually, when we graphed it out, the increasing efficacy did
not parallel the increase of the incidence of dyskinesias.  I would
agree with you that you can occasionally produce dyskinesias in
patients initially.  I don't doubt that at all.  I think denervation
hypersensitivity does play some role.  I think that sinemet does
shift the dose response curve, which raises a question, by the way,
whether we ought to be using sinemet; that is a very profound issue.
If the problem in levodopa is the chronic central side-effects,
if chronic high dose agonism has to do with the central side effects,
if the central side effects start earlier with sinemet, should we use
it?  I will leave that as an unanswered question.  On the other hand,
I think the dyskinesias are progressive in the individual patient,
and I think that's the strongest argument for the fact that more than
denervation hypersensitivity is playing a role.  The progression within the individual patient, I think, is very clear.

*Dr. Frigyesi*
     I am concerned by the extrapolation from rodents to man and in
particular with respect to the rotation.  The rotational phenomena
definitely is nonspecific. The other thing is a species difference;
it appears that after placing the nigral lesions, rodents rotate for
quite some time.  On the other hand, after placing nigral lesions in
cats,the behavioral effects last for not more than one or two days.
So I think the species differences ought to be considered in extra-
polation from rodents to man.

*Dr. Klawans*
     I have no other comment.  Roger, would you like to answer that?

*Dr. Duvoisin*
     Yes.  It's not so easy to get good rotating in animals, even
with rats.  There is no question that most people who have worked
with them a long time agree that there is an excellent correlation
between the location of lesion which should be in the rostro-medial
portion of the zona compacta of the substantia nigra; good rotational behavior is also obtained with lesions on the head of the
caudate and this is said to be topographically related to the
rostral part of the nigra.  It's true that there are many lesions
and many sites from which rotational behavior may be elicited, but
that doesn't invalidate the evidence that the nigro-striatal system

may be related to rotational behavior, and the evidence is quite
strong.  Moreover, there is a clinical analogy; human patients with
unilateral parkinsonism also rotate.  They have latero-pulsion, and
when they crawl on all fours as Purdon Martin observed some time ago,
they will rotate in the expected manner.  We haven't given the
patient amphetamine to see if it will drive the rotation but the
patients do spontaneously show analogous behavior and that surely
adds some significance to that animal model.

*Dr. Volkman*

Dr. Fahn made references to some patients who respond initially
to L-dopa therapy, who manifest choreic movements while they have
significant rigidity.  Do you think this indicates that a different
set of neurons are involved in the two phenomena or are different
receptors involved?

*Dr. Klawans*

One of the things that I had debated talking about today,
was the fact that we are normally taught that Parkinson's and chorea
are opposite ends of the same continuum; I don't believe that.  Even
though parkinsonism may be decreased dopamine effect and chorea may
be an increased dopamine effect, I don't think they are opposite
ends of the same continuum which would virtually make them initially
an exclusive phenomena, including you do see patients who still
have parkinsonian tremor who are on levodopa who are carrying that
arm with its tremor in a choreic posture; or a dystonic posture
or whatever you want to call it.  But clearly a levodopa induced
dyskinetic posture in the hand that has still got rigidity and
still got tremor in it.  And that they can co-exist in the same anatomical location and thereby in theory in the same caudatal locus
at the same time.  And I have felt that there are probably at least
two different caudatal systems; one which relates to rigidity and
akinesia, and one which relates to chorea, but co-exist at the same
time.  Whether that is true or not, whether you may have anatomical
correlations to that, I don't know.  But I think that they clearly
are not opposite and there must be two separate systems; they cannot be opposite ends of the same single system, for that to happen.

*Dr. Duvoisin*

I just wanted to second Donald's remark and repeat clinical
observations I have made to previous meetings of this sort.  I
have repeatedly said that, when we have looked at the laterality of
the dyskinesias, the choreiform dyskinesia is greater on the side
of the body that was the last to develop parkinsonism.  The dyskinesia on the side which was initially parkinsonian is apt to be more
dystonic in character; this holds up in something like two-thirds
of the patients, which would be consistent with an inverse or seesaw

relationship between choreoathetosis and parkinsonism in these patients. Descriptions of such an antagonism goes back to the days of encephalitis lethargica. We still occasionally see a few old time postencephalitics who commonly have some dyskinesia before they begin levodopa therapy, and a few have hemiparkinsonism on one side and hemichorea on the other. In these cases levodopa increases the hemichorea and reduces the hemiparkinsonism; neuroleptics do the reverse.

*Dr. Fahn*

Before your discussion time runs out, Harold, I just want to make a comment. It's a little off the subject that we are talking about right now, but it relates to what you initially spoke about: your dopa test for preclinical diagnosis of Huntington's disease. I don't think you mean to imply that this test should be done just because it may be positive, and I think you should be given a chance to perhaps emphasize it at this point, because it won't come out in the discussion otherwise.

*Dr. Klawans*

I actually thank you for that. No, I don't sell that in any way, shape or form. I look at that primarily as an exercise now in demonstrating the hypothesis of postsynaptic hypersensitivity in the pathophysiology of chorea. Obviously the patients and the patients' families and the subjects at risk all look at it as a means of preclinical diagnosis. I tried to point out very strongly that our incidents of false negatives may well be up to 50 percent, which would clearly limit, the clinical usefulness of this procedure. I don't think we will know whether it should be done or not for a long time. It was an interesting observation; I think it was worth doing the first time, and I understand the pressure from Huntington patients, but until we really know, I don't think this should be done under any circumstances other than collecting a large series where we can follow them. If somebody is going to do it in thirty more patients and follow them, we are going to get data within a few years that would give us some information. I think individual physicians doing it on individual patients is not justified in any way.

*Dr. Flores*

I was wondering if there were any studies or experiments done on the treatment of Parkinson's disease using tranquilizers or muscle relaxants together with L-dopa?

*Dr. Klawans*

Minor tranquilizers?

*Dr. Flores*
      Yes, like Valium®, for instance, or muscle relaxants?

*Dr. Klawans*
      I don't know of any reasonable double blind controlled studies.
We all know lots of patients get put on these; I have never seen any
particular efficacy from them, for a variety of reasons.  Is anybody
aware of any good studies on that?

*Dr. Flores*
      I brought this question up because I have a particular Parkin-
sonian patient, who is about a 65 year-old female, I found that ten
milligrams of Valium® about three times a day, together with L-dopa,
could control her tremors better.

*Dr. Klawans*
      Tremor of all the symptoms is probably most susceptible to level
of anxiety and there are patients who claim they feel better on a
variety of minor tranquilizers.  But I don't know of any good studies
that demonstrate any specific effect or a population effect on large
groups of patients.

*Dr. Flemenbaum*
      On the basis of animal data, I would very certainly look down
on using that kind of combination because I am aware of a few studies
that have shown an increase of receptor sensitivity to L-dopa and
amphetamine effects, when minor tranquilizers such as chlordiazepoxide are added.  There are several British papers that have shown a
clear increase of hyperactivity when given threshold doses of
amphetamine and chlordiazepoxide.  There are other papers showing
clear increases of stereotyped behavior when chlordiazepoxide is
given.  From that point of view (agonist-induced receptor hypersensitivity) I would consider minor tranquilizers contraindicated.
We are presently involved in testing that hypothesis.

*Dr. Hornykiewicz*
      I remember a short note in *Lancet* a few years ago in which,
if I remember correctly, the statement was made that concomitant
administration of Valium® with levodopa abolished levodopa's beneficial effect.

*Dr. Klawans*
      We have all seen patients who get put on Valium® by a variety of
physicians for a variety of reasons, in varieties of doses; and
clearly it doesn't abolish the levodopa effect.

*Dr. Duvoisin*

When we were at the dopaminergic symposium, that Donald Calne edited, Iverson stated that Valium® was a potent phosphodiesterase inhibitor, and we mentioned that it was our clinical impression that Valium® tended to make the bradykinesia of parkinsonism worse, while it was true it might reduce tremor somewhat. But I agree there is a risk of significantly increasing the bradykinesia, at least in some patients. It's an old observation that barbituates and other sedatives also share that risk, so that they should be avoided in Parkinson patients. There are cases of dyskinesia, I think Masland described one thirty years ago of chorea induced as a toxic effect by phenobarbital used as an anticonvulsant; but those are very rare cases. There are reports, however, of phenobarbital severely exacerbating the bradykinesia of parkinsonism.

# TREATMENT OF PARKINSONISM

D.B. CALNE, P.F. TEYCHENNE and R.F. PFEIFFER

Experimental Therapeutics Branch
National Institute of Neurological and Communicative
    Disorders and Stroke
National Institutes of Health
Department of Health, Education and Welfare
Bethesda, Maryland 20014

DECARBOXYLASE INHIBITORS

Over the last decade the treatment of Parkinsonism has under-
gone major developments.  Advances deriving from a logically struc-
tured series of laboratory experiments have been transferred to the
clinic to generate substantial therapeutic achievements.

The advent of levodopa led to dramatic improvement in neurological deficits in many patients; the appearance of unexpected, dose
dependent, reversible adverse reactions also resulted in important
hypotheses, such as the attribution of choreoathetoid movement
disorders to excessive dopaminergic transmission.  Some adverse
reactions, such as cardiac arrhythmias, are likely to be caused by
peripheral formation of catecholamines from levodopa.  It was therefore predicted that an improvement in the therapeutic index (ratio
of toxic dose/effective dose) might be achieved by concomitant
administration of a drug which supressed conversion of levodopa to
catecholamines (by inhibition of the relevant enzyme, dopa decarboxylase), provided a blocker could be found which did not itself
cross the blood-brain barrier.  This combination of drugs would be
expected to decrease all adverse reactions induced by catecholamine formation outside the central nervous sytem, while still allowing therapeutic efficacy to be attained by cerebral conversion of
levodopa to dopamine.

Two extracerebral inhibitors of dopa decarboxylase have been
introduced successfully into routine management of parkinsonism,
i.e carbidopa (combined with levodopa in the proprietary preparation "Sinemet") and benserazide (combined with levodopa in the
branded product "Madopar").   There is no convincing evidence that
either one of these decarboxylase inhibitors is therapeutically
superior to the other (*Greenacre, et al., 1976*).   The main advan-
tages gained by the use of extracerebral decarboxylase blockers are:
1) reduction of anorexia, nausea and vomiting, probably achieved
by inhibition of catecholamine formation in the region of the area
postrema, which is close to the emetic center and, although located
in the central nervous system, is outside the blood-brain barrier;
2) reduced risk of cardiovascular toxicity, in particular cardiac
arrythmias and orthostatic hypotension; and 3) decreased risk of
inducing glaucoma.
       Since the usual early adverse reactions to levodopa (emesis
and orthostatic hypotension) are decreased, dosage can be built up
to optimal levels over a shorter period than is possible with levodopa alone.   For the same reason, there is a higher risk of encoun-
tering more severe centrally induced adverse reactions, such as
dyskinesia and psychiatric disturbance.   This is simply an "over-
shoot" phenomena which is corrected by reduction of dosage, but it
is a sufficiently real problem to justify some caution in the rate
of increment of dosage at the start of therapy.
       From these viewpoints, it is evident that when starting patients
on treatment with levodopa, it is normally best to give this drug
in combination with a decarboxylase inhibitor.   However, in those
patients who are already stabilized on levodopa, there is no reason
to give a decarboxylase inhibitor unless the patient is experiencing
emesis, or orthostatic hypotension, or is particularly vulnerable
to the risk of cardiac arrythmia or glaucoma.
       Having decreased the "peripheral" adverse reactions to levodopa,
the major therapeutic task is amelioration of "central" unwanted
effects, such as dyskinesia.   In recent years this problem has been
recast with the emergence of "on-off" phenomena, in many of which
patients fluctuate abruptly from severe exacerbations of parkinsonism
to florid choreoathetosis.

DOPAMINERGIC AGONISTS

       In this review, drugs which mimic a transmitter by acting
directly upon postsynaptic receptors will be described by the simple
term "agonist" (which will be employed as a synonym for "direct
agonist" or "receptor agonist").   It is probable that the next
important step in the treatment of parkinsonism will be the development of a dopaminergic agonist which has a predeliction for the
receptors at those synapses in the striatum which are primarily

disturbed by degeneration of the nigrostriatal pathway.  It is clear
that different types or conformational states of dopaminergic receptors exist from the categorization of such varied properties as:
1) receptor binding to different ligands (Creese, et al., 1976);
2) dopaminergic responses involving depolarization or hyperpolarization (McLennan and York, 1967); 3) dopaminergic formation of cyclic
adenosine monophosphate at striatal postsynaptic receptors but not
at striatal presynaptic receptors (Mishra, et al., 1974); and 4)
dopaminergic induction of changes in neuronal membrane permeability
which may be short (less than 10ms) or long (over 100ms) (Libet and
Tosaka, 1970).

       With accumulating evidence it is already possible to start
defining the different types of dopamine receptor (Cools and VanRos-
sum, 1975), and the task of developing selective agonists for one
form of receptor is quite feasible.  In this context, it is of considerable interest that an ergoline agonist of dopamine (9,10-Dide-
hydro-6-methyl-8β-[2pyridylthiomethyl] ergoline: CF25-397) has been
shown to induce contralateral turning in rats with unilateral nigral
lesions (an analogue for the efficacy of drugs employed to treat
parkinsonism) without causing stereotypic behavior (usually considered a paradigm for choreoathetosis) (Jaton, et al., 1975).  Such
an agonist might be anticipated to improve parkinsonism without
producing the major dose limiting adverse reaction - dyskinesia.
Unfortunately, CF25-397 has not proved effective as a therapeutic
agent (Teychenne, et al., 1976), possibly because its action in the
rat appears to depend upon formation of an active metabolite, which
may not accumulate in man (Silbergeld et al., 1977).

       Another promising ergoline dopaminergic agonist, lergotrile
(Lieberman, et al., 1975), has recently been found to produce abnormalities of hepatic function which may limit its value as an antiparkinsonian agent (Teychenne, et al., 1976).

       Up to now, the most encouraging results have been achieved with
an ergoline tripeptide, bromocriptine (Kartzinel, et al., 1976) and
an apomorphine derivative, N-propylnoraporphine (Cotzias, et al.,
1976).  With both of these compounds, optimal therapeutic results
are achieved by concomitant administration of levodopa (with an
extracerebral decarboxylase inhibitor).  This clinical observation
may perhaps be interpreted in terms of the recent demonstration that
certain agonists have additional presynaptic actions, in particular
releasing dopamine and inhibiting its active reuptake (Silbergeld,
and Pfeiffer, 1976).  An agonist with these properties could be
predicted to attain maximum dopaminergic effect when the nerve
endings are loaded with dopamine by administration of levodopa.

       With increasing study, it is probable that there will be ero-
sion of the specificity currently attributed to agonists.  For
example, changes in serotonin function have recently been reported
with bromocriptine (Kartzinel, et al., 1976).  At present, it is

not possible to predict with any precision whether the various profiles of activity for agonists on diverse receptors for different
transmitters will prove useful or deleterious. Previous suggestions
have proposed, for example, that concomitant activation of certain
norepinephrine or serotonin receptors might play a crucial role in
the induction of both therapeutic and adverse responses to treatment.

Other relevant points, in comparing precursor with agonist
therapy, include: 1) dopa decarboxylase is depleted in the brain of
parkinsonian patients (Lloyd, et al., 1973); unlike precursors, agonists do not require the presence of this enzyme; and 2) the plasma
half-life of levodopa is short (around 45 minutes by itself, about
3 hours with an extracebral decarboxylase inhibitor) (Reid, et al.,
1972), a fact which may account for some of the fluctuations in
clinical response encountered by patients receiving levodopa. Certain agonists, such as bromocriptine, appear to have a more prolonged
action than levodopa.

EARLY MANAGEMENT

The major problem now encountered in treating parkinsonism is
the development of "on-off" attacks, usually presenting as abrupt
changes from severe parkinsonism to florid dyskinesia with a corresponding reduction in the period of optimal response. This clinical
dilemma generally occurs after 3 to 6 years of treatment with levodopa.
No satisfactory method of managing "on-off" reactions has yet been
established. The best compromise can probably be reached by reducing
the dose of levodopa and adding bromocriptine (Kartzinel, and Calne,
1976) but some patients are refactory to every therapeutic maneuver.

The cause of "on-off" phenomena is not known; suggested mechanisms include: 1) pharmacokinetic variations leading to fluctuating
concentrations of striatal dopamine; 2) spontaneous alterations
in dopaminergic receptor sensitivity; and 3) abrupt changes of activity in neural pathways which modulate striatal input or output.
These proposals are not mutually exclusive; as currently, and rather
loosely defined, "on-off" reactions could be caused by a number of
different mechanisms (Marsden, and Parkes, 1976).

Whatever the neuropharmacological determinants of "on-off"
phenomena may prove to be, it is probable that the cumulative dose
of levodopa is an important element in their aetiology because:
1) they are more frequent in patients who have been taking levodopa
for several years and 2) their prevalence is higher in countries
where large doses of levodopa are prescribed, such as the United
States, compared to countries which employ smaller dose regimens,
such as Great Britain.

Two important conclusions derive from these premises. First, it
is desirable to treat patients with the lowest dose of levodopa that
will achieve a reasonable quality of life, rather than striving for
maximal therapeutic response. Second, it may be preferable to

start treatment of new patients with anticholinergic agents or amantadine unless their livelihood or psychological well-being demand
the most potent conventional therapy available - levodopa combined
with an extracerebral decarboxylase inhibitor *(Yahr, 1973)*.  Since
it appears that a substantial and unpredictable proportion of patients will only respond well to levodopa for a limited period of
time, it would seem reasonable to preserve this treatment until it
becomes really necessary *(Yahr, 1975)*.

In this context, an important question relates to the early
treatment of patients with dopaminergic agonists such as bromocriptine.  These drugs are the only experimental medications of comparable
potency to levodopa and at present we do not know whether their use
over several years, without levodopa, will lead to serious adverse
reactions such as "on-off" phenomena.  If they should prove to have
sustained efficacy without inducing the late problems of levodopa
therapy, they would become the best form of initial treatment for
parkinsonism.  However, until more information on the long term
human toxicology of agonists is available, early and prolonged treatment with these drugs alone should be limited to a few experimental
studies.  At present, the major role for bromocriptine in the treatment of parkinsonism is as adjuvant therapy, combined with submaximal
dosage of levodopa in patients with "on-off" reactions.

## SUMMARY

While many problems relating to the cause and treatment of
Parkinsonism are still unanswered, the striatal dopamine depletion
syndrome remains a dynamic area of study for those interested in
neurological pharmacology and therapeutics.  Over the last few years
at least three important developments have occurred with definite
implications for the practical management of patients: 1) the assimi-
lation of extracerebral decarboxylase inhibitors into routine treatment; 2) the recognition of certain limitations of levodopa therapy,
such as "on-off" reactions, which is leading to a reappraisal of
early management; and 3) the identification of certain dopaminergic
agonists as drugs which have profiles of efficacy and toxicity
comparable to levodopa.

## ACKNOWLEDGEMENTS

We wish to thank Mrs. P. Barnicoat and Miss V. Bergmeyer for
administrative assistance and Mrs. A. Miller for typing this manuscript.

## REFERENCES

Cools, A.R. and Van Rossum, J.M.  (1975).  Excitation-mediating and
    inhibition-mediating dopamine-receptors: A new concept towards

a better understanding of electrophysiological, biochemical, pharmacological, functional and clinical data. *Psychopharmacologia (Berl)*. *45*, 243-254.

Cotzias, G.C., Lawrence, W.H., Papavasiliou, P.S., Tolosa, E.S., Mendez, J.S. and Bell-Medura, M. (1976). Treatment of Parkinson's disease with aporphines, possible role of growth hormone. *New Engl J. Med 294*, 567-572.

Creese, I.N., Bunt, D.R. and Snyder, S.H. (1976). Dopamine receptor binding; differentiation of agonist and antagonist states with $^3$H-holaperidol. *Life Sci. 17*, 993-1002.

Greenacre, J.K., Coxon, A., Petrie, A. and Reid, J.L. (1976). Comparison of levodopa with carbidopa or benserazide in parkinsonism. *Lancet 2*, 381-384.

Jaton, A.L., Loew, D.M. and Vigouret, J.M. (1975). CF 25-397 (9,10-didehydro-6-methyl-8β-[2-pyridylthiomethyl] ergoline), a new central dopamine receptor agonist. *Proc B.P.S. 56*, 371.

Kartzinel, R. and Calne, D.B. (1976). Studies with bromocriptine Part I. "On-off" phenomena. *Neurology, 26*, 508-510.

Kartzinel, R., Perlow, M.J., Carter, A.C., Chase, T.N. and Calne, D.B. (1976). Metabolic studies with bromocriptine in patients with idiopathic Parkinsonism and Huntington's Chorea. *Trans Am Neurol Assoc*. In press.

Kartzinel, R., Perlow, M. Teychenne, P., Gielen, A., Gillespie, M., Sadowsky, D. and Calne, D.B. (1976). Bromocriptine and levodopa (with or without carbidopa) in Parkinsonism. *Lancet 2*, 272-275.

Libet, B. and Tosaka, T. (1970). Dopamine as a synaptic transmitter and modulator in sympathetic ganglia: A different mode of synaptic action. *Proc Nat Acad Sci USA 67*, 667-673.

Lieberman, A., Miyamoto, T., Battista, A. and Goldstein, M. (1975). Studies on the anti-Parkinsonian efficacy of lergotrile. *Neurol. 25*, 459-462.

Lloyd, K.G., Davidson, L. and Hornykiewicz, O. (1973). Metabolism of levodopa in the human brain. *In Advances in Neurology, Vol. 3, (Calne, D.B., Ed.)* pp. 173-188. Raven Press, New York.

Marsden, C.D. and Parkes, J.D. (1976). "On-off" effects in patients with Parkinson's disease on chronic levodopa therapy. *Lancet 1*, 292-296.

McLennan, H. and York, D.H. (1967). The action of dopamine on neurons of the caudate nucleus. *J. Physiol. (Lond). 189*, 393-402.

Reid, J.L., Calne, D.B., Vakil, S.D., Allen, J.C. and Davies, C.A. (1972). Plasma concentrations of levodopa in Parkinsonism before and after inhibition of peripheral decarboxylase. *J. Neurol Sci. 17*, 45-51.

Silbergeld, E.K., Adler, H., Kennedy, S. and Calne, D.B. (1976). Roles of presynaptic dopamine function and hepatic drug metabolism in effects of three dopamine agonists: bromocriptine, lergotrile and CF25-397. In press.

Silbergeld, E.K. and Pfeiffer, R.F. (1976). Differential effects of
    three dopamine agonists: apomorphine, bromocriptine and lergo-
    trile. In press.
Teychenne, P.F., Jones, A. and Calne, D.B. (1976). Changes in liver
    function induced by lergotrile. In preparation.
Teychenne, P.F., Pfeiffer, R.F. and Calne, D.B. (1976). Actions of
    CF25-397 in parkinsonism. In preparation.
Yahr, M.D. (ed.) (1973). *In Advances in Neurology, Vol. 2-Treatment
    of Parkinson's Disease-the Use of Dopa Decarboxylase Inhibitors.*
    pp. 303. Raven Press, New York.
Yahr, M.D. (1975). Levodopa. *Ann Intern Med. 83*, 667-682.

## DISCUSSION

*Dr. Frigyesi*
    Have you had an opportunity to try bromocriptine in patients
with coma, and compare the effects with L-dopa?

*Dr. Calne*
    What kind of coma?

*Dr. Frigyesi*
    Patients with traumatic coma.

*Dr. Calne*
    No. Could you tell us a little bit Dr. Frigyesi about the
rationale and the experience in treating patients with traumatic
coma?

*Dr. Frigyesi*
    Dello Oro administered it first with success. Hassler con-
firmed it. I induced coma in monkeys by twisting their mediastinum.
They developed cardiac problems first, then a flat EEG. Following
administration of L-dopa, spindles appeared on the EEG. I am just
curious whether bromocriptine may be more effective in such cases.

*Dr. Calne*
    Well, thank you very much. That is very interesting, and I
am not aware of anyone having used bromocryptine up to now, in that
context.

*Dr. de la Torre*
    I was a little confused about your statement that bromocrip-
tine increases flow rather than decreases it. I wonder if you could
elaborate on that, if any blood flow tests were done in view of the
fact that most ergot alkaloids will constrict cerebral blood vessels?

*Dr. Calne*
        We were gratified that we hadn't seen any vasoconstriction any-
where.  We were disturbed to find that other people had encountered
digital vasospasm.  When one encounters the peripheral hyperemic problems one feels ethically impelled to stop treatment quickly; and we
just weren't geared up to do blood flow studies over the critical
phase, because they do get better quickly when you stop the treatment.
You may occasionally see profound reduction of blood pressure; we have
had one patient who fainted on 2.5 mg of bromocryptine.  We thought it
was coincidence, so we brought him into the hospital and repeated the
dose; this was clearly drug induced syncope.  The majority of patients
on bromocriptine do display some hypotension but this is mild: maybe
less troublesome than with levodopa.  The patients adjust to it as
time goes on.

*Dr. Fahn*
        I would like to come to your point that you raised about how
to best treat newly diagnosed parkinsonism, because this is a topic
that I have been thinking about for some time, and I have advocated
for over a year now more or less the same line that you are advocating.

*Dr. Calne*
        You have been saying this for a long time and certainly long
before I have, and I fully agree with you.

*Dr. Fahn*
        I would like to elaborate a little bit about various factors.
First of all, it's true in our hands also, that many patients on
levodopa therapy, tend to have less benefit over the years, and maybe five years is a reasonable average median time for maximum benefit.  I should, however, point out that one does see patients who
go six or seven years, and who really still do very very well.  So
one cannot generalize.  But then there are patients who, after two
years, do very poorly.  I think we have all seen patients who started out with the unilateral mild parkinsonism and who, in the very
early days of levodopa trials, were given levodopa and deteriorated
terribly over the years, and are now very difficult to control.
That is certainly one reason why one should perhaps delay levodopa,
that is the lack of benefit with time.  Second, there is the development of toxic manifestations; the choreic movements as we have mentioned, which one could perhaps live with; but then the on-off effect
is so difficult to control today, that it's another important factor
which one has to think about before starting treatment.  In our
experience patients with parkinsonism, 30 to 40 year range, let's
say, they have all done terribly badly with on-off effects.  They
are very difficult to control.  They are the ones who really are

devastated by the on-off effect.  They become unable to work and carry
out a normal life.  A third type of problem that I think we should
mention here, although nobody really has proof that it's related,
is the increasing memory impairment and intellectual difficulties in
patients with long-term treatment.  One is always concerned if
perhaps the drug we are using is partly causing this, even though
one is aware that even before treatment, some Parkinson patients
have difficulties in this sphere.  Nevertheless, dementia becomes
almost untreatable when a Parkinson patient does develop this on dopa.
If the drug is in any way causing dementia one would have liked to
have delayed its use.

*Dr. Calne*

I agree with everything you say.

*Dr. Duvoisin*

I must enter a dissenting note.  I don't agree that you can
make a flat rule that you should not use the drug of choice first.
Each case should be individually evaluated.  I don't believe that
we have good evidence that the response the patient will have five
years from now is any different whether you start them on levodopa
today or next year or the year after.  I think you have to balance
what the patient's difficulties are now and the side effects of the
other drugs, which are quite substantial.  We tend to underrate the
significant side effects of the anticholinergics and amantadine.
Finally, many of the things that are reported are artefacts of observation.  As Hippocrates said, life is short, art is long, experience
fallacious.  I think we are having a good deal of difficulty in
understanding or separating the effects of progression of the disease,
its interaction with the patient's life, and the effects of our
treatment.

*Dr. Calne*

I am not quite sure how you are dissenting, because I agree
entirely that you must judge every patient individually; that the
patient whose life depends on maximal dexterity of the hands must
be treated from the first time you see him, with the most powerful drug that you have available.

*Dr. Duvoisin*

Yes; but I detected a note in what you were saying and particularly what Stanley was saying that you prefer to reserve your best
arrow, if you will, your best weapon, for later on.  And I agree
that there is mileage in that and patient rapport, but there are
many situations in which I would prefer to use our best drug initially.  Maybe I misunderstood you, but I thought that you meant
that you prefer to delay those things.

*Dr. Calne*
     I prefer to delay it if the disease is not really making an important difference to the patient's life.

*Dr. Duvoisin*
     Then we agree.

*Dr. Fahn*
     Well, I must say the same thing, that it is depenent on what is needed for that particular patient, when you decide whether or not to start.  The person who is already retired and is not doing much except daily exercises at home doesn't need to be started right away when he only has his first symptom of tremor; you can wait.  But the person who obviously is occupationally handicapped needs it; and there is no question about his treatment with levodopa.  You have to take into consideration each individual patient.  It was mentioned that one should always use the best drugs, but I would like to point out the most potent drug isn't always the best drug at that particular moment.  One should think about what the best drug is for that specific individual.  Perhaps a little amantadine would go a long way for a couple of years to help a person until the symptoms develop with his disease.

*Dr. Mars*
     I want some clarification, first.  Did I understand you to say that the period of clinical effectiveness of the levodopa preparation was five years, and then you have a loss of effect and a catch up of symptomatology?

*Dr. Calne*
     I was giving average impressions.

*Dr. Mars*
     Next question.  Does this apply for levodopa alone or levodopa combined with the decarboxylase inhibitors?

*Dr. Calne*
     You just induce therapy quicker; that's a matter of a month or two, and is of no significance.  Perhaps we are also tending to over-treat our patients more, when they are taking a decarboxylase inhib-itor, because they are not dose limited by emesis and anorexia.

*Dr. Mars*
     I am asking whether there is a loss in the anti-bradykinetic anti-rigid effect in five years.  I am not talking about dyskinesia.

*Dr. Calne*
     As time goes on your therapeutic index deteriorates; that is

to say, the balance between efficacy and toxicity changes adversely.

*Dr. Mars*
     Well, I think I can go along with that.  But it's certainly
very variable from one patient to another, and you will have patients
who do demonstrate a very rapid onset of brittleness in response.

*Dr. Calne*
     Yes.

*Dr. Mars*
     And others can go for an awfully long time without getting to
that difficulty?

*Dr. Calne*
     Yes, the problem is prediction; if only we could predict how
an individual is going to change.

*Dr. Hunt*
     Several of the speakers here today have alluded to this, but
I think somebody ought to answer the question more directly:  Does
any of the treatments that we use now influence the natural course of
the disease?  It seems to me that is a basic problem in making a
decision on how vigorously we should treat early and mild parkinsonism.

*Dr. Calne*
     Well, I think that life is extended by the administration of
levodopa.  Now, that does not mean that the underlying pathology is
in any way modified.  There may simply be palliative amelioration
of symptoms and signs.

*Dr. Volkman*
     There have been a number of recent reports about the effects
of bromocriptine which raised questions about its mechanism of action
in alleviating symptoms of Parkinson's disease.  Trabucci *et al. (Life
Sciences 19: 225-232, 1976)* reported that bromocriptine does not
stimulate adenyl cyclase activity of striatal homogenates, and in
fact, inhibits the dopamine-induced increase in striatal cyclase.
Johnson *et al. (British Journal of Pharmacology 56: 59-68, 1976)*
reported that the effects of bromocriptine in producing contralateral turning in unilaterally substantia nigra-lesioned rats and increasing locomotor activity are blocked by pimozide, but require intact catecholamine stores, suggesting a dopamine-releasing action
of bromocriptine.  Dray and Oakley *(Journal of Pharmacy and Pharmacology 28: 586-588, 1976)* reported that bromocriptine reduced
apomorphine-induced turning behavior in unilaterally substantia
nigra-lesioned rats, but enhanced the actions of amphetamine,

suggesting that bromocriptine is a dopamine-releasing agent or
perhaps a partial agonist at dopamine receptors.  In a model
system for a peripheral vascular dopamine receptor, both bromocriptine and lergotrile are inactive in the production of renal
vasodilation *(Volkman and Goldberg, Pharmacologist 18: 130, 1976)*.
All of the above may indicate that bromocriptine is not a directly-
acting dopamine agonist.  In further support of this concept is the
fact that the maximum therapeutic benefit from bromocriptine was in
conjunction with L-dopa therapy.  This is probably the case with
lergotrile as well.

*Dr. Calne*

I think what you say is further evidence that there are probably
several categories of dopamine receptor.  Furthermore, we are not just
dealing with a dopamine agonist, we are dealing with a drug that has
presynaptic effects on dopamine and that probably has actions on
serotonin mechanisms as well.

*Dr. Fahn*

As a person who has never used an ergoline to treat parkinsonism,
I would like to get a better feeling as to its potential value for
our patients.  What I would like to ask in this regard is: Assuming
it was now readily available on the market and with the same cost factor as levodopa or sinemet, and a patient comes to you who needs to
be treated with a fairly potent agonist drug, whether levodopa or
ergoline derivative, how would you rate bromocriptine?  Would you say
that would be your first drug of choice and if so, why?

*Dr. Calne*

I think a critical piece of information which we do not yet have,
to answer the question whether we should treat all patients this way
if we could, is what happens if you take a patient who has never been
given levodopa; you treat him with bromocriptine for years. Will he
get on-off reactions?  Since the biggest problem in handling patients
is these on-off reactions, the single most important piece of information that we need to have is: does bromocriptine by itself induce
on-off reactions?  I don't think that a patient who is doing well on
dopa or sinemet should be changed to bromocriptine.  But if a patient
is getting on-off reactions, then you should reduce his dose of dopa,
and build up an intake of bromocriptine; this is a difficult manipulation, requiring frequent attendances in the clinic.  I would say
that seventy-five percent of patients with on-off reactions derive
improvement from this maneuver.

*Dr. Potter*

Since you are proposing perhaps the chronic use of bromocriptine, is it like methysergide in that it can produce a retroperitoneal fibrosis?

*Dr. Calne*

There have been no reports of retroperitoneal fibrosis induced by bromocryptine.

*Dr. Potter*

Is there any idea as to the mechanism of the hypotensive effect; is this believed to be central or peripheral?

*Dr. Calne*

I think there are two elements to the hypotensive action. One is that the set of the blood pressure is modified by a central dopaminergic effect. By the set of the blood pressure, I mean the blood pressure that you record with a patient recumbent. Now in addition to that, the baroceptor adjustment to postural change is impaired by a peripheral dopaminergic mechanism.

*Dr. Franz*

Earlier you made passing reference, in discussing the on-off effect, to a pharmacokinetic problem. I wonder if you would expand on that, because the pharmacokinetic problems we can usually handle better than the pharmacodynamic ones.

*Dr. Calne*

There has been conflicting reports in the literature about, for example, the correlation of blood levels with on-off fluctuations. Some have found that the exacerbation of parkinsonism, the off phase of the on-off reaction, is associated with a low plasma level of dopa. Others have reported an exacerbation of parkinsonism with a high blood level of levodopa. Some say that you can improve the fluctuations, the on-off reactions, by more frequent administration of levodopa. In some patients, maybe you can. But in some patients, you certainly can't.

*Dr. Franz*

Wouldn't you see it much earlier if it was a pharmacokinetic problem?

*Dr. Calne*

That's quite right, there is some change of metabolism of the drug or absorption of the drug after prolonged therapy, and prolonged not in terms of months but in terms of years.

# PARKINSONISM AND EPILEPSY*

TAMAS L. FRIGYESI

Department of Physiology
Texas Tech University School of Medicine
Lubbock, Texas 79409

Clinical observations indicate that parkinsonians do not, or
only exceptionally, exhibit epileptic phenomena and *vice versa*
(*Scholz, 1957; Klee, 1975*). Yakovlev reported *(1928)* that when
epileptic patients develop parkinsonism, the epilepsy *pari passu*
disappears. The exact neurophysiological mechanisms underlying
these pathological conditions are poorly understood. Yet, it is
apparent, that both of these diseases dominantly involve the
sensorimotor system. Thus the question appears to be of more than
heuristic importance as to why these two disease states are mutually exclusive. Whereas epilepsy readily lends itself to experimental approaches in the domain of electrophysiology, parkinsonism
does not, because only its morphological and biochemical features
but not its clinical symptomatology can be reproduced in experimental animals. The normal integration of sensorimotor activities,
and the electrophysiological consequences of caudatal and nigral
damage (established sites of pathology in parkinsonism) to such
integrative processes, have extensively been explored in felines
and subhuman primates *(Frigyesi, 1975a, 1975b)*; these studies
yielded data which, when extrapolated to parkinsonism, suggested
the nature of elementary processes which underlie, at least some
symptoms of, parkinsonism *(Frigyesi, 1971; Frigyesi, et al., 1974)*.

The present report gives a succinct account of three series of
experiments which together provide an answer to the posed question
of what basic mechanisms preclude the coexistence of parkinsonism
and epilepsy in man. While data are presented and various

---

*In Memoriam, Dr. Albert J. Dinnerstein

possible neurophysiological mechanisms are described, the inter-
pretations are justified on the grounds of parsimony and on successful experimental tests rather than on the ground of excluding alternative hypotheses.  Although there is a striking disparity between
the first and the subsequent series of experiments, the common
denominator in all three is that they are addressed to the propo-
sition that the sensorimotor system is comprised of a hierarchy of
circuits (feedback and feedforward loops) in which timing plays a
significant role.

## 1. DELAYED PROPRIOCEPTIVE FEEDBACK AS A POSSIBLE MECHANISM IN PARKINSONISM

Parkinsonism with identical symptomatogy is produced by diverse
etiologic factors: encephalitis (von Economo, 1929), syphilis (Wilson and Cobb, 1924), mercury (Kulkow, 1930), CO (Beretervide and
Carrega-Casaffousth, 1933), manganese (Edsall and Drinker, 1919),
and cyanide poisoning (Buzzo and Guerra, 1930), brain tumor (Hunt
and Lisa, 1927), drugs (Steck, 1954) and maybe trauma [for discussion, (see Schwab and England, 1968)].  A unifying process, A.P.U.D.
cell deficiency, was recently proposed for the etiology of the
disease (Barbeau, 1976).  Why should so dissimilar events produce
similar symptoms?  To account for this, a unifying process may be
found in the hypothesis that a simple perceptual malfunction, an
abnormal delay in proprioceptive feedback, could account for some
of the symptomalogy of parkinsonism (Dinnerstein and Frigyesi, 1962).
Variable delays in the normal perceptual processes are well
established phenomena (Boring, 1950).  They were first noted in
the early 1800's by astronomers.  They appeared as a disagreement
between different observers in attempts to compare the time of the
transit of a star across a point in the telescope field with the
beat of a clock.  Laboratory research eventually showed that if
stimuli of different sensory modalities were presented simultaneously, either one or the other was experienced as occurring first.
The intermodal difference in perceptual speed varied among obervers,
and varied within a single observer as a function of direction of
attention (Angell and Pierce, 1892), and an inverse function of
stimulus intensity (Cattell, 1885).
Parkinsonian tremor has been compared with oscillations found
in electromechanical feedback systems (Weiner, 1950).  Oscillations
in such systems may be induced by a variety of factors; relevant
to the present disucssion is that oscillation occurs if the feedback system has a lagging characteristic, the load change does
not come in a secular manner and the compensation system fails
(Weiner, 1961).  Sensory delay should induce oscillations in the
effectors with respect to postural feedbacks, i.e. proprioceptive
delay should induce oscillations in the motor-effectors.  An
important aspect of this concept is that it lends itself to human
experimentation.

The behavioral disabilities in parkinsonism have analogies
in the speech disabilities in stuttering.  The tremor in parkinsonism
is superficially similar to syllable repetition of stuttering speech.
Bradykinesis (the slowness and the tardy initiation of movements)
in parkinsonism are somewhat analogous to the explosive speech after
the tense pauses in the stuttering speech.  While the neurophysiological mechanisms leading to stuttering are yet to be explained,
stuttering can be induced experimentally by delayed auditory feedback *(Lee, 1950):* dramatic disruption of speech is produced by
having the subjects speak or read aloud while listening to their
own speech which has been recorded and played back via earphones
after a delay of 100-400 msec.

Equally relevant to the present concern are the data that show
the vacillation, repetitions and pauses in writing and other visuo-
motor tasks can be experimentally induced by delayed visual feedback *(Kalmus, Fry and Denes, 1960).*  The situation involved procedures similar to those employed in auditory delay.  The subjects
could not directly see what they were writing; a visual display
presented information to the subjects concerning their movements
but the display lagged behind the subjects' movements.  Again, the
disruption of motor behavior was dramatic.

The effect of auditory delay on a task normally utilizing
auditory feedback, and the effect of visual delay on a task normally
utilizing visual feedback suggest that a general proprioceptive
delay would produce analogous disruption of those motor tasks which
involve general proprioceptive feedback, i.e. all sensorimotor
activities.

*The test of deductions from the theory.*  Parkinsonism here is
hypothesized to involve longer than normal delay of impulses in the
ascending pathways which provide proprioceptive  feedback to those
forebrain structures which control limb position and muscle tone.
(Proprioception here is distinguished from kinesthesia; the former
refers to sensibility mediated by ascending systems which arise
in the muscle spindle, tendon, joint and skin, procede toward the
cerebellum and hence to the ventrolateral thalamus and terminate
in the motor cortex; the latter, to the sensibility mediated by a
system which arises at the same sites, but proceeds in the dorsal
columns toward gracile and cuneate nuclei, and hence to the ventro-
basal nucleus of the thalamus, and terminates in the somato-sensory
cortex; the former contributes to processing of motor activities,
whereas the latter to perception of the moment-to-moment spatial
position of the body and its parts).  The simplest mechanism of
delay would be non-specific, involving all of the ascending proprioceptive tracts.  Parkinsonisms should, therefore, exhibit delays
of activities initiated in the muscle spindle, tendon, joint and
skin relative to their speed of perception in modalities *not*
involving the *ascending* proprioceptive tracts (audition and vision).

The subjects were 18 parkinsonian and 14 non-neurological
patients; the age groups were matched (40-82 years).

An apparatus was designed to present pairs of stimuli for judgements of subjective sequence. The basic unit was a turntable which rotated at 30 rpm. A 13mm high flexible plastic tab was attached perpendicularly to the surface of the turntable; the subjects hand was supported above the turntable in such a manner that the rotating tab could flex the distal phalanges of his forefinger.

The visual stimulus was presented by a white bar which, while passing behind a slit in a screen, become momentarily visible to the subjects. The auditory stimulus was a click.

Adjustable microswitches were mounted around the edge of the turntable; these permitted the prevention of any pairs of these three stimuli either simultaneously or at ± 167 and ± 333 msec time separation.

Pairs of stimuli were presented at temporal distances of -333, -167, 0, +167 and +333 msec. The subject was required to answer the appropriate question: "Which occurred first, the sound or the touch?"; or "the flash or the touch?"; or "the sound or the flash?". Each of the five temporal distances were presented, in random, twenty times, thus yielding 100 judgments. The three series of intermodal comparisons usually occurred on separate days.

The point of subjective equality (PSE) was computed for each subject on each of the three intermodal test series. The PSE between modalities is that temporal distance between the stimuli at which the subject judges one or the other stimulus occurring first in 50% of the trials; i.e. PSE denotes miliseconds between stimuli presented at different times and judged as occurring simultaneously.

Figure 1 illustrates the data obtained from 12 parkinsonian and 12 control subjects. (Data from 9 subjects had to be discarded because they either did not permit computation of the 50% point or yielded more than one such point on one or more of the test series).

The data illustrated were obtained by comparing pairs of PSE and expressing them as a deviation from that of the subject's average speed of perception. The group averages of these deviation scores are displayed so that a minus sign indicates that perception in that modality was faster, and a plus sign that it was slower, than the average speed. Proprioception (denoted as touch in the Figure 1) was slow in parkinsonians and fast in the control group. The difference in perception speed pattern, between the parkinsonians and controls, was significant with $p < 2$ according to Wilcoxon's nonparametric analysis of variance test (*Wilcoxon, 1949*); excluding the parkinsonians on medication (6 patients) (Artane and barbiturates), the difference was even more reliable ($p < .001$).

Figure 1 also shows that antiparkinsonian medication reduced the proprioceptive delay in the parkinsonian patients significantly ($p < .01$). Thus, the data show that an extensive proprioceptive delay operates in parkinsonism. The relevance of co-variation of audition with proprioception has as yet been undetermined.

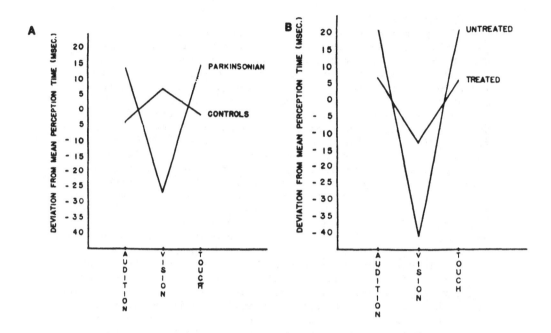

Figure 1. A. *Relative speeds of perception in audition, vision and touch (proprioception) for parkinsonians and a control group of matched-aged, non-neurological patients. There were 12 subjects in each group. The difference in perception speed pattern between the two groups was significant with p < .02.*
*B. Comparison of perception speed patterns for six parkinsonians who did, with six parkinsonians who did not, receive antiparkinsonian medication. The difference between groups was significant with p < .01. (Modified from Dinnerstein, Frigyesi, and Lowenthal, 1962).*

Both the data and the theory, that parkinsonism involves a proprioceptive delay, gain in relevance that a specific perceptual delay (auditory) operates in another population of patients: in schizophrenics; these two disease conditions are not unrelated: effective pharmacotherapy of the latter may induce the former *(Haase and Jansen, 1965)*; similar biochemical abnormality with different polarities have been postulated for these two diseases *(Yariura-Tobias, et al. 1970; Axelrod, 1976, Nauta, 1976; Mettler, 1955; Heath, 1959; Groves, et al. 1975)*. Schizophrenics, when compared to normal controls, have been shown to exhibit a delay in auditory perception by virtue of prolonged response times under conditions of cross modality triggering *(Sutton, Hakerem, Zubin and Portnoy, 1961).*

The proprioceptive delay theory may account for a number of generally puzzling aspects of parkinsonism. The shortcomings of the theory are also evident. It was first reported by *Meyer-Koenigsbery (1923)* that many parkinsonian patients who can no longer walk, can march or dance to music. This was confirmed in my laboratory *(Pineland Hospital and Training Center, 1959).* Further, parkinsonians examined in our laboratories *(N.Y. Medical College, 1960-61),* whose bradykinesia and rigidity prevented them from feeding themselves could often catch a ball. These apparent paradoxes in the behavior of patients with parkinsonism become meaningful when viewed in the context of present theory. During activities of daily living, the moment-to-moment information of position of the body or its parts through proprioceptive feedback serves as a signal for the next stage during the execution of a movement; consequently, a proprioceptive delay would distort the sequence, timing and balancing of a movement. On the other hand, ball catching involves a brief movement in response to a visual signal, in marching and dancing, the beat of the rhythm signals each step. That is, under certain conditions, the bradykinesia and rigidity of parkinsonians may temporarily subside: the conditions being when extra-proprioceptive stimuli provide an alternative to proprioception. However, it is noted that this explanation is also an over simplification because we observed that parkinsonians, who could catch a ball, would not (or could not) catch a burning cigarette thrown toward them in the same fashion as the ball was. These and other observations (such as wheelchair bound parkinsonians may become fully ambulatory, for a period, under the influence of anger: in one reported instance, he pursed and knifed someone who insulted him) indicate that selective limbic influences, via nucleus accumbens *(Frigyesi, Purpura, 1967; Hornykiewicz, elsewhere in this volume)* may also play a role. The efferent projections *(Powell and Leman, 1976)* and particularly the fronto-limbic-n. accumbens and nigro-hypothalamic-n. accumbens projections *(Domesick and Nauta, 1975)* subserve and provide structural basis for the linkage between mood, motivation, and affective, ideational and visceral sensations and perceptions as well as fixed action patterns and motor behavior.

In summary, the proprioceptive delay theory may provide a unifying concept to explain how dissimilar etiologic factors produce similar symptomatology in parkinsonism. The data presented provides some support for the theory. Yet the theory has its shortcomings, primarily the lack of crucial experimentation, i.e. the direct measurements of the delay in parkinsonians.

The current unfeasibility of obtaining such data from parkinsonian patients necessitated seeking the putative proprioceptive delay in animals. Such studies, however, have another shortcoming, namely, that only the anatomical and biochemical abnormalities of parkinsonians can be reproduced in experimental animals *(Frigyesi, et al., 1971 and 1974)* but not all the clinical signs *(Frigyesi, 1975a; Duvoisin, 1976).*

## 2. NORMAL AND ABNORMAL INTEGRATION OF ACTIVITIES IN THE CEREBELLO-CORTIOSPINAL PROJECTION SYSTEM

Operational properties of the sensorimotor system may be regarded as analogous to electromechanical feedback systems in which unwanted oscillation may be induced by delayed input or sped-up output signals or underdamping *(vide supra)*. Evidence was presented in the preceeding part of this communication which has revealed that delayed input (proprioceptive feedback) may be a part of the pathomechanism of parkinsonism. The major output systems connected to proprioceptive inputs are the corticospinal and rubrospinal tracts (only these major descending, long-tract systems receive excitatory input from "the head ganglion of proprioception", the cerebellum). Positive feedback (proprioception) tend to destabilize electromechanical feedback systems (sensorimotor organization). To prevent large and destructive overshorts in such a system (where signals are all-or-none, frequency coded activities) means are needed to absorb energy which induce the oscillations. Extrapolating these to the sensorimotor organization, in general, and parkinsonism (where the pathological process involves systems between the caudate nucleus and substantia nigra), in particular, the damping has to take place at neuraxial levels above the cerebellum, and operationally, ought to be a device which, according to the Nyquist criteria, decreases input signals to the effectors (only corticospinal neurons meet the Nyquist criteria) *(Nyquist, 1932)*; cerebellofugal activities are capable of producing sinusoidal input signals only to the motor cortex [and not to the red nucleus] by exciting different population of thalamic neurons with different conduction velocities and varying number of interposed synapses *(Frigyesi, Purpura, 1965; Frigyesi, 1971; and Frigyesi, Schwartz, 1971)*. Accordingly, the animal experiments 1. scrutinized activities in the corticospinal tract elicited by electrical stimulation of the cerebellar ascending output system (superior cerebellar peduncle = brachium conjunctivum [BC]); and 2. were aimed at determining the mechanism which altered the frequency and the timing of BC evoked activities to corticospinal neurons. Since there are (optimally) only two synapses interposed between neurons in the deep cerebellar nuclei and the cortiospinal tract, and large diameter, fast-conducting axons are in between, there is little room for freedom of sped-up action in this system; in fact, BC evoked activities in the medullary corticospinal tract exhibited minimal variations in latencies *(Frigyesi, Purpura, 1964)*. Attention was paid to detect delays in the input side of the system; this search focused on BC evoked activities in the thalamus and in the thalamo-cortical radiation *(Frigyesi, Purpura, 1965 and 1966)*. This issue

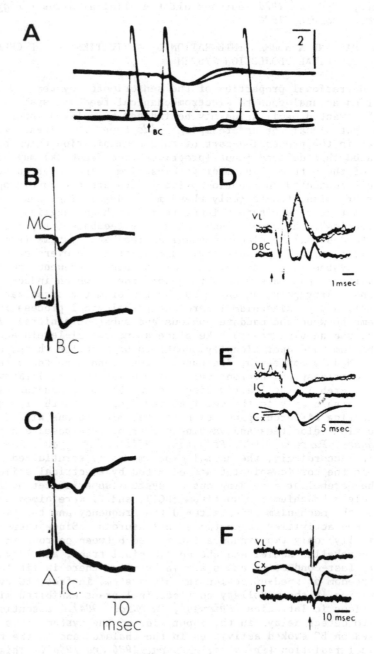

Figure 2A

Figure 2A. *Functional continuity in the cerebello-corticospinal projection system. A. Upper trace, surface recording from the motor cortex; lower trace, intracellular recording from a VL neuron. BC stimulus is applied at the upward arrow. The BC stimulus elicits in the VL neuron a small EPSP (0.7 msec latency) which triggers a single spike discharge. The dashed horizontal line is drawn through the firing level of this neuron. Following the evoked spike discharge, a prolonged IPSP is noticeable. In the motor cortex, the BC stimulus elicits a positive-negative evoked potential. Preceding the cortical evoked potential, two small positive deflections are seen; the evoked spike in VL coincides with the second of these two positivities in the cortex. B. and C. Recordings from an identified VL relay neuron (lower traces). Upper traces are from the motor cortex. BC stimulus elicits a monosynaptic EPSP and a superimposed spike discharge (B, at upward arrow), internal capsule stimulus an antidromic spike discharge (C, at the open triangle) in this VL neuron. D. Upper trace, recording from VL; lower trace, from the decussation of brachium conjunctivum. A BC stimulus is applied at the upward arrow. A compound action potential is seen in the decussation. A positive-negative wave followed by a high-amplitude negativity is seen in VL. Early components of the compound action potential are coincident with the positive-negative wave in VL; this diphasic wave in VL reflects presynaptic activity. The large amplitude negativity in VL reflects postsynaptic activity. E. Recordings from VL (upper trace), internal capsule (middle trace) and the motor cortex (lower trace). BC stimulus is applied at the upward arrows. Evoked activities at the progressively more rostral recording sites show progressively longer latercies. F. Recordings from VL (upper trace), motor cortex (middle trace), and corticospinal tract (lower trace). BC stimulus is applied at the upward arrow. The BC evoked potentials exhibit progressively longer latencies at the three recording sites. Voltage calibrations are 25 mV and refer to the intracellular recordings: in A to A, in C to B and C. Time marker in C refers to B and C. (A-C, modified from Frigyesi, Machek, 1970; D unpublished from Frigyesi and Purpura, 1966; E, F, unpublished from Frigyesi and Purpura, 1964).*

will be discussed in detail in the following chapter of this communication. The damping mechanism (as defined above) has been identified as recurrent, evoked inhibitory postsynaptic potentials (IPSPs) in neurons in the ventrolateral thalamus (VL) (*Frigyesi, 1975b*).

The discussion, which follows in this chapter, relates only to these IPSPs in VL neurons.

The recordings of evoked activities in the decussation of brachium conjunctivum, VL, thalamo-cortical radiation, motor cortex and medullary corticospinal tract, which were elicited by electrical stimulation of the deep nuclei or brachium conjunctivum (Fig. 2A),

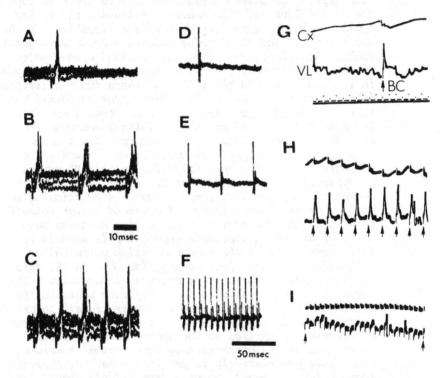

*Figure 2B. Following capability of postsynaptic potentials in VL neurons to frequency stimulation of brachium conjunctivum. A-C, Focal potentials in VL (superimposed traces) follow BC stimulation at 1 Hz in A, 50 Hz in B, and 100 Hz in C (unpublished from Frigyesi, Purpura, 1965). D-F, single unit discharges in VL follow BC stimulation at 1 Hz in D, 50 Hz in E, and 100 Hz in F (unpublished from Frigyesi, Purpura, 1966). A-F, recordings are from the cat. G-I, recordings from the squirrel monkey; upper traces are from the surface of motor cortex; lower traces are from VL. BC stimulation (at upward arrows) at 1 Hz in G, and 100 Hz in H; in I, between the arrows, at 250 Hz. Focal potentials in VL follow BC stimulation up to 100 Hz, at higher stimulus frequencies, focal potentials are only occasionally seen (unpublished from Frigyesi, Cohen, 1973).*

has established that in the cat *(Frigyesi, Purpura 1964; Frigyesi, Macheck, 1970)* and the monkey *(Frigyesi, Schwartz, 1972)* that evoked activities followed the stimulation over a broad range of frequency (1-100 Hz).  At the two interposed relays, in the thalamic nuclei (especially in VL) and in the motor cortex, for each incoming volley one outgoing volley was demonstrable; intracellular recordings have revealed that, for each presynaptic potential, a singleton postsynaptic spike discharge was generated in VL and in the motor cortex.  That is, the basic operational property of the cerebello-corticospinal projection system is that there are one-to-one synaptic relations in its thalamic and motor cortical relays *(Frigyesi, 1975b)*.

Such synaptic relations are profoundly affected by activities arising in a variety of systems: medial thalamus, basal ganglia, substantia nigra and motor cortex *(Frigyesi, Purpura, 1964; Frigyesi, Rabin, 1971; Frigyesi, Machek, 1971; Frigyesi, Schwartz, 1972)*. Eight-to-12 Hz stimulation of medial, midline and intralaminar thalamic nuclei elicited short-latency (5-10 msec), short-duration (10-20 msec) negativities and following prolonged (up to 100 msec) positivities in VL *(Frigyesi, Purpura, 1964)*.  Intracellular recordings from VL neurons have revealed that such negativities are extracellular reflections of excitatory postsynaptic potentials (EPSPs) of comparable latencies and durations generated in large population of VL neurons *(Purpura, Cohen, 1962)*.  Similarly, the prolonged positivities reflect underlying inhibitory postsynaptic potentials (IPSPs).  Further, stimulation of the head of the caudate nucleus *(Frigyesi, Machek, 1971)* (Fig. 3), putamen *(Frigyesi, Rabin, 1971)*,

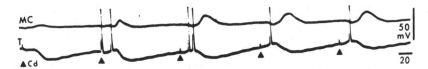

*Figure 3.  Caudate stimulation evoked synaptic potentials in the thalamus and motor cortex.  Cat.  Upper Trace: motor cortex; lower trace: intracellular recording from a thalamic neuron.  Stimulation of the head of the caudate nucleus (at 8 Hz, at the closed triangles).  Following each stimulus, a recruiting response is seen in the cortex, and an EPSP-IPSP sequence in the thalamic neuron.  (Modified from Frigyesi, Machek, 1971).*

globus pallidus internal segment *(Frigyesi, Schwartz, 1972)*, or its feline homologue: entopenduncular nucleus *(Frigyesi, Rabin, 1970)* and substantia nigra *(Frigyesi, Machek, 1971; Frigyesi, Schwartz, 1972)*, elicited similar, frequency specific EPSP-IPSP sequences in VL neurons (Fig. 4).  EPSP-IPSP sequences of different temporal characteristics were elicited in VL neurons by electrical stimula-

tion of the motor cortex, the underlying corona radiata and the
internal capsule: *(Frigyesi, Machek, 1971; Frigyesi, Schwartz, 1972).*
When stimulation of BC (at frequencies of 1-100 Hz) was paired
with stimulation of either the medial thalamus, or various components of basal ganglia or substantia nigra (at 8-12 Hz), interactions
were demonstrable in VL (neurons): BC evoked action potentials

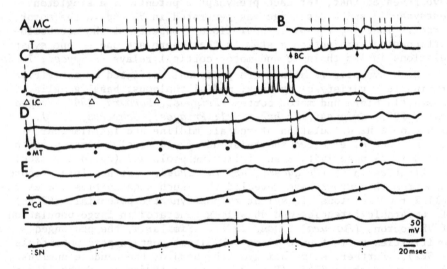

*Figure 4. EPSP-IPSP sequences in a thalamic neuron elicited by 8 Hz
stimulation of converging synaptic pathways. Cat. Upper
traces: recordings from the surface of the motor cortex;
lower traces: intracellular recordings from a medial
thalamic neuron. A, background discharges of the neuron.
B, BC evoked monosynaptic EPSPs without superimposed
spike discharges are seen. EPSP-IPSP sequences are noticeable in the thalamic neuron during internal capsule
(in C), medial thalamus (in D), caudate nucleus (in E)
and substantia nigra (in F) stimulation. Note the essential similarities in the EPSP-IPSP sequences in the thalamic neuron, and the differences in the evoked potentials
in the cortical traces. (From Frigyesi, Machek, 1971).*

which reached the VL (neurons) coincident with the evoked negativities
(EPSPs) did, whereas those which reach the VL (neurons) coincident
with the evoked positivities (IPSPs) failed to elicit spike discharges
in VL (neurons) and resultant activities in the thalamocortical radiation (which, in turn, triggered discharges in the corticospinal neurons) *(Frigyesi, Purpura, 1964; Frigyesi, Rabin, 1971; Frigyesi,
1975b; Purpura, 1976).* That is, 8-12 Hz stimulation of medial thal-

amus, basal ganglia and substantia nigra effectively converted in
VL a tonic input volley arriving via BC to a phasic output pattern
in the thalamocortical radiation (Fig. 5, 6, 7).  Under these conditions, significant, additional, evoked PSPs in identified cortiospinal
neurons were not observed; and, the one-to-one synaptic relationships
between activities in the thalamocortical radiation and corticospinal tract were maintained (*Frigyesi, 1971; 1975b*).  In essence,

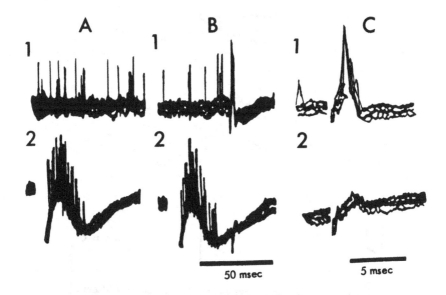

*Figure 5.  Internuclear interactions in the thalamus.  Cat.  Record-
ings of focal potentials from the ventrolateral thalamus;
superimposed traces.  A1, characteristics of background
activities.  B1, BC evoked large amplitude focal potentials are followed by a positivity of 20-30 msec duration.
Spontaneous activities in VL are abolished following the
BC stimuli.  C1, BC evoked potentials are shown on a
faster time-base: early, diphasic, presynaptic potentials
are followed by high-amplitude, postsynaptic negativities.
A2, medial thalamus stimulation evoked negative-positive
waves are seen; unit discharges override the negativities.
B2, BC stimuli are timed to occur coincident with the
medial thalamus evoked positivities: inhibitory interactions are seen.  C2, the BC evoked focal responses from
B2 are shown on a faster time-base: the early diphasic
potentials are unchanged (cf. C1); the postsynaptic focal
negativities are virtually abolished.  (Modified from
Frigyesi, Purpura, 1966).*

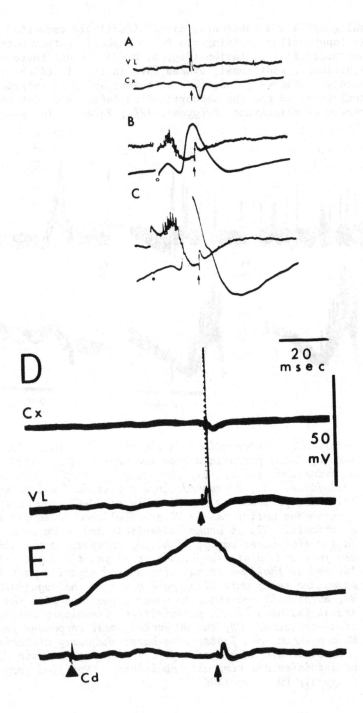

*Figure 6*

*Figure 6. Interactions in VL between cerebellofugal and medial thala-
mic basal ganglia projection activities. Cat. A-C, upper
traces, recordings from the motor cortex, lower traces:
recordings from VL. At the upward arrows, BC stimuli are
applied. A, control: BC evoked focal potential in VL, and
a somewhat longer latency relayed potential in the motor
cortex are seen. B, conditioning entopenducular nucleus
(internal pallidal segment), C, conditioning medial thalamic stimulus precede the BC stimuli: both modes of stimuli
elicit in the cortex long-latency, high-amplitude negativities and, in VL, negative-positive waves. BC evoked focal
potentials in VL and relayed potentials in the cortex are
abolished; small, residual negativities are seen in VL
following the BC stimuli. D, E, cat, upper traces: recordings from the surface of the motor cortex, lower traces:
intracellular recordings from a VL neuron. BC stimulus in
D elicits a monosynaptic EPSP and a superimposed spike discharge in the VL neuron; (the spike is truncated at 70 mV);
a BC evoked relayed potential is seen in the motor cortex
approximately 1 msec after the spike discharge. E, a conditioning stimulus is applied to the head of the caudate
nucleus (at the closed triangle) 60 msec prior to the BC
stimulus. The caudate stimulus elicits a recruiting double
negativity in the motor cortex, and low-amplitude prolonged
EPSP and a following prolonged IPSP in the VL neuron. The
BC stimulus coincides with the caudate evoked IPSP; the
BC stimulus elicits a monosynaptic EPSP that fails to
trigger a spike discharge under this condition. Comparison
of E to B and C reveals that the residual negativities in
the extracellular records reflect EPSPs without spike discharges generated in a population of VL neurons by the
BC stimulation (A, C, modified from Frigyesi, Rabin, 1971;
D, E, modified from Frigyesi, Machek, 1971).*

the major site of interaction between the cerebello-corticospinal
projection system and the medial thalamic system, basal ganglia and
substantia nigra was observed to be in the thalamus (VL); the activity
patterns in the thalamocortical radiation were replicated in the
corticospinal tract. In summary, the data show that the medial
thalamic system, basal ganglia and substantia nigra regulate transmission in the cerebello-corticospinal projection system by generating
frequency-specific IPSPs in the VL neurons.

To the extent that the medial thalamic-VL functional linkage
alters the input (proprioceptive) to the forebrain by virtue of guid-
ing the corticospinal contribution (output) to obtain a desired condition of a limb, the medial thalamic system may be regarded as a con-
troller *(Dewan, 1969)* which functions to reduce the error to an

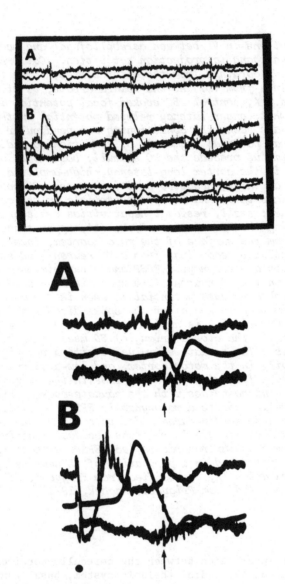

*Figure 7. Functional consequences of internuclear thalamic inter-*
*actions in the cerebello-corticospinal projection system.*
*Cat. Simultaneous recordings from the VL (upper traces),*
*motor cortex (middle traces) and medullary corticospinal*
*tract (lower traces). A, B, C, in the black frame, time*
*marker: 50 msec. In A and C, BC stimuli, 125 msec apart,*
*elicit focal potentials in the VL, and relayed potentials*
*in the motor cortex and corticospinal tract. In B, 8 Hz*

acceptable value in the shortest possible time consistent with stable
operation of the system.   Such controllers operate on an error signal
*(Braitenberg, 1973)*.   A noteworthy feature of neurons in the CM-Pf
complex is that they receive brachium conjunctivum input (proprioceptive = error signals) which, in these neurons, commonly elicit only a
small EPSP without a superimposed spike (Fig. 8).   Such EPSPs in CM-Pf
neurons are coincident with BC evoked EPSPs, which trigger spike
discharges, in VL neurons (thus establishing functional connectivity
between the cerebellum and the motor cortex).   That is, BC evoked
IPSPs in CM-Pf neurons do not appear to directly contribute to the
maintenance of functional connectivity between the cerebellum and
motor cortex, they signal to CM-Pf neurons the time of arrival of
the BC evoked excitation to VL neurons.   The CM-Pf neurons, in turn,
initiate activities that determine which BC evoked EPSPs will generate a spike discharge, thus determine the temporal pattern of VL-
input to corticospinal neurons.   Similar EPSPs to caudate, globus
pallidus and substantia nigra stimulation have not yet been reported.
It can be readily appreciated that in the sensorimotor system, where
there is no true equilibrium position *(Burns, 1968)*, the medial
thalamic, basal ganglia-substantia nigra systems operate as oscillatory controllers *(Walter, 1953; Dewan, 1969)*: under normal conditions,
limb positions oscillate at constant amplitude around an intended
position (physiological tremor, inherent in the peripheral loop
delays: alpha-gamma, and agonist-antagonist).   The frequency of
physiological and parkinsonian tremors are unidentical.   Therefore,
it is assumed that the oscillation in parkinsonism does not involve
these peripheral loops but their supraspinal control: increased
delay between the initiation of controlling signal and its effect
on the controlled parameter is to be sought for in the supraspinal
mechanisms.

The recurrent IPSPs in VL neurons which regulate transmission
in the cerebello-corticospinal projection system may be elicited
by stimulation of the medial thalamus, basal ganglia and substantia

---

*medial thalamic stimuli precede the BC stimuli by 50 msec.*
*Typical recruiting responses are seen in the cortical*
*traces.   At this conditioning testing interval, inhibitory*
*interactions are seen.   Lower A and B, the BC evoked poten-*
*tials (at the upward arrows) and the medial thalamus (at*
*the dot)-BC interactions are shown at greater detail (A*
*and B, in the lower half of the figure correspond to A and*
*B in the inset).   (Unpublished from Frigyesi, Purpura, 1964).*

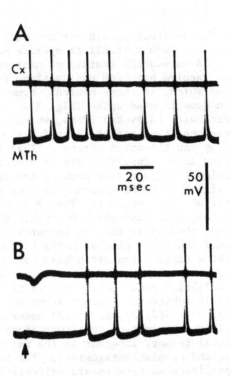

*Figure 8. Brachium conjunctivum evoked excitation in the CM-Pf complex. Cat. Upper traces: recordings from the motor cortex; lower traces: intracellular recordings from a CM-Pf complex neuron. A, background discharge of the neuron. B, BC stimulation (at arrow) evoked monosynaptic EPSP is noticeable in the medial thalamic neuron which does not trigger a spike discharge, though no detectable spontaneous or induced hyperpolarization is evident. This is in sharp contrast to observations on BC evoked EPSPs in VL neurons (cf. Fig. 2A: A, and B; Fig. 2B; Fig. 6D). (Modified from Frigyesi, Machek, 1971).*

nigra at specific frequencies (8-12 Hz). Stimulation of these structures outside this range of frequency fails to elicit recurrent IPSPs (*Purpura, 1972*). Further, high-frequency (above 25 Hz) stimu-

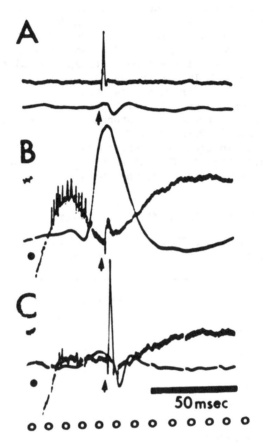

*Figure 9. The selective inhibitory effect of high-frequency pallidal
stimulation on the inhibitory components of evoked rhythmic
activities in VL. Cat. Upper traces: recordings from VL;
lower traces: surface recordings from the motor cortex.
BC stimulations at the upward arrows. A, BC evoked focal
potential in VL and relayed potential in the cortex are
shown. B, conditioning medial thalamic stimulus inhibits
the BC evoked focal potential in VL and abolishes the relayed potential in the cortex. C, 70 Hz stimulation of the
entopeduncular nucleus abolishes the 8 Hz medial thalamus
evoked recruiting response in the motor cortex, and blocks
the medial thalamus-BC inhibitory interactions in VL by
suppressing the medial thalamus evoked positivity in VL;
under this condition, the amplitude of the BC evoked focal
potential in VL is larger, and the relayed potential in the
cortex is enhanced. (Modified from Frigyesi, Rabin, 1971).*

lation of any of these structures selectively abolishes the IPSPs
component of the EPSP-IPSP sequences in VL neurons generated by 8-12
Hz stimulation of any of the other structures (Fig. 9) *Frigyesi,
Rabin, 1971; Purpura et al., 1966).* The stimulation of the brainstem reticular formation not only at high but also at low frequencies
also selectively abolishes the evoked (from all sources) recurrent
IPSPs in VL neurons *(Frigyesi, Purpura, 1964).*

Experiments in animals which exhibited sleep spindles in the
motor cortex have revealed an abundance of underlying IPSPs in VL
neurons *(Frigyesi, Purpura, 1965).*

Following intracarotid administration of atropine and L-Dopa,
rhythmic activities in VL increased and, following similar administration of acetylcholine and reserpine, decreased *(Frigyesi, Purpura,
1966).*

*TABLE 1. RECURRENT IPSP's IN VENTROLATERAL THALAMIC NEURONS*

| STIMULATION OF | INDUCED | ABOLISHED |
|---|---|---|
| Caudate Nucleus | At 8-10 Hz | Over 25 Hz |
| Substantia Nigra | "     " | "     " |
| Globus Pallidus | "     " | "     " |
| Medial Thalamus | "     " | "     " |
| Motor Cortex | "     " | |
| Reticular Formation | | Over 5 Hz |
| | Slow Sleep | Behavioral Arousal |
| | Atropine | Acetylcholine |
| | L-DOPA | Reserpine |

Table 1 tabulates some of the conditions under which a quantitative increase and a quantitative decrease of rhythmic activities
(recurrent IPSPs) are demonstrable in VL neurons. The Table shows
that certain conditions (sleep, atropine and L-Dopa) which induce
quantitative increase of recurrent IPSPs in VL neurons are also

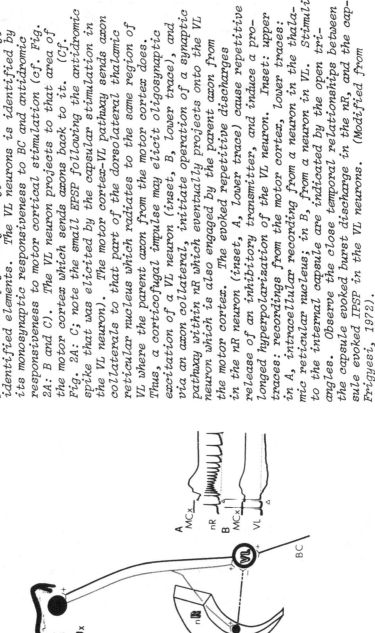

Figure 10A. Diagrammatic illustration of the monosynaptic relationship between neurons in the thalamic reticular nucleus (nR) and neurons in VL. Pathways and neurons here represent electrophysiologically, and not anatomically, identified elements. The VL neurons is identified by its monosynaptic responsiveness to BC and antidromic responsiveness to motor cortical stimulation (cf. Fig. 2A: B and C). The VL neuron projects to that area of the motor cortex which sends axons back to it. (Cf. Fig. 2A: C; note the small EPSP following the antidromic spike that was elicited by the capsular stimulation in the VL neuron). The motor cortex–VL pathway sends axon collaterals to that part of the dorsolateral thalamic reticular nucleus which radiates to the same region of VL where the parent axon from the motor cortex does. Thus, a corticofugal impulse may elicit oligosynaptic excitation of a VL neuron (inset, B, lower trace), and via an axon collateral, initiate operation of a synaptic pathway within nR which eventually projects onto the VL neuron which is also engaged by the parent axon from the motor cortex. The evoked repetitive discharges in the nR neuron (inset, A, lower trace) cause repetitive release of an inhibitory transmitter, and induce a prolonged hyperpolarization of the VL neuron. Inset: upper traces: recordings from the motor cortex, lower traces: in A, intracellular recording from a neuron in the thalamic reticular nucleus; in B, from a neuron in VL. Stimuli to the internal capsule are indicated by the open triangles. Observe the close temporal relationships between the capsule evoked burst discharge in the nR, and the capsule evoked IPSP in the VL neurons. (Modified from Frigyesi, 1972).

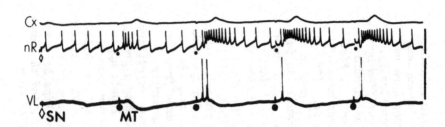

*Figure 10B. Close temporal relationships between recruiting responses
in the motor cortex (upper trace), bursts in thalamic
reticular neurons (middle trace) and IPSPs in VL neurons
(lower trace) elicited by low-frequency (8 Hz) stimulation of the medial thalamus. Stimuli are 125 msec apart.
Shock artefacts are denoted by symbols: the lozenge-
shaped symbol denotes substantia nigra, the dots medial
thalamus. Both neurons are unresponsive to nigral
stimulation. During stimulation of the medial thalamus,
there is a gradual development of burst discharges in the
nR neuron; the IPSPs in the VL neuron, and the recruiting
responses in the motor cortex develop* pari passu. *(Modified from Frigyesi, 1972).*

known to ameliorate the parkinsonian tremor. Conversely, conditions
(behavioral arousal, acetylcholine) which induce quantitative decrease
of recurrent IPSP in VL neurons are also known to aggravate the parkinsonian state. Further, both reserpine and behavioral arousal
(excitement) can reversibly disrupt normal functioning of the sensorimotor system and induce transient tremor. Taken together, there is
a positive correlation between the quantitative increase of recurrent
IPSPs in VL neurons and alleviation of the parkinsonian symptomatology;
conversely, a quantitative decrease in the recurrent IPSPs in VL

neurons and aggravation of the parkinsonian condition as well as
disruption of normal integretion of sensorimotor activities. It is
inferred that the generation of recurrent IPSPs in VL neurons is
a necessary, but not sufficient, condition for normal central integration of sensorimotor activities.

Finally, it is noted that the recurrent IPSPs in VL neurons are
functions of activities of neurons in the thalamic reticular nucleus
(nR), i.e. nR neurons, when activated by medial thalamic, pallidal,
nigral or motor cortical projection activities, monosynaptically
generate prolonged IPSPs in VL neurons by inducing repetitive (per-
sistent) release of an inhibitory transmitter (Fig. 10). *(Frigyesi,
1972)*.

## 3. INDUCED PAROXYSMAL ACTIVITIES IN THE CEREBELLO-MOTORCORTICAL
PROTECTION SYSTEM

In the foregoing discourse, it was established that the ventrolateral and some medial thalamic nuclei are integral parts of the
sensorimotor organization. Activity patterns were specified which
in these thalamic nuclei positively correlate with normal and abnormal motor behavior. Therefore it was considered that it might be
of interest to study activity patterns in these nuclei during experimentally induced paroxysmal activities in cats and monkeys. The
data, in essence, showed that the cerebello-thalamocortical system
is involved not only in central integration of sensorimotor activities
but also in several varieties of experimental epilepsies.

Paroxysmal activities were induced in cats, squirrel and Cebus
(Alba) monkeys by several well established techniques: penicillin
focus, strychnine, metrazol, bicuculline, etc. This communication will
be concerned only with the penicillin induced effects in the thalamocortical circuit.

Acute penicillin foci were established in the motor cortex. A
point-to-point reciprocal relationship has earlier been established
between the VL and motor cortex *(vide supra)* *(Frigyesi, Machek, 1970,
Frigyesi, Schwartz, 1972)* (Fig. 10A, diagram). This relationship
permitted recordings to be obtained from populations of VL neurons
which were reciprocally linked with those restricted areas of the
motor cortex where the penicillin foci were established and the surface activities were recorded from. (Fig. 2A:C, note the small EPSP,
immediately after the antidromic spike, both elicited by capsular
stimulation in the VL neuron.) Additional simultaneous recordings
were obtained from those medial thalamic regions where BC stimulation
also elicited focal potentials.

In general, the major finding in these studies was the demonstration that after placement of the penicillin onto the motor cortex,
the first detectable paroxysmal events occurred in the thalamus: both

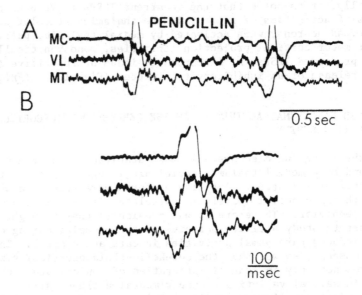

Figure 11A. Interictal episodes in the thalamocortical circuit in a
             cat with a penicillin focus in the motor cortex.
             Upper traces: recordings from the motor cortex, middle
             traces: from VL, and lower traces: from medial thalamus.
             Mature penicillin focus. A, two interictal spikes are
             seen in the motor cortex; both of these spikes are pre-
             ceded by prominent activities at both thalamic recording
             sites. B shows in greater detail that the interictal
             spike in the VL precedes that in the cortex by approxi-
             mately 50-60 msec, and that in the medial thalamus by
             10-15 msec. The interictal episode in the thalamus
             lasts about one second. The cortical interictal spikes
             appear only at the beginning and at the end of the
             thalamic episode; the cortical spikes appear to be
             appended to the thalamic episode as quasi "on" and "off"
             responses. (Unpublished from Frigyesi, Tsukamoto, Grimm).

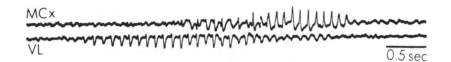

*Figure 11B. Thalamo-cortical relationships in hypoxic seizures.
Upper traces are recordings from the motor cortex;
lower traces from VL. The thalamic interictal episode
is conspicuous for more than one second before interictal
spikes are recordable from the closely coupled motor
cortical area.*

VL and medial thalamic nuclei exhibited interictal spikes before cortical manifestation of any seizure activity *(Hess et al. 1974; Frigyesi, et al. 1976)*. Essentially similar observations were made by
Rosen *(1976)* in the lateral geniculate body in cats with pencillin
foci in the association cortex (marginal gyrus). Regarding the later
interictal episodes, the thalamic interictal spikes generally preceded those in the motor cortex by 50-100 msec  (Fig. 11). The VL
interictal spikes were either coincident with or preceded the medial
thalamic spikes by 5-10 msec. Thalamic interictal spikes without
ensuing motor cortical interictal spikes were observed but not *vice
versa* (a few exceptions to this were observed only in the Cebus (Alba)
monkey). Further, thalamic interictal spikes were commonly seen at
a time separation of 500-1500 msec, during which smaller amplitude
but prominent thalamic activities of various configurations were
recordable; under these conditions, interictal spikes in the cortex
were seen only at the beginning and at the end of the thalamic episodes; thus, the cortical spikes frequently appeared as quasi-
"on and off" responses appended to the thalamic processes (Fig. 11A).
Data of apparent practical significance are those which showed that
the thalamic interictal episodes were demonstrable in the absence
of recordable seizures in the neocortex (Fig. 11B).
    The experimental demonstration of thalamic dependence of motor
cortical seizure activities in connection with motor cortical penicillin foci raises the question as to the nature of the effects of
activities generated by the major input-system, brachium conjunctivum,
in the thalamic neuron on the paroxysmal activities in the thalamus-
cortical circuits. The data show that high frequency (2-500 Hz)
stimulation of BC drives seizure activities at the thalamus and motor
cortex in cats and squirrel and Cebus (Albus) monkeys with motor
cortical penicillin foci (in 28/33 cats, 10/11 squirrels and 7/9
Cebus (Albus) monkeys) (Fig. 12).
    Regarding the exact nature of this BC drive, species differences
were encountered; this issue is considered in detail elsewhere. For
the nonce, suffice it to look closely into the generation of thalamic

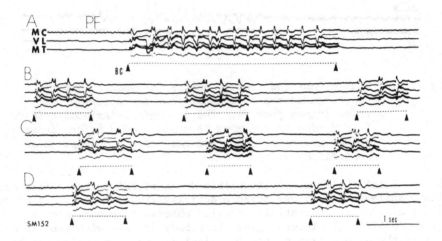

*Figure 12. Brachium conjunctivum drive of interictal discharges in
the thalamocortical circuit. Squirrel monkey. Upper
traces: surface recordings from the motor cortex, middle
traces: focal recordings from VL; lower traces: focal
recordings from the medial thalamus. Mature penicillin
focus in the motor cortex. High-frequency (500 Hz) stimulation of the BC is indicated by the dashed horizontal
lines between the upward arrow-heads. High-frequency
BC stimulation drives interictal discharges at the three
recording sites during the entire period of stimulation.
After effects are not seen.*

potentials in VL and some medial thalamic neurons *(vide supra)*. The
salient properties of the cerebello-VL (and, largely similarly, medial
thalamic) potentials are as follows: 1. the vast majority of EPSPs
exhibit 0.7-1.2 msec latencies, trigger single spike discharges
and are followed by IPSPs; 2. focal potentials: initial, positive-
negative (presynaptic) potentials are followed by prominent negativities (postsynaptic potentials) which show latencies and durations
comparable to those of the EPSPs; focal positivities are seen following the focal negativities; and 3. both extra- and intracellularly,
BC evoked excitatory potentials are recordable at 1-100 Hz frequencies
of stimulation; stimulus frequencies over 100 Hz generally fail to
elicit postsynaptic potentials in VL and medial thalamic neurons
*(Frigyesi, Purpura, 1964; Frigyesi, Machek, 1970; Frigyesi, Schwartz,
1972)*. In the epileptic animals, the cerebello-VL and cerebello-
medial thalamic potentials exhibited properties different from
those in the non-epileptic animals: 1. latencies and duration of the
presynaptic potentials were frequently significantly longer than in

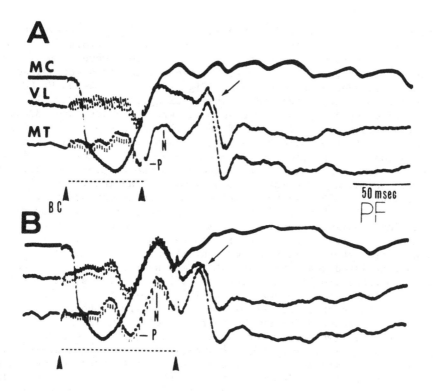

*Figure 13. Characteristics of brachium conjunctivum evoked focal
thalamic and relayed motor cortical potentials during
interictal lulls in the squirrel monkey with penicillin
focus in the motor cortex. Upper traces: surface recordings from the thalamus. High-frequency BC stimulation
(500 Hz) coincident with the dashed horizontal lines
between the arrow-heads. A and B, BC stimulation elicits
short-latency relayed potentials in the motor cortex. BC
evoked monosynaptic potentials in the thalamus are not
seen. Long-latency (50 msec) positive (p)-negative (N)
waves are followed by large-amplitude negativities (at
arrows). Although the sequence, direction of changes of
potentials and the relative amplitude of the components
of the evoked potentials are the same as in the control
animals, the latencies and durations of the various components are 20-90-fold longer than in the control animals.
BC stimulation lasts longer in B than in A. Comparison of
potentials in A and B indicate that prolonged BC stimulation potentiates the evoked responses. (Unpublished from
Frigyesi, Tsukamoto, Grimm, 1977).*

the controls (Fig. 13), 2. latencies and duration of postsynaptic
potentials are significantly longer than in the controls (latencies
as long as 50-60 msec were encountered; durations were commonly 20-30
msec) (Fig. 13), 3. the BC evoked cortical potentials were dissociated
from the BC evoked VL potentials; (Fig. 13), and 4. 4-500 Hz BC
stimulation elicited thalamic postsynaptic potentials (Fig. 13).
These effects in the epileptic animals were fully developed 30-50
minutes after the application of penicillin onto the motor cortex.
In essence, in the epileptic animals, the BC evoked monosynaptic
excitation was displaced by BC evoked polysynaptic excitation in VL.
The question arises as to what happened to the BC evoked monosynaptic
excitation in VL?  The most parsimonious explanation is that it
was inhibited by BC excited intrathalamic inhibitory neurons.   Similarly, the BC evoked multisynaptic focal excitation was generated
by an intrathalamic synaptic system.  Since evidence for the operation of these thalamic neurons is apparent a short period (10-
30 minutes) after application of penicillin onto the motor cortex,
it is postulated that these intrathalamic neuronal chains are under
tonic cortical inhibition in the non-epileptic animals, and one of
the functional consequences of penicillin application is the removal
of this cortico-thalamic inhibition.  The observed phenomenon can
readily be accounted for by the operation of an intrathalamic multisynaptic chain,(which may very well be dendro-dendritic *(Harding,*
*1971, Rinvik, 1972; Frigyesi; Schwartx, 1972)*, that is activated by
BC fiber collaterals, which exert early inhibitory and late excitatory
effects on the target neuron of the parent BC axon.  At present, it
is open to speculation what the physiological role of these intrathalamic (intra-VL?) synaptic pathways are.  Such synaptic mechanisms
have already been described and many of their functional properties
elaborated *(Scheibel and Scheibel, 1970; Schiebel et al. 1972;*
*Schiebel et al. 1973).*  A physiological role must be postulated
because natural selection during phylogenesis eliminates systems
which no longer secure adaptation to the changes of milieu, yet,
such interneuronal machinery exists in the non-epileptic animals
in an apparently non-operative fashion.  To comply with the biogene-
tic law of Heckel, it is postulated that they are operative in the
infancy and become suppressed during maturation.  Data are currently
unavailable on the nature of BC evoked PSPs in the immature cats
and monkeys; developmental studies are needed to clarify this
phenomenon.  Machek *(1965)* has already elaborated on the issue that
ontogenetic factors are more important than phylogenetic ones in
determining the possible role of a structure in the genesis of the
seizure.

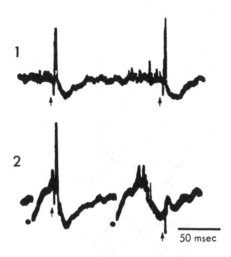

*Figure 14A. Criticalness of timing in intrathalamic internuclear
        interactions. Focal recordings from VL. BC stimulation
        at 8 Hz at upward arrows. 1. Both BC stimuli evoke focal
        potentials. 2. At the dots, 7.7 Hz medial thalamic
        stimuli are interacted with, at arrows, 8 Hz BC stimuli.
        The first interaction is facilitatory, the second is inhi-
        bitory. (Unpublished from Frigyesi, Purpura, 1964).*

## 4. PLASTICITY IN VL

Several lines of investigation in the foregoing electrophysiological studies were kindled by the interest in the putative delayed
proprioceptive feedback as a contributing factor in the pathomechanism
of parkinsonism. The electrophysiological data have revealed that
timing of evoked activities in VL is indeed a powerful factor in
determining discharges in the corticospinal tract. Figure 14 illustrates that slight differences in stimulus frequencies (0.3 Hz) may
induce opposite directional interactions in VL between cerebellofugal and medial thalamic projection activities during a short span
of time (125 msec).

Survey of data obtained from a large series of experiments
(1230 cats and 175 monkeys [squirrel and Cebus (Alba)]) have revealed
that evoked activities in VL in the unanesthetized encèphalè isolè
or the lightly methoxyflurane anesthetized animals exhibited remarkably constant ranges of intramodal latencies to stimulation of
the various input systems *(for details: Frigyesi, 1975a and b).*

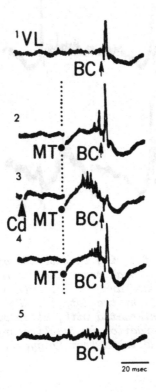

*Figure 14B.* *Conversion of facilitatory to inhibitory internuclear*
*thalamic interactions by preconditioning caudate stimula-*
*tion. Cat. Focal recordings from VL. BC stimulation*
*at the upward arrows. Medial thalamic stimulation (at*
*dots) are equidistant to and timed to occur 30 msec prior*
*to the BC stimuli. 1. BC evoked control focal potential.*
*2. Conditioning medial thalamic stimulation induces*
*facilitation of the BC evoked focal potential. 3. A*
*preconditioning caudate stimulus (at the upward triangle)*
*alters the time course of the medial thalamus evoked*
*excitatory-inhibitory sequence in VL; at the same time*
*separation between conditioning and testing stimuli as*
*in 2, now inhibitory interactions are demonstrable.*
*4. Following cessation of the caudate stimulations.*
*Medial thalamic stimulation, once again, facilitates*
*the BC evoked focal potential. 5. BC stimulus evoked*
*recovery focal potential is shown. (Unpublished from*
*Frigyesi, Purpura, 1964).*

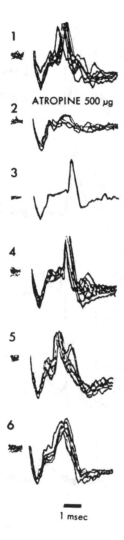

Figure 15. Prolongation of latency of brachium conjunctivum evoked
           focal potentials in VL following intracarotid administra-
           tion of atropine. Cat. Superimposed traces. 1. BC
           evoked control, monosynaptic potentials. 2. Depression
           of BC evoked focal negativity following intracarotid
           administration of atropine. 3. During early stages of
           recovery from the atropine effect, the BC evoked post-
           synaptic potential in VL exhibit approximately 2 msec
           latency; the control, in 1, show 1.2 msec latency.
           4 and 5, gradual reduction of latencies of the focal
           negativities are noticeable. 5, full recovery; the latency
           of the evoked focal negativity is once again 1.2 msec.
           (Modified from Frigyesi, Purpura, 1966).

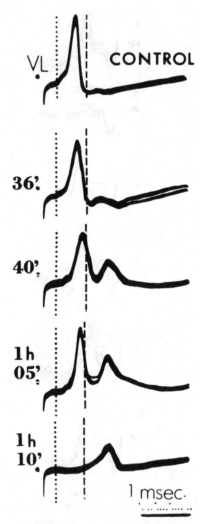

*Figure 16. Disappearance of caudate evoked monosynaptic and neoformation of polysynaptic potentials in VL. Squirrel monkey. Control: Superimposed traces; the caudate evoked monosynaptic potentials in VL are bracketed between the vertical lines. The vertical lines in the other traces are equidistant to the shock artifacts of caudate stimuli to emphatize the development of a caudate evoked polysynaptic potentials following a standard tetanus (the elapsed time between the tetanus and the recordings is indicated at the right of each trace). At 1 hour 10 minutes, caudate evoked monosynaptic potential is no longer seen, only the polysynaptic potential is observed. (Modified from Frigyesi, Cohen, 1974).*

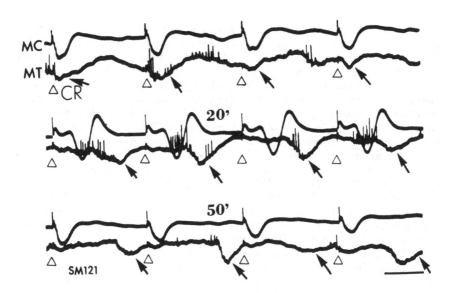

*Figure 17. Disappearance of short-latency positivities in VL elicited by stimulation of the corona radiata, and gradual development of long-latency positivities following systemic administration of L-DOPA. Squirrel monkey. Upper traces: recordings from the motor cortex; lower traces: from the thalamus. Corona radiata stimulation (at 8 Hz), immediately below the motor cortex, is applied at the open triangles. Short-latency positivities are elicited by the stimulation (indicated by the arrows in the control records, top). Twenty and 50 minutes after systemic administration of L-DOPA, the corona radiata evoked positivities exhibit progressively longer latencies (at arrows). In the control, the positivities follow, whereas at 50 minutes, precede the shock artifacts. This shift in latency is about 100 msec. Time marker: 50 msec. (Unpublished from Frigyesi, Yahr, Schwartz, 1974).*

Prolongation of latencies (not only beyond the control values in a given animal, but beyond the established range in the series) were encountered only under a few experimental conditions. Delayed PSPs and focal potentials were observed in VL during stimulation of BC, caudate nucleus, medial thalamus and the motor cortex provided that such stimulations were applied in combination with another experimental variable. Delayed evoked activities were demonstrable in VL 1. during BC stimulation following intracarotid administration

of atropine (Fig. 15) and in animals which had a penicillin focus
in the motor cortex (Fig. 13); 2. during caudate stimulation, following tetanization (Fig. 16); and 3. during motor cortical stimulation,
following systemic administration of L-Dopa (Fig. 17). The most
prominent delays (over tenfold prolongation of latencies) were
observed in experimental epilepsies and following systemic administration of L-Dopa *(Frigyesi, et al. 1974)*. The conditions under
which delayed activities were observed in VL were apparently diverse;
yet, they have a common denominator: with the exception of atropine,
they are sensitive to diphenylhydantoin *(antiepileptic effects:
Merritt and Putnam, 1939; anti-posttetanic effects: Esplin, 1957;
and anti-L-Dopa effects: Mendez et al., 1975)*.

These delayed PSPs in VL reflect some plastic capabilities of
the intrathalamic neuronal organizations. Under the experimental
conditions listed in the foregoing, VL neurons behave as if they
were wired differently *(vide supra)*.

The major implication of these experiments in animals with
penicillin focus is that factors leading to the electrical manifestations of the interictal states in the thalamocortical circuit are
organizational ones. It has been reported that neurons in the penicillin focus function normally *(Matsumoto et al. 1969)*. It has been
proposed that motor cortical neurons develop abnormal discharge patterns without being anything wrong with these neurons if they receive
abnormal inputs *(Ayala et al. 1973)*. It has been estimated that if
1% of the input to neocortical neurons is abnormal that can induce
epileptic bursting firing patterns in normal cell populations *(Calvin,
1972)*. Data here are consistent with the concept that one of the
mechanisms which can lead to interictal paroxysms in the motor cortex
is a reactivation of intrathalamic circuits which normally (presumably)
are operative during infancy and are suppressed during ontogenesis
by an inhibitory corticothalamic reflux. This mechanism does not
call for development of qualitative changes in the participating
thalamocortical neurons *(Ajmone-Marsan, 1961; Ayala, et al. 1973)*.

The penicillin in the motor cortex affects neurons which exert
tonic inhibition on thalamic interneurons. This interference with
corticothalamic inhibition results in that the thalamopetal impulses
are diverted to intrathalamic interneuronal systems which are disused
in normal adult animals. This conclusion is consonant to the concept
of centrencephalic epilepsy of Penfield and Jasper *(1954)* in that
neocortical epileptic activities are driven by abnormal mechanisms in
the upper brainstem.

Implicit in the foregoing is that essentially similar mechanisms
are involved not only in experimental epilepsy but also in the other
experimental conditions which indicated plastic capabilities of VL
neuronal organizations. Germane data were reported by *Racine et al.
(1972)* from limbic structures in the rat during epileptiform discharges
induced by electrical stimulation. They observed evidence for plasti-

city in these structures involved in the development of seizures.
Curiously, however, their data in epilepsy exhibit close similarity
to our data on posttetanic potentiation (cf. their Figure 3 with
Figure 16 in this paper). Similar findings were reported from the
cat limbic structures with penicillin foci (*Lebovitz, 1974*); in this
species, however, development of new components were associated with
prolongation of latencies of fornix evoked potentials in the hippocampus.

## 5. CONCLUSIONS

Two questions were posed here: 1. does a proprioceptive delay
operate in parkinsonism as a factor in the pathomechanism of the
disease, and 2. why parkinsonism and epilepsy do not coexist? These
questions appear to be tangential; however, the experimental findings
show that they are intimately related.

First, prominent delays in central projections of proprioceptive
input systems (brachium conjunctivum) indeed occur. Curiously, however, the most prominent delays are seen in the predicted pathway but
in the "wrong" disease, i.e. in epilepsy.

Second, the same forebrain circuits, reciprocal thalamocortical
projections, are involved in both the genesis of parkinsonsim and
epilepsy. The dominant functional defect in parkinsonism appear to
be correlated with abnormal temporal patterning of thalamic activities
which provide the major input to corticospinal neurons. The functional defect, which so far has been identified in the thalamic input
system to corticospinal neurons in epilepsy, is a plastic phenomenon
in VL: diversion of brachium conjunctivum impulses, which normally
monosynaptically excite VL neurons, to intrathalamic polysynaptic
chains.

Third, the profoundly different intrathalamic elementary processes in the two diseases apparently effectively preclude the simultaneous generation of the respective specific abnormal inputs to
corticospinal neurons.

## ACKNOWLEDGEMENTS

Much of the data summarized here were obtained in joint studies
with Drs. A.J. Dinnerstein, D.P. Purpura, J. Machek, A. Rabin, M.D.
Yahr, R. Schwartz, L. Cohen, R. Hess, Y. Tsukamoto, and J.J. Grimm.
I am indebted to these colleagues for kindly permitting publication
of data obtained in collaborative studies. The original data reported
here were obtained at the Dept. Neurosurgery, University of Zurich,
Switzerland; it was supported, in part, by grants from the Slack-Gyr
Foundation and the Swiss League Against Epilepsy. Additional grant
support is from TTUSM # 12-A550-400 000. I gratefully acknowledge
the assistance of Mss. Paula Gazaway, Sherry Sterwart and Cendy
Philips during the preparation of the manuscript.

## REFERENCES

Ajmone-Marsan, C. (1961). Electrographic aspects of "epileptic" neuronal aggregates. *Epilepsia 2*, 22-38.

Angell, J.R. and Pierce, A. (1982). Experimental research upon the phenomena of attention. *Amer. J. Psychol. 4*, 528-541.

Axelrod, J. (1976). Discussion In: *Basal Ganglia*. M.D. Yahr, Ed. Raven Press, New York, pp. 178-179.

Ayala, G.F., Dichter, M., Gumnit, R.J. Matsumoto, H. and Spencer, W.A. Genesis of epileptic interictal spikes. New knowledge of cortical feedback systems suggests a neurophysiological explanation of brief paroxysm. *Brain Res. 52*, 1-17.

Barbeau, A. (1976). Parkinson's Disease: Etiological considerations. In: *The Basal Ganglia*. M.D. Yahr (ed). Raven Press, New York, pp. 281-282.

Beretervide, J.J. and Carrega-Casaffousth, C.F. (1933). Parkinsonism: case with hemiplegia and psychic disturbances following carbon monoxide poisoning. *Hosp. Argent. 4*, 239-243.

Borina, E.G. (1950). *A history of experimental psychology*. Appleton-Century, New York.

Braitenberg, V. (1973). *Gehirngespinste*. Springer, Berlin.

Burns, B.D. (1968). *The uncertain nervous system*. Edward Arnold, London.

Buzzo, A. and Guerra, C. (1930). Secuelas de la intoxication cianhidrica prentado uno de ellos parkonsonismo y otro polineoritos. *Rev. esp. Oto-neuro-oft. 1*, 243-253.

Calvin, W.H. (1972). Synaptic potential summation and repetitive firing mechanisms: input-output theory for the recruitment of neurons into epileptic bursting firing patterns. *Brain Res. 39*, 71-94.

Dewan, E.M. (1969). Cybernetics and attention. In: *Attention and Neurophysiology*. Ed. C.R. Evans and T.B. Mulholland. Appleton-Century-Crofts, New York, pp. 323-347.

Dinnerstein, A.J., Frigyesi, T.L. and Lowenthal, M. (1962). Delayed feedback as a possible mechanism in parkinsonism. *Perc. Mot. Skills 15*, 667-680.

Domesick, V.B. and Nauta, W.J.M. (1976). Some ascending and descending projections of the substantia nigra and ventral tegmental area in the rat. *Neurosci. Abstr. 2*, 61.

Duvoisin, R.C. (1976). Parkinsonism: animal analogues of the human disorder. In: *The Basal Ganglia*. M.D. Yahr (ed.) Raven Press, New York, pp. 293-303.

Edsall, D.L. and Drinker, C.K. (1919). The clinical aspects of chronic manganese poisoning. *Contrib. Med. biol. Res. ded. to Sir W. Osler 1*, 447-449.

Esplin, D.W. (1957). Effects of diplenylhydantoin on synaptic trans-
    mission in cat spinal cord and stellate ganglion. *J. Pharmac.*
    *Extl. Therap. 120,* 301-323.
Frigyesi, T.L. (1971). Organization of synaptic pathways linking the
    head of caudate nucleus to the dorsal thalamus. *Int. J. Neurol.*
    *8,* 111-138.
Firgyesi, T.L. (1972). Intracellular recordings from neurons in the
    dorsolateral thalamic reticular nucleus during capsular, basal
    ganglia and midline thalamic stimulation. *Brain Res. 48,* 157-
    172.
Frigyesi, T.L. (1975). Structure-function relationship of the inter-
    connection between the caudate nucleus, globus pallidus, sub-
    stantia nigra and thalamus. In: *Subcortical Mechanism and*
    *Sensorimotor Activities.* T.L. Frigyesi (ed.) Hans Huber Publ.,
    Bern, pp. 13-45.
Frigyesi, T.L. (1975b). Basal ganglia-thalamus interface. In:
    *Subcortical Mechanism and Sensorimotor Activities.* T.L. Frigye-
    si (ed.) Hans Huber Publ., Bern, pp. 251-288.
Frigyesi, T.L. and Cohen, L. (1974). Appearance of plasticity in
    caudato-thalamic relationships in the primate. *Ergeb. exp.*
    *Med.,* 271-297.
Frigyesi, T.L., Ige, A., Iulo, A. and Schwartz, R. (1971). Denigra-
    tion and sensorimotor disability induced by ventral tegmental
    injection of 6-Hydroxy-Dopamine in the cat. *Exptl. Neurol. 33,*
    78-87.
Frigyesi, T.L. and Machek, J. (1970). Basal ganglia-diencephalon
    synaptic relations in the cat. I. An intracellular study of
    dorsal thalamic neurons during capsular and basal ganglia stimu-
    lation. *Brain Res. 20,* 201-217.
Frigyesi, T.L. and Machek, J. (1971). Basal ganglia-diencephalon
    synaptic relations in the cats. II. Intracellular recordings
    from dorsal thalamic neurons during low-frequency stimulation
    of the caudato-thalamic projection system and the nigrothalamic
    pathway. *Brain Res. 27,* 59-78.
Frigyesi, T.L. and Purpura, D.P. (1964). Functional properties of
    synaptic pathways influencing transmission in the specific
    cerebello-thalamocortical projection system. *Exptl. Neurol. 10,*
    305-324.
Frigyesi, T.L. and Purpura, D.P. (1965). Diencephalic distribution
    of evoked responses to brachium conjunctivum stimulation.
    *Proc. VIII. Int. Congr. Anatomists.* Wiesbaden, p. 41.
Frigyesi, T.L. and Purpura, D.P. (1965). Alterations in activity of
    a thalamic relay nucleus (VL) during motor cortex spindle waves.
    *Electroenceph. clin. Neurophysiol. 19,* 533.
Frigyesi, T.L. and Purpura, D.P. (1966). Acetylcholine sensitivity
    of thalamic synaptic organizations activated by brachium con-
    junctivum stimulation. *Arch. int. pharmacodyn. 163,* 110-132.

Frigyesi, T.L. and Purpura, D.P. (1967). Electrophysiological analy-
    sis of reciprocal caudato-nigral relations. *Brain Res. 6,*
    440-456.
Frigyesi, T.L. and Rabin, A. (1971). Basal ganglia-diencephalon
    synaptic relations. III. An intracellular study of ansa
    lenticularis, lenticular fasciculus and pallido-subthalamic
    projection activities. *Brain Res. 35,* 67-78.
Frigyesi, T.L. and Schwartz, R. (1972). Cortical control of thalamic
    sensorimotor relay activities in the cat and the squirrel mon-
    key. In: *Corticothalamic Projections and Sensorimotor Activities,*
    Ed. T.L. Frigyesi, E. Rinvik and M.D. Yahr. Raven Press, New
    York, pp. 161-196.
Frigyesi, T.L., Tsukamoto, Y., and Grimm, J.J. (1976). Species
    differential effects of cerebellar stimulation on topical
    penicillin induced paroxysmal activities in the reciprocal
    thalamocortical projections (cat and squirrel monkey).
    *Anat. Rec. 180:* 407.
Frigyesi, T.L., Tsukamoto, Y., Ige, A., Szabo, J. and Cohen, L.
    (1974). Substantia nigra and the sensorimotor system. (Chemoni-
    grectomies induced by intrategmental administration of the
    paraquinone of 6-hydroxydopamine and 6,7-dihydroxytryptamine
    in the cat and monkey). *Int. J. Neurol. 10,* 98-114.
Frigyesi, T.L., Yahr, M.D., and Schwartz, R. (1974). Electrophysio-
    logical analysis of the effects of L-DOPA on reciprocal cortico-
    thalamic projections in the squirrel monkey. I. Iatrogenic
    coma and disinhibition of medial thalamic neurons. *J. Neural
    Transm. 35,* 151-173.
Groves, P.M., Wilson, C.J., Young, S.J. and Rebec, G.V. (1975).
    Self-inhibition by dopaminergic neurons. *Science 190,* 522-
    529.
Haase, J.-J. and Jansen. P.A.J. (1965). *The action of neuroleptic
    drugs.* North-Holland Publ. Co., Amsterdam.
Harding, B.N. (1971). Dendro-dendritic, including reciprocal, synapses
    in the ventrolateral nucleus of the monkey thalamus. *Brain Res.
    34,* 181-185.
Heath, R.G. (1959). *Studies in Schizophrenia.* Harvard U. Press,
    Cambridge.
Hess, R., Tsukamoto, Y., and Frigyesi, T.L. (1974). Electrophysiolog-
    ical analysis of cerebello-thalamocortical relations to paro-
    xysmal discharges in the motor cortex (Penicillin focus).
    *Experientia 30,* 679.
Hunt, E.L. and Lisa, J.R. (1927). Frontal lobe tumor. A case simu-
    lating epidemic encephalitis with Parkinson's syndrome. *J.
    Amer. Med. Assoc. 89,* 1674-1676.
Kalmus, M., Fry, D.B., and Denes, P. (1960). Effects of delayed
    visual control on writing, drawing and tracing. *Lang. Speech
    3,* 96-108.

Klee, M. (1975).  Increased excitability of interneurons vs. enhanced
    positive feedback; possible mechanisms of epileptic activity.
    In: *Subcortical Mechanism and Sensorimotor Activities*.  Ed. T.L.
    Frigyesi Hans Huber Publ. Bern.

Kulkow, R. (1930).  Ueber Quecksilberencephalopathie.  Paralysis
    agitans. *Z. ges. Neurol. Psychiat. 125*, 52-57.

Lebovitz, R.M. (1974).  Inhibitory phasing of penicillin interictal
    discharge. *Brain Res. 79*, 301-305.

Lee, B.S. (1950).  Effects of delayed speech feedback. *J. Acoust.
    Soc. Am. 22*, 824-826.

Machek, J. (1965).  Macrostructural Generators in Seizure Origin
    and Spread. *Excerpta Medica*, Congress Series 124, 183-191.

Matsumoto, H. (1964).  Intracellular events during the activation of
    cortical epileptiform discharges. *EEG. clin. Neurophysiol. 17*,
    294-307.

Mendez, E.S., Cotzias, G., Mena, I. and Papavasiliou, P.S. (1975).
    Diphenylhydantoin. *Arch. Neurol. 32*, 44-46.

Merritt, H.M. and Putnam, T.J. (1939).  Sodium diphenyl hydantoinate
    in the treatment of convulsive seizures, toxic symptoms and
    their prevention. *Arch. Neurol and Psychiat. 42*, 1053-1058.

Mettler, F.A. (1955).  Perceptual capacity, functions of the corpus
    striatum and schizophrenia. *Psychiatric Quant. 29*, 89-111.

Meyer-Koenigsberg, E. (1923).  Die Beeinfluessung der Bewegung
    Stoerungen bei der Encephalitis Lethargica durch ritmische
    Gefuehle. *Muench. Med. Wchnschr. 70*, 459-469.

Nauta, W.J.M. (1976).  Discussion in: *Basal Ganglia*.  M.D. Yahr, Ed.
    Raven Press, New York, pp. 179-180.

Nyquist, H. (1932).  Regeneration theory. *Bell Syst. tech. J. 11*,
    126-142.

Penfield, W. and Jasper, H. (1954).  *Epilepsy and the functional anatomy
    of the human brain*.  Little, Brown and Co., Boston.

Powell, E.W. and Leman, R.B. (1976).  Connections of the nucleus
    accumbens. *Brain Res. 105*, 389-403.

Purpura, D.P. (1972).  Synaptic mechanism in coordination of activity
    in thalamic internuncial common paths.  In: *Corticothalamic
    Projection and Sensorimotor Activities*.  Ed. T.L. Frigyesi, E.
    Rinvik and M.D. Yahr.  Raven Press, New York, 1972, pp. 21-56.

Purpura, D.P. (1976).  Physiological organization of the basal ganglia.
    In: *The Basal Ganglia*.  M.D. Yahr (ed.) Raven Press, New York,
    pp. 91-114.

Purpura, D.P. and Cohen, B. (1962).  Intracellular recordings from
    thalamic neurons during recruiting responses. *J. Neurophysiol.
    25*, 621-635.

Purpura, D.P., Frigyesi, T.L., McMurtry, J.G. and Scarff, T. (1966).
    Synaptic mechanisms in thalamic regulation of cerebello-cortical
    projection activity.  In: *The Thalamus*.  D.P. Purpura and M.D.
    Yahr (eds.) Columbia U. Press.  New York, pp. 154-170.

Racine, R.J., Gartner, J.G. and McIntyre Burnham, W. (1973).
    Epileptiform activity and neural plasticity in limbic struc-
    tures. *Brain Res.* *47*, 262-268.
Rosen, A.D. (1976). Influence of association cortex on penicillin
    discharges in the primary visual cortex. *EEG. clin. Electro-
    physiol.* *41*, 571-579.
Rinvik, E. (1972). Organization of thalamic connections from motor
    and somato-sensory cortical areas in the cat. In: *Corticothala-
    mic Projections and Sensorimotor Activities.* Ed. T.L. Frigyesi,
    E. Rinvik, and M.D. Yahr. Raven Press, New York, pp. 57-90.
Scheibel, M.E., Davis, T.L. and Scheibel, A.B. (1972). On dendritic
    relations in the dorsal thalamus of the adult cat. *Exptl.
    Neurol. 36*, 519-529.
Scheibel, M.E., Davies, T.L. and Scheibel, A.B. (1973). On thalamic
    subtrates of cortical synchrony. *Neurology 23*, 300-304.
Scheibel, M.E. and Scheibel, A.B. (1970). Elementary processes in
    selected thalamic and cortical subsystems-the structural sub-
    strates. In: *The Neurosciences.* Second study program. Ed.
    A.C. Quarton et al. Rockefeller U. Press. New York, pp. 443-
    457.
Scholz, W. (1957). An nervose Systeme gebundene (topistische)
    Kreiscaufschaden. In: *Handbuch Der Speziellen Pathologischen
    Anatomy und Histologie.* Vol. XIII. 1. A. Ed. O. Ludarsch,
    F. Henke and R. Roessle, Springer-Verlag, Berlin. pp. 1328-1383.
Schwab, R.S. and England, A.C. (1968). Parkinson syndromes due to
    various specific causes. In: *Handbook of Clinical Neurology.*
    P.J. Vinken and G.W. Gruyn (eds.), vol. 6 *Diseases of the Basal
    Ganglia.* North-Holland Publ. Co. Amsterdam., pp. 227-247.
Steck, H. (154). Le syndrome extra-pryamidal et di-encephalique au
    cors des traitments au largactil et au serpasil. *Ann. med.-
    psychol. 112*, 737-743.
Sutton, S., Hakerem, G., Zubin, J. and Portnoy, M. (1961). The effect
    of shift of modality on serial reaction time: a comparison of
    schizophrenics and normals. *Am. J. Psychol. 74*, 224-232.
Von Economo, C. (1929). *Die Encephalitis Lethargiga.* Urban and
    Schwarzenberg, Wien.
Walter, G.W. (1953). *The living brain.* Norton, New York.
Wiener, N. (1950). *Human use of human beings.* Houghton Mifflin,
    Boston.
Wiener, N. (1961). *Cybernetics or Control and Communication in the
    Animal and the Machine.* Second Edition, M.I.T. Press and John
    Wiley and Sons, New York.
Wilcoxon, F. (1949). *Some rapid approximate statistical procedures.*
    Am. Cyanamid Co., New York.
Wilson, S.A.K. and Cobb, S. (1924). Mesencephalitis Syphilitica.
    *J. Neuro. Psychopath. 5*, 44-60.

Yakovlev, P. (1928).  Epilepsy and parkinsonsim.  *N.E.J. Med. 198*,
    629-638.
Yariura-Tobias, J.A., Diamond, B., and Merlis, S. (1970).  The action
    of L-Dopa on schizophrenic patients.  (A preliminary report).
    *Curr. Ther. Res. 12*, 528-

## DISCUSSION

*Dr. Barnes*

Obviously part of the pathological condition in parkinsonism
is a disruption involving the caudate nucleus.  If you are proposing
that the caudate nucleus disruption results in disruption of the
pathway cerebellum-thalamic-cortex, how is it that this influence on
conversion takes place?

*Dr. Frigyesi*

The essential point I tried to show was that these recurrent
excitatory-inhibitory sequences in the thalamus, converting the
tonic input to phasic output are necessary though not sufficient
conditions for maintaining normal motor activity.  According to the
electrophysiological data, low frequency-stimulation of all components of the basal ganglia would produce this type of excitatory-
inhibitory sequences.  It appears that for normal sensory motor
integration, the thalamic relays need the sum total of these recurring
inhibitory sequences coming from various sources.  If the caudate is
diseased, there is going to be a quantitative deficit of these recurrent IPSP's: those recurrent IPSP's which normally would come from
the caudate.  This particular condition is associated with parkinsonism.  What happens if these recurrent IPSP's which come from globus
pallidus are missing?  Well, it may be associated with chorea or other
abnormal movements.  One can make neuropathological correlations.
Low-frequency stimulation structures where anatomical damage has been
shown in various abnormal movements, produces excitatory-inhibitory
sequences in VL.  What does L-dopa do?  What does atropine do?
Apparently they induce a quantitative increase of recurrent IPSP's
in the VL.

*Dr. Messiha*

If I understood you correctly, you hinted that phenytoin
interfers in the dopaminergic system.  The first question is: what
is the mechanism of action if it is known?  The second question
is on the 20-year old slide, as you have described it, are the data
significant and what is the age bracket of the subjects shown?  And
thirdly, what is the anti-parkinsonian medication which was available 20 years ago?

*Dr. Frigyesi*
   The anti-parkinsonian medications of those patients were Artane®
and Panparnit®.

*Dr. Messiha*
   So the sample is mixed medication, or is it a single anti-
parkinson agent?  I realize it is perhaps too late, 20 years later,
to ask.

*Dr. Frigyesi*
   Yes.  I must admit I did not check last night on the old papers.
The age group in the parkinsonian patients was 40-82; the control
group, who were chronically hospitalized patients, was matched.
Lastly, the dopamine-Dilantin® relationship.  Costzias reported
recently that Dilantin® decreases the efficacy of L-dopa in parkinsonian patients.

*Dr. Messiha*
   Is there any speculation on the mode of action in this regard?
Does it deplete dopamine?

*Dr. Frigyesi*
   Yes.  Dilantin® altered the uptake and binding of catecholamines
in rat brain slices.  Dilantin® can inhibit cerebral protein
synthesis and inhibitors of protein synthesis can block the cerebral
effects of L-dopa.

*Dr. Pirch*
   Are there connections from the basal ganglia or substantia
nigra to other cortical areas, and could these, if they exist,
explain some of the sensory deficits that are seen in Parkinson
patients?

*Dr. Frigyesi*
   Well, yes, probably there are.  But we don't know any of those.
As a matter of fact, input-output properties of the nigra are poorly understood.  What is known today, simply cannot be the entire
story.  For example, inasmuch as caudate self-regulates its dopaminergic input from the nigra, and the major input to the nigra is
from the caudate, and its major output is to the caudate, the
machine could be simpler without the nigra and the dopamine manu-
factured in the caudate.  Another example is the caudato-nigro-
thalamic projection system.  Why not direct caudato-thalamic linkage?  Obviously, these questions will be answered when the input-
output properties of nigra will be better understood.

*Dr. Lake*

Yesterday we heard all about the nigral-striatal projections, and their importance in parkinsonism. Could you discuss some of the neurophysiological aspects of nigral-striatal projections in the context of what you talked about today, that is the nigral-striatal inputs to the caudate?

*Dr. Frigyesi*

Are you asking is dopamine an excitatory transmitter or inhibitory transmitter?

*Dr. Lake*

I am specifically interested in the effects of dopaminergic inputs and their interactions with other inputs on the caudate output that you discussed.

*Dr. Frigyesi*

The major input to the caudate is from the cortex and media thalamus. The output systems are to the globus pallidus and substantia nigra. Caudate effects could reach the thalamus via the globus pallidus-ansa lenticulanis system or via the caudato-nigro-thalamic projection system. Since the major effect of the caudate in ansa-lenticulenis projection neurons is hyperpolarization, and sin caudate evokes EPSP's in many nigral neurons, I believe the primary route for establishing caudate-thalamic functional linkages is via the substantia nigra. In answer to the transmitter question, neither Kitai nor myself found IPSP's in non-traumatized caudate neurons during nigral stimulation. But we found EPSP's. These other data indicate that dopamine is a putative excitatory transmitter in the caudate.

*Dr. Lake*

Do you have any insight as to the neurochemistry of the caudate nigral and nigral-thalamic projections? Specifically what transmitters are involved in those two pathways?

*Dr. Frigyesi*

The data do not permit me to speculate on this matter.

*Dr. Duvoisin*

It's always been my impression that there is an inverse relationship between parkinsonism and epilepsy. A large series of patients seem to have a lesser incidence of seizure disorders than one would expect in them. I gather that is similar to your own view. Many years ago, a fellow name Cavat administered Dilantin® in toxic doses to Parkinson patients, on the theory of a cerebellar striatal antagonism. I repeated that about fifteen years ago and could demonstrate no anti-Parkinson effect of Dilantin® itself. Yesterday Dr. Klawans and I were comparing notes. We both have some Parkinson patients who have seizures and were placed on Dilantin®. Neither he nor I have seen any reduction of the levodopa efficacy on Dilantin® treatment, despite the Cotzias observation. We did not have to increase levodopa dosage at all; the effect was well maintained. On the other hand, it appears that there was some difficulty controlling the seizures, in that if one removes the levodopa, the seizures are better controlled; and if one increases them, they are worse.

*Dr. Frigyesi*
        Thank you. On the one hand you have an argument with Cotzias; I don't want to get into that point. On the theory you had seen a number of parkinsonian patients with epilepsy. I guess because you see a selected sample; in a random sample, the coincidence is very low.

*Dr. Duvoisin*
        That is what I am saying.

*Dr. Frigyesi*
        Further, your patients had extensive but undertermined pathology. My remarks were related to pathologically simpler situations. The integrity of so far undermined systems may be necessary for the manifestations of the described phenomenon.

*Dr. Fahn*
        To continue this type of discussion, I have no personal experience on Dilantin® and parkinsonism, except that many years ago I did try to use Dilantin® as an anti-parkinsonian agent, but it was not successful. But I do want to comment about my experience with Dilantin® and chorea. I have tried this with about three patients with Huntington's disease. The chorea became much worse and more difficult to control, and the family stopped the drug because of that. I think Cotzias has also shown that. The second comment I would like to make in regards to your slide showing the input from the caudate to the thalamus via the substantia nigra, and I suspect you are referring to the pars reticulata fibers that Carpenter showed goes from that region to the ventrolateral nucleus. But you didn't include in that slide the globus pallidus. Are you excluding it for a reason?

*Dr. Frigyesi*
        The electrophysiological data show that stimulation of the caudate is followed by evoked responses in the thalamus. The anatomical data suggest that there is no major caudate-thalamic

pathway. Thus, caudate effects must relay through structures. Caudate projects to globus pallidus where its major effect is inhibitory. Caudate projects to the nigra where in some neurons it generates EPSP's, in others IPSP's. Both the globus pallidus and nigra send axons to the thalamus. But, in view of the foregoing, globus pallidus is not likely to be the major relay; nigra is. In earlier studies, I destroyed the globus pallidus, and could elicit in these animals caudate responses in the thalamus. When subsequently, I destroyed the nigra also (by 6-OHDA), the caudate-evoked thalamic potentials were abolished. These indicate that the major trajectory for caudate-thalamic projection activities is via the substantia nigra. This also shows that it is difficult to determine the functional property of an axonal system from purely morphological studies.

# NEUROPHYSIOLOGY OF MOVEMENT DISORDERS

J.C. DE LA TORRE


Institute of Neurological Surgery
Brain Research Institute
University of Chicago Pritzker School of Medicine
Chicago, Illinois 60637

## ABSTRACT

The relation of the cortex, cerebellum, and basal ganglia and their participation in movement disorders is presented. Studies have shown that lesions to the cortex will produce contralateral paralysis while damage to the basal ganglia or cerebellum will result in movement abnormalities. These data provide support for the view that subcortical but not cortical structures initiate and control movement activity. It would appear that the basal ganglia and cerebellum receive signals from the auditory, visual, and somatosensory cortex integrate this information, and relay signals back to the motor cortex, which in turn sends out efferent fibers to the motor neurons of the spinal cord. The electronic and neurophysiological basis of the somatosensory evoked responses (SER) test following peripheral nerve stimulation and sensory recording in human cortex is given. Control values of SER peak to peak latency waveforms from 66 normal volunteers show the practicality of this test. Preliminary results using SER in patients are discussed from clinical case reports. The subjects had mild to marked movement disorders secondary to Parkinson's disease, vascular occlusion, multiple sclerosis, and spino-cerebellar degeneration. The potential of the SER as a clinical and experimental tool in evaluating movement abnormalities and other neuropathological conditions is presented.

## INTRODUCTION

Movement is an essential part of function because it affects an organism's capability to assume some activity in its search for self-survival. When movement is impaired in non-human animals, survival is generally compromised. To understand movement abnormalities, one must first classify them as to location, rhythmicity, frequency, and form. I would like to dwell for a moment on the types and causes of some of these movement abnormalities.

*Athetosis*, or athetoid movements, is a form of involuntary movement involving the skeletal muscles. They are characterized by their irregular, slow, and writhing, somewhat rhythmic movements. They may involve the trunk, neck, face, and the extremities especially the fingers, hands, and toes. Athetosis can be produced by lesions in the caudate nucleus and putamen.

*Chorea* consists of sudden, jerky, and involuntary movements. They are nonrhythmic and explosive in character. Choreiform movements may involve one or all extremities, one half of the body or the entire body. They are characteristic in the upper extremities but can affect the lower extremities and can also involve the vocal cords, tongue and the mouth. They are frequently observed in the neck muscles.

When the movements are slow, rhythmic, and alternate with rapid jerky motions, the condition is known as *choreo-athetosis*. Choreo-athetosis may be produced experimentally by lesions in the anterior column of the spinal cord or in the internal capsule which results in hemiplegia as well. It has been reported that athetosis can be temporarily abolished by severing the efferent extrapyramidal fibers from the subcortical ganglia.

*Tremors* are defined as involuntary, rhythmical, alternating movements. The alternation of movement results when there is contraction and relaxation by the same muscle or group of muscles. The oscillatory rate of tremors may be slow from 3-5 oscillation/ second, medium ranging from 6-10 oscillations/second, or rapid ranging from above 10-20 oscillations/second. Parkinson's disease has been estimated to have 5.5 oscillations/second on the average which places it between slow and medium in rate.

There are three general types of tremors: a) static, b) intention, and c) postural. Static, resting, or non-intention tremors are characterized in Parkinson's disease and involve the skeletal musculature supported by involuntary contractions. Intention, or action tremors, result when the muscles are put in motion and are generally not seen when the muscle is at rest. Postural, or intension tremors, occur when there is an increase in muscle tonus, as, for example, when the hands or arms are outstretched, or the head is maintained in a certain posture. They are usually absent when the body is completely at rest. Destruction of the dentato-rubro-thalamic tract can result in intention tremor while lesions

of the globus pallidus and the substantia nigra can produce the
resting tremors.

*Ballismus* is another movement abnormality that is characterized
by involuntary, purposeless movements and is seen in the form of
*hemiballism*. It resembles chorea but is much more rapid and force-
ful, generally involving the proximal portions of the extremities.
*Hemiballism* may appear when the subthalamic nucleus of Luys is dam-
aged. Such a lesion affects the vasculature of the subthalamic
nucleus producing hemorrhage and the characteristic hemiballistic,
irregular and violent movement on the contralateral extremity.

*Torsion dystonia* or dystonic movements are characterized as a
spontaneous, slow, and involuntary movement which can become exaggerated following voluntary motion. The movements resemble athetosis except that they involve the trunk more than the limbs, and
show a bizarre twisting, writhing and turning of the body, particularly the shoulder muscles, trunk and hip girdle. The movements of
the spine show a torsion of the vertebral axis with tilting of the
shoulder and pelvic area resulting in lordotic and scoliotic pos-
turing. The movements cease while the patient is asleep but return
upon awakening. The pathology of this movement disorder consists
of degenerative changes in the putamen and caudate nucleus. Changes
in the dentate nuclei, substantia nigra, cerebral cortex, and thalamus have also been found. The etiology may either be infectious,
vascular, neoplastic, toxic, or idiopathic.

The last type of movement disorder is termed *bradykinesia* which
is characteristic of Parkinson's disease. Bradykinesia implies
poverty of movement, slowness in walk and little or no arm swinging
or other associated movements.

When bradykinesia is severe, it is termed *akinesia* which involves complete loss of power resulting in paralysis. The loss of
expressive and associated movements gives rise to the typical mask-
like facies and infrequent blinking so typical in Parkinsonism.
Parkinsonian patients usually suffer from *rigidity* of the muscles
characterized by marked hypertonia affecting the proximal and flexor
groups of the extremities and the spinal muscles. Often the rigidity is of the *cogwheel* type seen when an observer passively moves
the patient's limb and resistance is encountered leading to a series
of rapid fluctuations causing an alternating contraction and relaxation of the muscle being stretched. A second type of rigidity,
the *lead pipe*, shows no fluctuations and the resistance is uniform.
There are many other variations and types of abnormal movement disorders, but the above are of particular interest here because they
involve the basal ganglia structures.

There are numerous ways of studying these movement disorders
in both animals and man using a variety of tools and experimental
models (*Liles and Davis, 1969; Cools, 1961; Forman and Ward, 1957;
Chandler and Crosby, 1975; Yu, 1974; Denny-Brown, 1960; Klüver and
Bucy, 1937; Twitchell, 1965*).

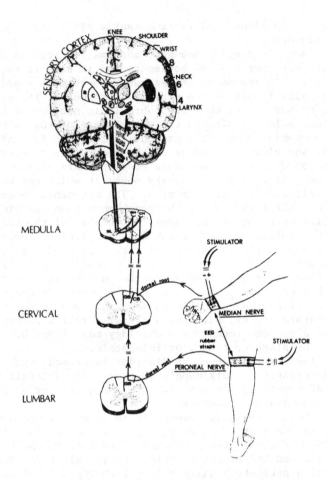

*Figure 1.*   *Schematic representation of the spinal cord, medulla and brain shows the postulated sensory conduction pathway arriving at the dorsal horn from the dorsal roots following cutaneous stimulation of the median (wrist) and peroneal (leg) nerves. The pathways ascend from first-order neurons (receptors) and proceed via the cuneate bundle (CB) from the wrist and the gracilis bundle (GB) from the leg. After reaching the cuneate (CN) and gracilis (GN) nuclei in the lower medulla, the fibers cross immediately to the contralateral medial lemniscus (ML) from second-order neurons and continue to ascend passing through the reticular formation (H). At this point, the exact pathway of the ascending afferents becomes less clear, but ultimately they reach the ventroposterolateral thalamic nucleus (D) where third-order neurons relay the impulses (dashed lines) to the postcentral sensory cortex in the*

Stimulation and ablation studies have revealed much of the functional localization and participation of cortical structures. In the frontal lobe, there are three areas which are important in the evolution of movement: areas 4, 6, and 8 (Fig. 1). Area 4 is the primary motor projection area and lies anterior to area 6. The two form part of the extrapyramidal tract system. Area 8 is concerned with volitional control of conjugate eye movements and with pupillary dilatation. It is also considered a suppresor region with functions similar to those of area 4. Damage to the frontopontine fibers which rise just anterior to areas 6 and 8 can cause contralateral ataxia (cerebellar damage causes ipsilateral ataxia). Surgical removal of either area 6 or 4 has been used to eliminate certain types of hyperkinesia and interruption of the U fibers between areas 4 and 6 have been tried neurosurgically for the relief of intention tremor, dystonia, hemiballism, athetosis, choreo-athetosis and Parkinsonism (*Hersley, 1908; Klemme, 1942; Bucy, 1951 Meyers, 1953*). Neuropharmacological agents have replaced many of these surgical interventions, the most successful being the use of L-dopa in combination with a peripheral dopa decarboxylase inhibitor for the treatment of Parkinson's disease (*de la Torre, 1968; Tissot et al, 1969*).

The scope of this paper would hardly do justice to even briefly discussing the experimental and clinical techniques concerned with motor activity. We will review instead two ways of analyzing cerebral function using neurophysiological recording equipment. The first method is to test the motor output of specific brain regions or neurons. The second method is to test the sensory input arriving at the brain from afferent sensory pathways.

One of the earliest writings on the mechanistic theory of brain function was advanced by Rene Descartes in his book, De Homine *(1662)* which demonstrates the basic process of the reflex as an involuntary and automatic reaction. This primitive theory is the beginning of the concept of afferent and efferent components of nerve-muscle

*cingulum (knee) and parietor region (wrist) where the somatosensory evoked responses are recorded from scalp electrodes. The cerebral cortex is then thought to send fibers to the caudate nucleus (A) and the cerebellum. These two structures may process and then relay the received sensory information via caudo-thalamo-cortical and dentato-rubro-thalamic connections to the motor cortex from where the information descends to the spinal cord motor neurons and finally the muscles. The participation of other extrapyramidal structures (putamen [B], globus pallidus [C], subthalamic nucleus [E]) in normal movement is less well understood. The numbers to the right of the cortical schema represent the more anterior precentral cytoarchitectonic location of some motor regions: areas 8, 6, and 4 (see text for details).*

reaction resulting in motion.  Although Descartes' theories were
based on speculation and incorrect anatomical observations, his in-
genious representation of a heuristic model to explain nervous function led to centuries of debates and speculation in the field of
brain research.  Descartes' ideas became a primary influence in subsequent investigations by Willis (1664) who placed the functional
center of the brain in its tissue substance and not in the humoral
element of the ventricles as previously assumed by the ancients.
Cartesian thinking also influenced to a large extent the work of
Sherrington (1906) who placed more emphasis on how volitional movement could control spinal reflexes.  At this time, Sherrington also
proposed his *law of reciprocal innervation* which states that innervation to one muscle group is accompanied by an inhibition of an
antagonistic muscle group.  Thus, when extensors of the arm are
contracted, there is a reciprocal relaxation of the flexors.

The revolutionary concept that the cerebral cortex controls or
regulates motor activity began with the work of Fritsch and Hitzig
(1870) who reported that electrical stimulation of the cortex in
dogs produced muscular contractions on the opposite side of the dog's
body.  This idea was further refined by J. Hughlings Jackson (1873)
who on the basis of clinical and pathological data showed that the
cerebral cortex was involved in specific motor activity.  Jackson's
work further led to descriptions of focal epilepsy where a localized
part of the body convulsed involuntarily, sometimes preceeding generalized body convulsions (Jacksonian seizure).  Although there were
seventy-five reports dealing with electrical stimulation of human
cerebral motor cortex between 1874 and 1914, none gave very accurate
information concerning the precise function of the motor strip.

Within the last fifty years, the work of Lashley (1929), Luria
1966), and Penfield and Boldrey (1937) have brought about our present
concepts on impairment of learning ability following ablation of cortical tissue.  Classification of the various motor areas, and the
functional significance of the motor and sensory strips were represented in the homunculus, an inverted graphic representation of the
human body stretching along the lateral surface of the perietal and
temporal lobes.  It has become increasingly evident following the
more recent work of Mountcastle (1966) and Denny-Brown (1966) that
although lesions to the motor cortex will generally result in paralysis to a contralateral portion of the body, similar lesions in the
basal ganglia and cerebellum will produce movement abnormalities,
such as those previously discussed in this paper.

A series of studies by Evarts (1967) on conscious monkeys whose
heads were immobilized and who had been trained to pull a lever
involving flexion and extension of the wrist as part of a reward, have
suggested that subcortical structures such as the basal ganglia are
responsible for the initiation and control of movement.  Moreover,
inputs received in these structures are relayed to the cerebral
cortex by way of thalamo-cortical projections which result in refined
control of motor activity.  In addition, damage to the cerebellum

results in practically opposite movement abnormalities as those found following lesions of the basal ganglia. It would seem then that simply stated, the motor cortex does not have the capacity to decide whether or not a movement, or the timing of such movement shall take place, but appears, rather, to be more concerned with the regulation, through complex somatosensory input systems, of those specific movements that require its participation (*Kornhuber, 1974; DeLong, 1974*).

Studies of single-unit activity in conscious monkeys support the view that the primary function of the basal ganglia is to generate slow rather than rapid movements. Thus, the bradykinetic or akinetic loss in speed and spontaneity of movement which if often clinically observed in Parkinson's disease is a result of damage to the basal ganglia. By contrast, myoclonic movements which are frequently encountered in epilepsy and which result in frequent, sudden jerking attacks of the neck, arms, and legs generally result following damage to the cortex. This theory, however, does not explain the evolution of ballistic movements such as those seen in hemiballism. This disorder, as previously stated, involved the rapid swinging and twisting of the extremities in one half of the body following an isolated lesion to the contralateral, subthalamic nucleus or its pathways. It is clear that the synthesis of available information indicates that certain subcortical brain structures preferentially initiate movement and that this movement is refined and smoothed out by the cortex and cerebellum. The precise integration of afferent pathways to these structures in clinico-pathological conditions affecting movement remains to be discovered.

Besides the experiments that test the motor outputs in specific cell systems or single neurons in the brain, there is also a growing number of investigations dealing with the sensory inputs in respect to the processing of peripheral signals in the brain, particularly as they apply to clinical movement disorders. These experiments stem from some original observations made by Dawson (*1947*) using somatosensory evoked averaged responses. The somatosensory evoked responses is based on the principle that stimulation of a subject's sensory system will result in some electrical activity in a localized region of the brain. If then, one assumes that the cerebral response always follows the stimulus after a fixed delay, then computer averaging a wanted signal can separate this signal from bioelectric background or unwanted noise. "Noise" is defined as any unwanted mechanical or biological signal that may be present in the system. Somatosensory evoked responses (SER) can be obtained by stimulating a peripheral nerve, for example, at the wrist or in the leg (see Figure 1) and recording on the scalp overlying the somatosensory cortex. If the stimulus pulse is locked into the signal, then it initiates a scanning device which samples the signal at fixed intervals in the memory locations of the computer averager. Each channel then collects data over a small time segment, and when the stimulus is repeated, the responses are added to values stored in each memory location. The

final signal, then, reads out the sum of all the previous samples fed
into it.  In this way, random activity such as background EEG or other
unwanted noise will not add linearly with the responses being averaged.
Figure 2 also illustrates the equipment generally used for averaging
evoked responses.  In our laboratory we use a Fabri-Tek 1052 computer

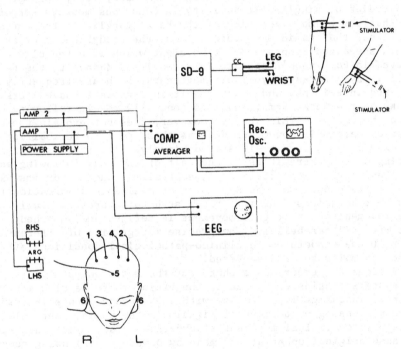

Figure 2.   *Schematic diagram showing the equipment used for recording
somatosensory evoked responses (SER).  A computer averager
(Comp. Ave.) receives amplified (Amp 1 and 2) evoked response signals from cup electrodes located over the somatosensory cortex strip, 5 cm from the midline (electrodes 1
and 2) and 1 cm from the midline (electrodes 3 and 4) for
wrist and leg respectively.  It was found that although
the projected area for the wrist is 7 cm from the midline
over the sensory cortex, electrodes placed 4.5 to 5 cm.
from the midline gave "cleaner" and more consistent waveforms.  A possible reason may be that the temporalis muscle causes myogenic interference when the recording electrodes are placed more laterally on the skull.  The signals are referenced to a forehead electrode (5) and the
subject is grounded with ear lobe clip electrodes (6).
Leads from electrodes 1 and 2 or 3 and 4 are connected to
head stages (LHS and RHS) input (A) for left and right*

averager which receives signals from two Grass P-511E amplifiers
powered by a Grass RPS 107 power supply which also drives a storage
oscilloscope for monitoring EEG.  The signals displayed in the computer are relayed to a second oscilloscope where the signals are
photographed with a polaroid camera for permanent records.  Stimulation is carried out using a Grass SD-9 stimulator coupled to a constant current unit producing squarewave pulses of 0.1 msec duration
and 0.1 msec delay every second.  Stimulation of regular monopolar
pulses are given until 128 responses are averaged by the computer.
The signals from the somatosensory cortex are amplified $10^5$ with a
cut-off at 0.3 Hz using a 60 cycle notch filter.  Although somatosensory evoked responses have been available for over 28 years, it
was not until about 5 years ago that their application in neuronal
trauma and neurological disorders was begun.  Since then, a number
of reports have appeared in the literature supporting the premise
that the SER can be an extremely useful clinical tool with far-
reaching potential applications, particularly in the diagnosis and
prognosis of neuropathological disorders.  Figure 1 shows the pathways thought to be involved in the transmission of afferent impulses
following bilateral stimulation of the common peroneal nerves and
median nerves in human subjects.  The signals arrive via the dorsal
roots and enter the dorsal columns where they ascend through the
gracilis bundle following stimulation of the leg, and through the
cuneate bundle (CB) following stimulation of the wrist.  At the
level of the lower medulla, the signals enter the nucleus gracilis
and the nucleus cuneatus respectively, then crossover immediately
into the medial lemniscus bundle passing through a series of brain
stem and mesencephalic structures until they reach the ventral pos-
terolateral nucleus of the thalamus and from there are relayed to
the somatosensory cortex,  The evidence showing the conduction of
such signals from the arm and leg can be found in the earlier works
of Giblin (*1964*), Halliday (*1967*), and Larson *et al.* (*1966*).  There
is more general agreement on the conduction pathways following sen-

---

*hemispheric recording.  Leads 5 and 6 are connected to the
reference (R) and ground (G) inputs and a banana plug is
used to bridge the two head stages for R and G.  Stimulation is carried out (see text for details) using a Grass
SD-9 stimulator connected to the computer and to a constant current (CC) unit.  Two leads with cup electrodes
on the ends are led to either the median or the peroneal
nerves from the CC unit and stimulation current is adjus-
ted until a thumb or toe twitch is elicited bilaterally.
The cathode stimulating electrode is 2 cm proximal to
the anode and both electrodes are filled with conducting
cream and held in place with a rubber strap.  The signals
that have been averaged on the computer are projected on
an oscilloscope for photograph recording and the EEG is
monitored from the scalp electrodes on the second memory
oscilloscope.*

sory stimulation than on the *origin* and *significance* of each waveform component following signal averaging from the somatosensory
cortex.  An important development in the use of the SER in recent
years has been to elucidate the origin of the waveform components
and relate these to specific sites or pathways in brain or spinal
cord.  This is complicated by the fact that the signal originating
from a sensory nerve following stimulation is relayed to the spinal
cord, and then proceeds through a complex series of steps as it is
propagated through a number of interrelated neuronal networks until
it arrives at the sensory cortex,  Our own studies have shown that
the presence of some or all components, their latencies, and amplitudes can be altered in the same subject by external sources such
as variable stimulus voltage applied to the peripheral nerve, the
position of the recording scalp electrodes overlying the somatosensory strip, and any mechanical noise in the recording equipment, or
from an external source in the testing room.  The SER waveform components can also be influenced by a number of biological factors
irrespective of the subject's neuropathological status, such as
level of consciousness, psychic mental state, muscular movements,
and medication being taken.  Although most of the SERs done today
are noninvasive, information as to the origin of the primary waveform component has been derived from stereotaxic thalamotomies on
patients suffering from intractable pain, and dyskinesia (*Larson and
Sances, 1968*), and from choreo-athetosis, intention tremor, intractable pain, and Parkinson's disease (*Fukushima et al., 1976*).  These
and other investigations (*Albe-Fessard and Bowsher, 1965; Guiot
et al., 1973; and Allison et al., 1962*) appear to support the view-
point that the first primary-wave peak response originates as a
thalamocortical response to sensory stimulation and ranges in latency
from 15-20 msec delay (*Fukushima et al., 1976*).

     One of the advantages of averaging responses from subcortical
structures as Fukushima and his group (*1976*) have shown, is that the
various thalamic nuclei can be identified for stereotaxic reference
points by their latencies following cutaneous sensory stimulation.
There is substantially less agreement on the origin and specificity
of the other waveform components in either animals or humans.  Our
own investigation has shown the value of the SER in human brain and
spinal cord trauma particularly in prognosing potential recovery from
the vegetative state (*de la Torre and Trimble, 1976*).  We began these
studies about four years ago in animals subjected to experimental
spinal cord trauma, and during the last two years have extended these
investigations into a number of neuropathological conditions in human
subjects.

     The French writer Andre Gide was once quoted as saying: "In order
to find out what is enough, one must first find out what is more than
enough".  By the same token, to find out what is abnormal, we first
had to know what was normal.  To do this, we examined 66 male and
female normal volunteer subjects ranging in age from 18 to 69 in order

TABLE 1.   NORMAL PEAK LATENCIES RECORDED OVER THE SOMATOSENSORY CORTEX
IN VOLUNTEER SUBJECTS FOLLOWING MEDIAN AND PERONEAL NERVE
STIMULATION.

### A. MEDIAN NERVE CONTROL PEAK LATENCIES (55 SUBJECTS)

| | Right Hemisphere Milliseconds | | | | Left Hemisphere Milliseconds | | |
|---|---|---|---|---|---|---|---|
| | Mean | SD | SE | | Mean | SD | SE |
| 1. | 11 | ± 3 | ±0.5 | | 11 | ± 3 | ±0.6 |
| 2. | 21 | ± 7 | ±1.4 | | 22 | ± 6 | ±1.1 |
| 3. | 44 | ± 9 | ±1.7 | | 43 | ± 12 | ±2.2 |
| 4. | 65 | ± 12 | ±2.3 | | 64 | ± 11 | ±2.2 |
| 5. | 82 | ± 16 | ±3.0 | | 82 | ± 16 | ±3.1 |
| 6. | 110 | ± 21 | ±4.0 | | 108 | ± 21 | ±4.0 |
| 7. | 131 | ± 24 | ±4.7 | | 130 | ± 25 | ±4.8 |
| 8. | 157 | ± 26 | ±4.9 | | 156 | ± 26 | ±5.0 |

### B. PERONEAL NERVE CONTROL PEAK LATENCIES (11 SUBJECTS)

| | Right Hemisphere milliseconds | | | Left Hemisphere milliseconds | |
|---|---|---|---|---|---|
| | Mean | SD | | Mean | SD |
| 1. | 20 | ± 2 | | 19 | ± 3 |
| 2. | 32 | ± 4 | | 32 | ± 4 |
| 3. | 46 | ± 6 | | 43 | ± 5 |
| 4. | 61 | ± 8 | | 62 | ± 8 |
| 5. | 73 | ± 11 | | 70 | ± 10 |
| 6. | 96 | ± 14 | | 94 | ± 13 |
| 7. | 137 | ± 17 | | 136 | ± 15 |
| 8. | 188 | ± 19 | | 191 | ± 17 |

For typical SER waveform activities, see Fig. 5a and b: Normal.  The
average current intensity required to elicit thumb-twitch was 1.3 mA
for median nerve.  The average for peroneal stimulation was 1.6 mA.

SD: standard deviation; SE: standard error of the mean.

to find the mean and standard deviation latencies after median and peroneal nerve stimulation in a control group.

Table 1 shows the mean peak averages following median and peroneal nerve stimulation in normal subjects. The distribution and standard deviation latencies as well as the frequency delays in this group are similar but not identical to those values previously reported by Giblin (1964) following median nerve stimulation. The mean peak latencies observed following peroneal nerve stimulation are in agreement with the values reported by Tsumoto (1972).

I would like to present four cases from our files of patients showing SER waveform alterations which fall outside the control range of values. I want to emphasize that these are preliminary case report presentations and as such they are not meant to typify a particular disorder at least until these waveform altencies can be confirmed in a larger group of patients showing similar symptomatology. The first two cases may be functionally interrelated although for different reasons.

## METHODS AND RESULTS

*Case Report Number 1.* A 62-year old male was admitted to this hospital with walking problems and stiffness in the left arm and leg. Patient also complained of headache and blurring of vision. A neurological examination showed cogwheel rigidity of the arms more pronounced on the left side, weakness of triceps and biceps on the left side, bradykinesia, and shuffling gait. A fine tremor in both hands was seen. On the basis of the symptomatology, the patient was diagnosed as having Parkinson's disease.

A SER was done before treatment was initiated with Sinemet (carbidopa + L-dopa). The results of the SER are shown in Figure 3. If one compares the normal SER peak-to-peak latencies, it will be seen that the subject with Parkinson's disease shows a similar waveform pattern for the first two peaks (9 and 25 msec delays) but that subsequent components show a progressive *increase* in the latency delays ranging from 10 to 60 msec faster than the baseline controls. Although the right hemisphere was recorded simultaneously, it is not shown because it is practically identical with the left hemispheric recording shown in Figure 3.

*Case Report Number 2.* The subject is a 58-year old white female who was admitted to the hospital for tremors and weakness of the right arm, right leg pain, headaches, neck pain, and low back pain. A neurological examination showed restriction of movement of the neck, localized tenderness at $C_{4-6}$, spasticity of all extremities with proprioception and sensation intact, and a negative Romberg test. The EEG showed 7-10 cycles/sec resting occipital rhythm suppressed by eye opening. An asymmetric right temporal rhythm briefly appeared during drowsiness. The left anterior temporal and frontocentral areas

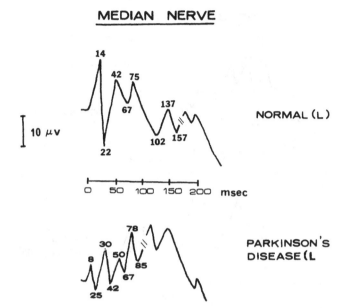

## MEDIAN NERVE

NORMAL (L)

PARKINSON'S
DISEASE (L

Figure 3. *Comparison of somatosensory evoked response (SER) traced from actual records in normal subject (left hemisphere, L) and patient with Parkinson's disease. First and second peak ($N_1$, $P_1$) latencies are similar in both subjects but subsequent latencies in parkinsonian patient were significantly increased. Numbers above and below peaks refer to msecond delay latencies. Right hemispheric recording (not shown) was similar to the left side. See also Table 1 for normal distribution and standard deviations of mean peak latencies and Case Report Number 1.*

showed sharp and slow activity in an unsustained fashion. Left carotid arteriogram showed a plaque on the posterior wall of the left common carotid at the bifurcation with the internal carotid artery. No narrowing of the internal carotid was noted. EKG, skull and cervical spinal x-rays were normal, and the ophthalmological exam was within normal limits. No evidence of multiple sclerosis was found. The static tremor seen on the right arm has recently been noted on the left arm also. A preliminary diagnosis indicated an old middle cerebral artery stroke which spared the speech area and a moderate spondylosis at $C_{5-6}$.

When compared to normal peak latencies, the SER showed a difference in the latency delay of the first component recorded over the left hemisphere. A significant decrease in amplitude was noted in

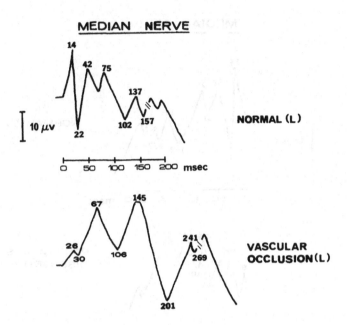

*Figure 4.*   *Comparison of SER in normal and patient with resting right*
           *hand tremors secondary to an old middle cerebral artery*
           *stroke.  Note the first primary negative peak ($N_1$) shows a*
           *10 msec delay from normal values.  The primary positive*
           *peak is within normal limits but subsequent peak latencies*
           *are slower than normal.  The right hemispheric recording*
           *(not shown) showed normal latencies of the first 4 peaks*
           *($N_1$-$P_2$) but delays in the late waveform components.  Peak*
           *5 ($N_3$) is flat only on left hemispheric recording.  See*
           *case report Number 2 for clinical details.*

the last waveform component of the left hemisphere but not in the
right hemisphere.  All SER waveform components in this patient were
symmetrical except for the first primary peak component which was
significantly delayed when compared to the right hemispheric peak latency.  The last negative peak was flat (Figure 4).

   *Case Report Number 3.*  Patient is a 26-year old white female who
was admitted for evaluation of recent weakness of the arm and leg
associated with blurred vision bilaterally.  Except for a slight
weakness in the right arm and leg, and a mild decrease in vibratory
sensation, the neurological examination was within normal limits.  The
EEG record showed resting occipital rhythm of 8-10 cycles/sec responsive to eyeopening.  Rare symmetric left-central, frontotemporal
spikes, and sharp activity during drowsiness and sleep was noted.  Lab-

oratory findings were normal. Ophthalmological exam revealed normal visual fields and fundi. There was a slight nystagmus on the right lateral gaze. Reflexes were normal and symmetric, and, except for a slight weakness on the sixth nerve, cranial nerves 2-12 were normal. CSF γ-globulin was 21% of the total protein. A visual evoked response test showed slowing of the latency responses.

Because of the possibility of multiple sclerosis, both the median and peroneal bilateral SER test was done. The results of the median nerve stimulation showed abnormal latency response but symmetric waveform components. Peroneal nerve stimulation showed a symmetry of all waveform components, and a normal primary waveform component, but delays ranging from 30-50 msec outside normal baseline involving the middle and late waveform components recorded over the right and left hemisphere (Figure 5).

*Case Report Number 4.* A 44-year old white female was admitted to the clinic for evaluation of a three-year history of difficulty with walking, particularly in the right leg. The patient's husband related that the patient suffered from short memory deficits accompanied by slurring of speech and occasional myoclonic jerks of the right leg. A neurological examination showed a thin, white female who alternated between laughing and crying. Sensory exam was within normal limits. The cranial nerves were intact from 2 to 12. Motor examination showed increased tone on the right side, with mild increased tone on the left side. There was a question of cogwheeling in the right hand. Ankle clonus was found bilaterally and all reflexes were hyperactive. Hoffmann's sign was positive bilaterally and Babinski was inconclusive. Cerebellar function showed that the patient had finger-to-nose, and heel-to-shin ataxia on the right side and minimally on the left side. The patient had difficulty with quick alternating movements. A computerized tomograph showed the ventricular volume to be normal but the cerebral sulci were abnormally wide particularly over the left parietal lobe. These findings were consistent with mild diffuse cortical atrophy. Ophthalmological examination showed no signs of retrobulbar neuritis. Visual evoked response showed slowing of waveform activity. EMI scan, myelogram and EEG were also normal. VDRL and laboratory findings were non-contributory. There appeared to be progressive ataxia with pyramidal tract and cerebellar dysfunction and on the basis of these findings, a discharge diagnosis of spinocerebellar degeneration of unknown etiology was made.

A bilateral SER following median nerve stimulation showed a slight asymmetric waveform component of the first and second negative peaks. The rest of the waveform components were symmetrical but the middle and late waveform components were found to be progressively delayed on both the left and the right hemispheres. These delays ranged from 33 to 41 msec from normal baselines. Bilateral peroneal nerve stimulation was not done (Figure 6).

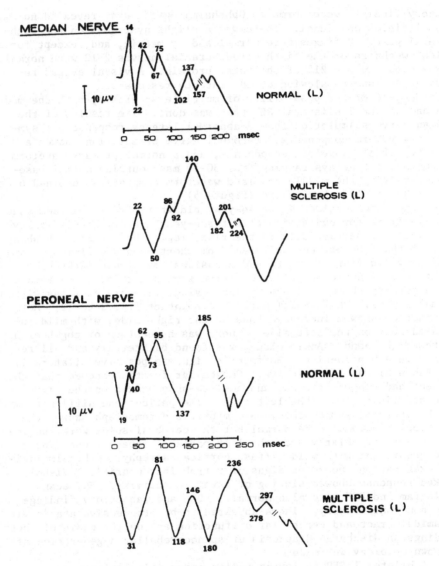

Figure 5.   *Somatosensory evoked response traces following median
(upper figure) and peroneal (lower figure) nerve stimulation in normal subjects and patient with multiple
sclerosis.   All peak latencies are delayed with a range
from 10-60 msec from baseline values.   Note that peroneal
nerve stimulation results in a primary positive peak (P₁)
unlike the primary negative (N₁) potential seen with
median nerve stimulation.   Right hemispheric recording
(not shown) demonstrated a similar SER pattern to the
left side.   See Case Report Number 3 for clinical details.*

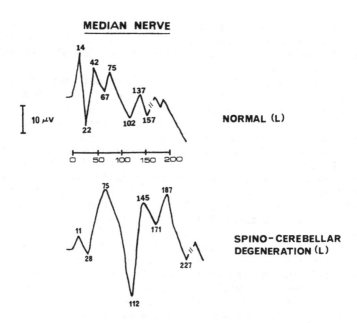

**Figure 6.** *Somatosensory evoked response traces of normal and patient with spino-cerebellar degeneration of unknown etiology (Case Report Number 4). Patient's trace shows that the first and second peaks are within normal limits but it appears that a waveform component (N₂P₂) with average peak latencies of 42 and 67 msec is missing. As a consequence, all subsequent peak latencies in this patient are delayed. The right hemispheric SER response (not shown) showed a small delay in the final (P₄) peak but all the right waveforms were present and had normal latency values.*

## DISCUSSION

It should be emphasized that these case reports are not presented to characterize these various neurological disorders since it is obvious that these investigations are still in the preliminary stages. Additional patients will be required to substantiate whether or not the waveform components seen in these SERs are specific or not. Consequently the cases are presented to slow brain and spinal alterations from normal baselines established in the course of our clinical studies

and simply confirm the fact that abnormalities of the central and
peripheral nervous system may exist.  As such, our impressions of
these SER waveform components must remain speculative until more
data becomes available.

Our studies do show, however, that there are at least three
variables involved in the interpretation and analysis of these waveform components.  These are: a) bilateral symmetry of peaks (including
absence of a specific peak; B) peak-to-peak latencies (as compared to
normal mean peak averages); C) peak amplitude.

Experience with normal subjects has shown us that the SERs recorded bilaterally should result in a right and left hemispheric symmetry
of the peak latencies.  Any differences in such symmetry of the peaks
should be no more than 5 msec of each other and the absence or flattening of a peak in one of the recorded hemispheres constitutes to us
an abnormality of the SER in that hemisphere.  From our established
mean peak latencies, we can classify as abnormal any latency that does
not conform to the established standard deviation pattern (Table 1).
Such latencies can be either faster or slower (delayed) than our control baseline.  Due to the variability of the amplitudes from subject
to subject and even within the same subject, this factor is generally
disregarded when the overall amplitude of the waveforms are analyzed.
However, *specific* amplitude changes of the waveform component that is
not similar or identical to its counterpart in the opposite hemisphere
is considered significant particularly if it is accompanied by a
latency delay outside the normal distribution.

The alterations in latency waveforms seen in the four cases presented are most likely due to local or diffuse damage of the peripheral
and/or central nervous system.

The most difficult SER interpretation is that of *Case Report* Number 1 where *faster* than normal latency delays are observed.  Since the
patient was not taking any medication that we were aware of including
L-dopa for his parkinson symptoms, it can be presumed, although not
totally excluded, that the increase in the latency waveforms is not due
to a pharmacological effect on the central nervous system.  One possibility may be, however, that some central damage has occurred in the
nigro-striatal system, and that such a system may participate or influence caudo-thalamo-cortical transmission or could somehow modulate
the frequency of the final SER recorded over the somatosensory cortex.
If the myelinated fibers, which are presumed to be undamaged, convey
the impulses following peripheral sensory stimulation, the conduction
to the sensory cortex would be expected to be faster especially if a
relay through slower unmyelinated portions of the nigro-striatal system is bypassed.

In discussing *Case Report* Number 2 (Fig. 4), a partial stroke of
the middle cerebral artery can be assumed to affect in part or totally
the parenchymal tissue of the basal ganglia, thalamus and cortex
(*Symon et al, 1974*).  Such damage would explain the delay or modifica-

tion of nerve conduction pulses following peripheral sensory stimulation. Local tissue necrosis could compromise caudo-thalamo-cortical relays on the left hemisphere. It must also be assumed that some right hemispheric involvement exists in view of the fact that SER delays are observed in late waveform components and b) the patient has recently developed tremors on the left arm. The flat negative peak ($N_3$) observed only on the left hemisphere has been noted in four other patients who had contralateral posterior root or cord compression. Flattening of this peak compliments the finding in this patient of a cervical spondylosis with osteophytic compression on the right side of the cord at $C_{5-6}$.

A demyelinating disease such as that described in *Case Report* Number 3 (Fig 5) may be responsible for the general and diffuse delay responses seen in the SER both after median and peroneal nerve stimulation. Because of the disseminating character of multiple sclerosis, such delays can affect *both* cerebral hemispheric recordings (*Namerow, 1968*).

The subtle differences in the right and left symmetry of the waveform responses seen in *Case Report* Number 4 (Fig. 6), and the pronounced peak latency delays seen over both hemispheres, would support a diagnosis of spino-cerebellar degeneration. However, at the present time, there appears to be little distinction between the pattern of these SERs and those where a probably multiple sclerosis has or is developing.

So far, I have taken the liberty of offering you a fishing expedition into an area which is highly controversial and complex. The next decade will see many more experiments, both clinical and experimental in our own and other laboratories, which hopefully will shed more light on this new but exciting field of research. For the moment, we can conclude, however, that the use of somatosensory evoked response testing, especially when coupled with the auditory and visual evoked responses, will become an extremely important ancillary tool in prognosing and possibly diagnosing a number of neuropathological disorders involving movement abnormalities.

## ACKNOWLEDGEMENTS

The author is grateful to Ms. Lydia Johns, Division of Neurosurgery, University of Chicago for the illustrations and artwork in this article. Supported by PHS-2-P01-NS-07376-08.

## REFERENCES

Albe-Fessard, D. and Bowsher, D. (1965). Responses of monkey thalamus to somatic stimuli under chloralase anaesthesia. *Electroenceph. Clin. Neurophysiol. 19*, 1-15.

Allison, T., Goff, W.R., Abrahamian, H.A. and Rosner, B.S. (1962)

*Electroenceph. Clin. Neurophysiol.* (Suppl. 24) 68–75.

Bucy, P.C. (1951). The surgical treatment of extrapyramidal diseases. *J. Neurol. Neurosurg. and Psychiat. 14*, 108–117.

Chandler, W.F. and Crosby, E.C. (1975). Motor effects of stimulation and ablation of the caudate nucleus of the monkey. *Neurology 25*, 1160–1163.

Cools, A.R. (1973). Chemical and electrical stimulation of the caudate nucleus in freely moving cats: the role of dopamine. *Brain Res. 58*, 437–451.

Dawson, G.D. (1947). Cerebral responses to electrical stimulation of peripheral nerve in man. *J. Neurol. Neurosurg. and Psychiat. 10*, 137–140.

de la Torre, J.C. and Trimble, J.L. (1976). *Progr. Abs. Soc. Neurosci. 2* (Part 2), 932. Toronto, Canada.

de la Torre, J.C. (1968). *Med. Hyg.* No. *1477*, 1–16.

DeLong, M.R. (1974). Motor functions of the basal ganglia: single unit activity during movement. In: *The Neurosciences, Third Study Program* (Schmitt, F.O. and Worden, F.G., Eds.) pp. 319–325. MIT Press, Cambridge, Mass.

Denny-Brown, D. (1960). Motor mechanisms – An introduction: the general principles of motor integration. In: *Handbook of Physiology: Neurophysiology*, vol. II. (Field, J., Magoun, H.W. and Hall, V.E., Eds.) pp. 781–796. American Physiological Society, Washington, D.C.

Denny-Brown, D. (1966). The Cerebral Control of Movement. Charles C. Thomas, Springfield, Ill.

Descartes, R. (1662). *De Homine*. Leyden, Moyardus and Leffen, Fol. 118.

Evarts, E.V. (1967). Representation of movements and muscles by pyramidal tract neurons of the precentral motor cortex. In: *Neurophysiological Basis of Normal and Abnormal Motor Activities.* (Yahr, M.D. and Purpura, D.P., Eds.) pp. 215–251. Raven Press, New York

Foreman, D. and Ward, J.W. (1957). Responses to electrical stimulation of caudate nucleus in cats in chronic experiments. *J. Neurophysiol. 20*, 230–244.

Fritsch, G. and Hitzig, E. (1870). Über die elektrische Erregbarkeit des Grosshirns. In: *The Cerebral Cortex* (von Bonin, G., Ed.) pp. 73–96. Charles C. Thomas, Springfield, Ill.

Fukushima, T., Mayanagi, Y. and Bouchard, G. (1976). Thalamic evoked potentials to somatosensory stimulation in man. *Electroenceph. Clin. Neurophysiol. 40*, 481–490.

Giblin, D.R. (1964). Somatosensory evoked potentials in healthy subjects and in patients with lesions of the nervous system. *Ann. N.Y. Acad. Sci. 112*, 93.

Guiot, G., Derome, P., Arfel, G. and Walter, S. (1973). *Progr. Neurol. Surg. 5*, 189–221.

Halliday, A.M. (1967). Changes in the form of cerebral evoked respon-

ses in man associated with various lesions of the nervous
  system. *Electroenceph. Clin. Neurophysiol.* (Suppl. 25) 178-
  192.
Horsley, V. (1909). The function of the so-called motor area of
  the brain. *Brit. Med. J. 2*, 125-132.
Jackson, J.H. (1873). Observations on the localization of movements
  in the cerebral hemispheres, as revealed by cases of convul-
  sion, chorea, and aphasia. In: *Selected Writings of John
  Hughlings Jackson*, I. (Taylor, J., Holmes, G. and Walsche,
  F.M.R., Eds.) pp. 77-89. Basic Books, New York.
Klemme, R.M. (1940). Surgical treatment of dystonia, Chapter XVII.
  *Assoc. Res. Nerv. and Ment. Dis.*, Proc. *21*, 596.
Klüver, H. and Bucy, P.C. (1937). *Amer. J. Physiol. 119*, 352.
Kornhuber, H.H. (1974). Cerebral cortex, cerebellum and basal gang-
  lia: An introduction to their motor functions. In: *The Neuro-
  sciences, Third Study Program* (Schmitt, F.O. and Worden, F.G.,
  Eds.) pp. 267-280. MIT Press, Cambridge, Mass.
Larson, S.J., Sances, A. and Christenson, P.C. (1966). Evoked somat-
  osensory potentials in man. *Arch. Neurol. 15*, 88-93.
Larson, S.J. and Sances, A. (1968). Averaged evoked potentials in
  stereotaxic surgery. *J. Neurosurg. 28*, 227-232.
Lashley, K.S. (1929). *Brain Mechanisms and Intelligence.* Univ. of
  Chicago Press, Chicago, Ill.
Liles, S.L. and Davis, G.D. (1969). Athetoid and chloreiform hyper-
  kinesias produced by caudate lesions in the cat. *Science 164*,
  195-197.
Luria, A.R. (1966). *Higher Cortical Functions in Man.* pp. 23-38.
  Tavistock Publications, London.
Mettler, F.A. (1967). Cortical, subcortical relations in abnormal
  motor functions. In: *Neurophysiological Basis of Normal and
  Abnormal Motor Activities* (Yahr, M.D. and Purpura, D.P., Eds.)
  pp. 445-496. Raven Press, New York.
Meyers, R. (1953). The Extrapyramidal System: An inquiry into the
  validity of the concept. *Neurology 3*, 627-655.
Mountcastle, V.B. (1966). The neural replication of sensory events
  in the somatic afferent system. In: *Brain and Conscious Ex-
  perience* (Eccles, C., Ed.) p. 86. Springer-Verlag, New York.
Namerow, N.S. (1968). Somatosensory evoked responses in multiple
  sclerosis. *Bull. L.A. Neurosurg. Soc. 33*, 74-81.
Penfield, W. and Boldrey, E. (1937). Somatic motor and sensory
  representation in the cerebral cortex of man as studied by
  electrical stimulation. *Brain 60*, 389-443.
Sherrington, C.S. (1906). Integrative Action of the Nervous System.
  Yale Univ. Press. New Haven, Conn.
Symon, L., Pasztor, E. and Branston, N.M. (1974). The distribution
  and density of reduced cerebral blood flow following acute
  middle cerebral artery occlusion: an experimental study by the

technique of hydrogen clearance in baboons. *Stroke 5*, 355-364.

Tissot, R., Gaillard, J.M., Guggisberg, M., Gauthier, G. and de
  Ajuriaguerra, J. (1969). Therapeutique du syndrome de Parkinson
  par la L-Dopa "per os" associée à un inhibiteur de la décarboxy-
  lase. *Presse Med. 77*, 619-622.

Tsumoto, T., Nonaka, S., Hirose, N. and Takahashi, M. (1972). Analysis of somatosensory evoked potentials to lateral popliteal nerve
  stimulation in man. *Electroenceoph. Clin. Neurophysiol 33*, 379-
  388.

Twitchell, T.E. (1965). Attitudinal reflexes. *J. Amer. Phys. Ther.
  Asso. 45*, 414.

Willis, T. (1664). *Cerebri Anatome*. Marlyn and Allestry, London.

Yu, M.K., Wright, T.L., Dettbarn, W.D. and Olson, W.H. (1974).
  Pargyline-induced myopathy with histochemical characteristics
  of Duchenne muscular dystrophy. *Neurology 24*, 237-244.

# PROBLEMS IN THE TREATMENT OF PARKINSONISM

ROGER C. DUVOISIN, M.D.

Department of Neurology
The Mount Sinai School of Medicine
The City University of New York
New York, New York 10029

## ABSTRACT

The progress achieved in our understanding of parkinsonism and
its treatment in the last decade has greatly improved the lot of
our patients but has also brought new sets of problems.  The very
effectiveness of levodopa therapy has modified the clinical spectrum
of symptomatology.  By suppressing tremor and rigidity and prolonging our patients' lives, we have uncovered other manifestations of
parkinsonism which were previously less prominent.  The greater
specificity of levodopa has rendered precise diagnosis more important, but at the same time the recognition of new entities has
changed the nosology of parkinsonism.  Although the diagnosis of
extrapyramidal disorders depends almost exclusively on clinical
observation, new diagnostic tools are beginning to alter the character of neurology and promise to have a significant impact on the
clinical evaluation of patients with basal ganglia diseases.

Our better understanding of the *modus operandi* of various
drugs used in treating extrapyramidal disorders has in some ways
complicated the physician's task.  In place of the simple empiricism
that prevailed a decade ago, there is now a body of knowledge and
theory which one must appreciate to obtain optimal therapeutic
results.

The remarkable relief of Parkinsonian symptomatology possible
in some patients has thrown into relief cases of treatment failure
and placed additional emphasis on manifestations of parkinsonism
which are either unresponsive to therapy or are actually exacer-

bated by it.  Finally, the diagnosis and management of intercurrent
illnesses in Parkinson patients on levodopa therapy has presented
additional new problems to the clinician.

## INTRODUCTION

The problems encountered in managing a chronic progressive
disease such as Parkinson's disease, whose progress extends over a
period of many years, are manifold, covering nearly the entire
range of clinical medicine.  It is only possible to point out here
some of the more common difficulties encountered in the diagnosis
and treatment of parkinsonism.

The first problem, of course, and one not to be minimized,
is that of recognizing parkinsonism in its initial symptomatic
phases and differentiating it from other disorders which it may
resemble.  It is also important to classify the type of parkinsonism to assess prognosis and reasonably estimate therapeutic possibilities.

The rationale and general principles of drug therapy in parkinsonism are now well understood and need not be detailed here.  However, the side effects and limitations of anticholinergic and levodopa therapy require consideration for they are encountered in
nearly all patients.  Success in therapy depends to a considerable
extent on the effective management of the various side effects,
the symptoms which are not responsive to current treatment and
those which may be exacerbated.  Finally, there are patients who
fail to respond to treatment or fail rapidly after a good initial
response.  They have come to represent an important problem in
clinical neurology.

The autonomic manifestations of Parkinson's disease merit special attention.  Although they are usually given scant consideration,
they are ubiquitous among parkinson patients and may on occasion
give rise to serious difficulties.  Other features of Parkinson's
disease such as behavioural changes, dementia, visual dysfunctions,
etc. which were generally overlooked prior to the levodopa era have
now become more prominent, probably due to the major impact of levodopa on the motor symptoms as well as on the patients' longevity.

## DIAGNOSIS

In the absence of chemical markers or pathognomonic signs, the
diagnosis of Parkinson's disease depends primarily on clinical
observation and therefore on clinical skill and experience.  Its
difficulty, especially in early phases of the disease, should not
be underestimated.  Because much of the early symptomatology lies
outside awareness, the patients' complaints often seem unrelated
to objective findings on examination.  The insidious onset and
slow progression make it difficult to obtain a clear chronological

history. As James Parkinson noted, "it rarely happens that the patient can form any recollection of the precise period of its commencement". Moreover, there is a marked pleomorphism in the symptomatology.

Although in retrospective histories, tremor is usually given as the initial symptom, in fact, many if not most patients have consulted their physicians some months or even one or more years before its advent with complaints of fatigue, weakness, restlessness, loss of dexterity or other general symptoms. These early symptoms, which might be termed prodromal, are often regarded as due to minor musculoskeletal disorders and treated with analgesics, various physical modalities and reassurance. The symptoms usually persist and when repeated laboratory examination and laboratory studies are normal, one is apt to consider the complaints to be "functional". The patients may indeed become depressed in this phase of apparently inexplicable difficulties and many are treated with tranquilizers and with antidepressant drugs. Depression usually responds well enough to appropriate therapy but the somatic complaints persist. Eventually, the telltale tremor or some other manifestation becomes apparent and the diagnosis is then obvious to all concerned.

If the patient has been on neuroleptic therapy, the question will arise whether the parkinsonism is iatrogenic. The only certain recourse is to withdraw the neuroleptic agent and observe the patient for a period of time. The iatrogenic syndrome should subside within a few weeks, whereas Parkinson's disease will persist. Subclinical Parkinson's disease may become overt during a period of neuroleptic therapy and apparently subside when the neuroleptic drug is stopped only to gradually re-emerge in the course of the following year or two. Such a sequence of events may also occur in hypertensive patients treated with reserpine or alphamethyldopa (Duvoisin, 1975). Care should be taken to properly explain these phenomena to the patient and his family for some are apt to harbor a lingering suspicion that their disease was caused by the neuroleptic agent.

In addition to the common prodromal phase of vague symptomatology during which proper recognition of the patient's real problem may be difficult, there are several frankly misleading presentations which merit specific comment. Bradykinesia occurring as the predominant clinical feature may be confused for hypothyroidism or the psychomotor retardation of depression. The patients are unaware of their bradykinesia until it is quite prominent and interferes with their lives. They then experience it as fatigue, weakness or simply as a loss of motor skills. When bradykinesia appears unilaterally, the differential diagnosis from a mild hemiparesis may prove troublesome as was recently noted by Gilbert (1976). The patient may be thought to have had a "stroke" or to have a brain tumor and invasive diagnostic procedures may be undertaken. Unilateral facial hypomimia, not uncommon in such patients, may mimic a central facial

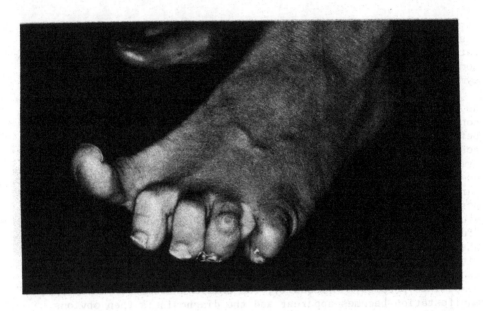

*Figure 1. "Striatal Toe" in case of Parkinson's disease, simulating Parkinson's disease.*

paresis.  The finding of a dorsiflexed first toe simulating a Babinski sign on the affected side may further complicate the probelm.  This "striatal toe" (Figure 1) has not been generally recognized, yet is is a common finding in Parkinsonian patients.  It also occurs in athetosis *(Denny-Brown, 1966)*, in dystonia musculorum deformans and other extrapyramidal diseases.  It may usually be differentiated from the Babinski sign (the "pyramidal toe") by observing a normal flexor response to plantar stimulation, however, in some cases the flexor response may still leave the toe dorsiflexed and one will remain suspicious of a pyramidal tract lesion. Observation of the patient's posture may help arouse suspicion that one is dealing with hemiparkinsonism rather than hemiparesis. In the latter, there is often a mild scoliosis which is usually concave ipsilaterally to the neurological deficit.  In contrast, in hemiparkinsonism, the scoliosis is concave contraleterally *(Duviosin & Marsden, 1975)* (Figure 2).

Another misleading presentation is characterized by painful cramps in the foot and sometimes the calf *(Duvoisin, Yahr, & Lieberman, 1972)*.  With cramp, the toes are flexed, though in some cases the first toe is dorsiflexed, sometimes to a remarkable degree.  The cramps are usually precipitated by walking which may suggest intermittent claudication and lead to treatment with peripheral vasodilators.  They may also occur at night as a form of nocturnal cramp.  Treatment with quinine may sometimes be helpful.

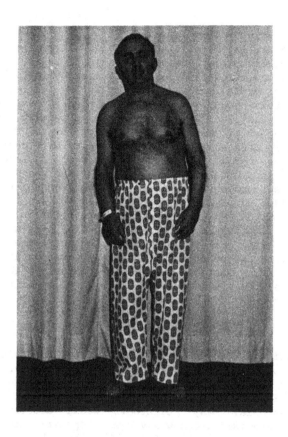

*Figure 2. Scoliosis in case of left hemiparkinsonism; patient leans away from side of parkinsonism symptoms.*

The thermal paresthesiase of Parkinson's disease, originally described by Charcot *(1871)* may sometimes be the initial symptoms. The patient complains of an unpleasant burning sensation affecting a large body area - a limb, the mouth and tongue, the perineal region or the entire body. Patients presenting this complaint in the extremities may be suspected of having peripheral vascular disease. Treatment with vasodilator drugs may be attempted but is usually ineffective. In one case which I observed, a lumbar sympathectomy was performed; it failed to provide relief of the symptom. It was only three years later that tremor developed and the clinical diagnosis of Parkinson's disease became apparent. A review of the tissue removed at surgery in this case revealed the presence of Lewy bodies in some neurones of the lumbar sympathetic chain *(Stadlan, Duvoisin, & Yahr, 1966)*.

A less common early symptom may be edema.  Edema of one or
both lower limbs in parkinsonism is not unusual.  It may suggest
congestive heart failure or be ascribed to varicose veins.  Its
genesis is unknown, but it seems plausible to ascribe it to hypo-
stasis, especially since it improves, often markedly, on levodopa
therapy.  However, this phenomenon occurred in an upper extremity
in a personally observed case.  The patient presented with marked
edema of the right upper extremity.  Occlusion of the veins drain-
ing the limb was suspected and angiographic studies were carried
out.  The vessels were normal.  It was only after the passage of
time that it became apparent that Parkinson's disease was developing.  This patient subsequently responded well to levodopa therapy
and the edema subsided completely.

Still another misleading early symptom is anterior chest pain
which may be confused for angina pectoris of cardiac origin.
Patients presenting this complaint have often received extensive
cardiac investigations and treatment with coronary vasodilators
with uncertain results.  Eventually, when progressive symptomatology
renders it clear that the patient has Parkinson's disease it is
found that the chest pains disappear with levodopa therapy.

## DIFFERENTIAL DIAGNOSIS

Once Parkinsonism is suspected, there remains the problem of
differential diagnosis: that is, of differentiating disorders which
may resemble it and then of classifying the type of parkinsonism.
Increased interest in parkinsonism over the past decade has resulted
in more precise diagnosis.  Many patients who would formerly have
been labelled "parkinsonism" are now given more specific diagnoses.
Some of these diagnoses represent entities which have been recognized
only in recent years;others were known but were frequently identified
only postmortem.

Perhaps the disorder most commonly mistaken for Parkinson's
disease is Benign Essential Tremor.  Although typically, the hand
tremor is usually postural in that condition in contrast to the
resting tremor of Parkinson's disease; in practice, there is
considerable variability in the morphology of these tremors.  The
unwary clinician may be misled by the fact that the tremor may be
felt as a cogwheel effect.  Attention should be paid not to the
cogwheel phenomenon itself but to the quality of muscle tone; it
is usually normal or "hypotonic" in essential tremor whereas a
plastic rigidity characterizes Parkinson's disease without a cogwheel effect.  This error will be avoided if one is careful to
diagnose parkinsonism only when all three cardinal elements -
tremor, rigidity and akinesia - are present.

Classifying the patient with regard to the type of parkinsonism is not always an easy task at a time when concepts are changing.

Barely more than a decade ago, parkinsonism was usually

divided into three main types: Postencephalitic, arteriosclerotic
and idiopathic.  The last named type was considered to be more or
less the disease described by James Parkinson in his essay on the
shaking palsy *(1817):* i.e. Parkinson's disease or paralysis agitans.
Then a large variety of extrapyramidal dysfunctions were loosely
included under the rubric of parkinsonism including CO and Mn intoxication and post-traumatic syndromes.  To many, it seemed that
parkinsonism was merely a syndrome of multiple etiology without a
consistent pathology.

        Parkinsonism is now considered a pathophysiologic state reflec-
ting primarily a dysfunction of the nigro-neostriatal dopaminergic
neuronal system.  Although it must be recognized that this view
ignores involvement of other important brain structures commonly
found in Parkinson's disease, e.g. the locus coeruleus, it has
served as a useful unifying concept.  We can thus recognize that a
number of diseases, principally neuronal system degenerations, can
involve the substantia nigra as part of a more widespread multi-
system degenerative process.  The variability from case to case in
these disorders makes a clinical differentiation very difficult
for a satisfactory diagnosis cannot always be made on clinical
grounds.  Finally, it must be recognized that a number of disorders
may mimic Parkinson's disease which do not directly involve the
nigro-striatal dopaminergic systems.

        The concept or arteriosclerotic parkinsonism has been largely
abandoned and postencephalitic parkinsonism has now virtually
disappeared.  The great bulk of parkinson patients presently seen
in practice are classifed as Parkinson's disease.  This entity, now
sharply defined in both its clinical and morphologic features,
serves as the point of departure for current classifications.  It
is the prototypic form of parkinsonism, the essential or primary
parkinsonism.  However, it must be recognized that certain cases
which from their pathology must surely be due to a different etiology, may be clinically indistinguishable from Parkinson's disease,
for several years or more in the course of their evolution.  These
include striato-nigral degeneration, progressive supranuclear palsy
and in some cases, olivo-ponto cerebellar degeneration.  In our
present ignorance of the etiology of these neuronal-system degenerations, nosology must remain uncertain and some cases will be difficult to classify, appearing to bridge the gaps between them.  It
has been suggested that failure of response to levodopa therapy
in a somewhat atypical primarily bradykinetic syndrome may suggest
the ante-mortem diagnosis of striato-nigral degeneration *(Rajput
et al., 1972).*  A pneumoencephalographic demonstration of putaminal
atrophy may support this suspicion.  Similarly, demonstration of
an enlarged fourth ventricle and atrophy of the pons in contrast
studies may suggest an olivo-ponto cerebellar atrophy.  The meager
therapeutic benefits derived make one hesitant to perfrom invasive
contrast studies in these patients.  Computerized axial tomography
offers promise of being helpful in these circumstances.  Experience

is still too limited to offer definite guidelines.  It is likely,
however, that the next few years will see numerous efforts to
analyze basal ganglia diseases by this new diagnostic technique.
    More recently, arteriosclerotic parkinsonism *(Parkes, et al,
1974)* has been the subject of renewed interest.  The resemblance of
patients with bilateral cerebral vascular disease, i.e. Marie's
lacunar state, to Parkinson's disease has long been recognized.
The term "arteriosclerotic parkinsonism" was applied to these
cases *(Critchley, 1929)* at a time when the concept of parkinsonism
had broadened widely in the wake of encephalitis lethargica.
Critchley's detailed description of the clinical features (summarized
in Table 1) would seem to render the differentiation of this condition from Parkinson's disease rather unlikely.  However, in practice
it must be admitted that at least in some cases it may be very difficult.

*TABLE 1.  CLINICAL FEATURES DIFFERENTIATING ARTERIOSCLEROTIC
          PARKINSONISM FROM PARKINSON'S DISEASE (FROM CRITCHLEY,
          1929)*

---

onset usually over 70
tremor uncommon
Gegenhalten instead of rigidity
dysarthric speech
more rapid course, stepwise progression
facial expression preserved, frontalis overactive
pseudobulbar dysarthria
pyramidal signs
cerebellar signs
dementia more common
gait apractic, armswing preserved
spasticity
pallilalia.

---

    The pathophysiologic disorder characterized as gait apraxia is
unrelated to dopaminergic dysfunction.  It is a manifestation of
frontal lobe disease and may be found in association with arterio-
sclerosic lesions, tumors, degenerative disease and the ill-defined
syndrome of low pressure hydrocephalus.  Gait apraxia itself, is a
poorly understood clinical entity.  It is often described as frontal
lobe ataxia *(Meyers & Barron, 1970)*.  The gait disturbance is sug-
gestive of parkinsonism.  This appears to be the nature of the
gait disturabnce in "arteriosclerotic parkinsonism".  It does not
appear to be responsive to any therapeutic modality.

SELECTING TREATMENT

Having made a diagnosis of parkinsonism or even more specifically, of Parkinson's disease, the clinician must now decide on a
therapeutic approach.  There is some disagreement as to which drug
to use initially.  If levodopa were curative or arrested the progression of the neuronal degeneration, then one would be obliged to
institute levodopa therapy as soon as the diagnosis is made.  But,
levodopa is only a symptomatic palliative therapy.  Thus some argue
that it should be reserved for use later on in the course of the
illness after the less effective agents have been tried.  Others
feel that only the best drug available should be used first, adding
adjunctive drugs later in an attempt to supplement the dopa effect
when an optimal dosage has been attained.  The former fear that
levodopa therapy may have some long term chronicity but, on the
other hand, the toxicity of the central anticholinergic agents is
also considerable.  It is impossible to resolve this controversy
with a general rule applicable to all cases.  Each patient must be
evaluated individually, taking into account the entire medical
situation, previous drug experience and the side effects of the drug
under consideration.

Any drug possessing some central anticholinergic properties
will have some mild anti-parkinson effect.  The therapeutic effect,
however, is relatively limited and is not so marked in early as in
more advanced cases.  Moreover, some degree of anticholinergic
intoxication must usually be accepted as the price of that limited
benefit.  The toxic mental effects in particular, can be significant.
Although often overlooked in retired or elderly individuals and
ascribed erroneously to senility or dementia, they are in fact
rather common.  In surveys carried out before the advant of levodopa therapy, significant disturbances requiring reduction of dosage or withdrawal of anticholinergic agents were found to occur in
about 20% of patients (Duvoisin & Yahr, 1972).  Less severe mental
changes, notably impairment of recent memory, occur more frequently.
There is a striking age correlation, adverse mental changes being
much more common in older patients.  One would thus hesitate to
start treatment with an anticholinergic agent in a patient over
65 years of age, especially if the patient is still actively
employed or already has some evidence of organic mental changes.

Although the antiparkinson action of amantadine is believed
to be due to enhancement of dopaminergic function, from a clinical
standpoint, it rather resembles the anticholinergic agents in its
side effects and in the limited nature of its therapeutic benefits.
The occurrence of livido reticularis and edema of the lower extremities has not so far been a major problem.  However, the edema
can sometimes be very marked and both the patient and the physician
may understandably have some anxiety about this phenomenon.  Though
no serious effects have been reported, one is usually tempted to

withdraw the drug in such cases.  A disturbing feature is that a
surprisingly long time, sometimes several months, may be required
for the edema and the livido reticularis to subside.

The limitations of levodopa therapy have become a major problem especially in view of the high expectations patients commonly
hold for good results and when initially excellent results are
marred by the subsequent appearance of dyskinesias, the "on-off"
effect, behavioral disturbances and other side effects.  These
limitations reflect the fact that our treatment essentially consists
of modifying the clinical expression of a progressing pathophysiologic state with a pharmacological agent which in turn induces another
abnormal state.  The goal of treatment is to balance the two to the
patient's maximal benefit.

LEVODOPA

Levodopa therapy is most conveniently undertaken today with a
combination of levodopa and a dopadecarboxylase inhibitor such as
Sinemet® (levodopa plus carbidopa) or Madopar® (levodopa plus bensari-
zide).  The combination has the great advantage of largely elimina-
ting the nausea and vomiting which are so common during the initial
phases of treatment with levodopa alone.  Thus a full therapeutic
response can be obtained in several days, rather than in several
months.  Normally, a new patient may be started on the 10/100mg
tablet of carbidopa/levodopa three times daily and observed.  In
hospital, the dosage can be increased every day or two until a
satisfactory response is obtained.  In outpatient practice, the
dose may be increased at weekly intervals.

Nausea, even vomiting may still occur in some patients.  The
10mg dose of carbidopa in the small combination tablet is not
sufficient to protect all patients from the central emetic effect
of levodopa.  The problem may be managed with the same measures
which were found useful in treatment based on levodopa alone.  That
is, care is taken to assure that the patients take the drug after
food, preferably solid food containing some protein, and, if the
patient was on treatment with an anticholinergic agent such as
trihexyphenidyl, it is continued.  Additionally, anti-emetics may
be given concurrently with each dose of levodopa or at least with
the first dose of the day.  The phenothiazine derivatives such as
prochlorperazine (Compazine) cannot be used for this purpose
because they will block dopamine receptors in the striatum as well
as in the vomiting center and thus block the desired therapeutic
effect as well as the emetic effect of levodopa.  Diphenidol (Von-
trol®), (Duvoisin, 1969) an analogue of trihexyphenidyl is preferred.
Trimethobromide (Tigan®) has also been useful.  If the patient can
tolerate the large tablet of Sinemet® containing 25mg carbidopa and
250mg levodopa, the nausea and vomiting may abruptly stop.  The
reason is that the larger dose of carbidopa can more effectively

block the decarboxylation of levodopa to dopamine in the medullary
vomiting center.

The next major problem to appear is the occurence of dyskinesias.
These usually appeared after a month or more of treatment with
levodopa alone but with Sinemet® therapy develop much earlier, often
as soon as the full therapeutic dosage is reached in the first few
days of treatment.

The dyskinesias reflect not only the drug and its efficacy
but the pathologic substate upon which it acts.  Put another way,
the dyskinesias appear to be an expression of Parkinson's disease
which is not usually evident unless revealed by levodopa treatment.
Dyskinesias can be produced by other agents including anticholinergic drugs, amphetamines, dopamine receptor agonists, etc.  No means
of blocking the genesis of the involuntary movements while preserving
the desired relief of the parkinsonian state has yet been developed.
In cases of post-encephalitic parkinsonism patients who already have
some dyskinesia in addition to parkinsonism before commencing levodopa therapy, the dyskinesias are usually exacerbated and often
preclude a satisfactory therapeutic result.  Occasionally, one still
sees a patient who has some mild athetosis or dystonia persisting in
one limb as a complication of stereotaxic thalamotomy.  In these
cases, the dyskinesia may be markedly exacerbated by levodopa and
may also preclude a satisfactory result.  Unfortunately, tolerance
does not develop and the only recourse when dyskinesia is excessive,
is to lower the dosage of levodopa.  Some degree of dyskinesia will
usually have to be accepted and may be seen in up to 80% of patients
in chronic treatment.  Patients usually do not mind mild dyskinesia,
preferring the involuntary movements to being parkinsonian.  The
patient's spouse and family however may be alarmed by the involuntary movements.  Careful explanation of their significance should
be made to the patient and the family before beginning treatment to
avoid such distress.

The "on-off" effect occurs in approximately 15-20% of patients
on chronic treatment.  It is more frequent in patients whose disease
is of longer duration and can be observed to increase gradually
year by year as the underlying disease progresses.  The therapeutic
response is not maintained through the day but lasts only one or
two hours after each dose then decays rapidly, sometimes abruptly,
before the next dose takes effect.  The patient may vary from periods of profound akinesia to periods of near normal mobility which,
however, are usually marked by choreiform dyskinesia.  This variability, often unpredictable, is an important cause of distress and
disability in itself.  The physician's only recourse is to decrease
the interval between doses, adjusting the size of individual doses
to the patient's response and adding an adjunctive drug to maximal
tolerated dosages.

There remain a number of unresolved questions regarding the
chronic toxicity of levodopa.  It was noted early in the initial

trials of levodopa that a slight anemia developed in the initial
months of treatment which appeared to diminish with the passage
of time. Several cases of autoimmune hemolytic anemia developing
on chronic levodopa treatment have now been described. *(Joseph,
1972; Territo, Peters & Tanaka, 1973; Wanamaker et al; 1976)* and
a mechanism similar to that observed in the rare hemolytic anemia
complicating methyldopa therapy has been postulated. In addition,
a number of patients are found to have a mild chronic normocytic
anemia with values ranging from 9-11 grams of hemoglobin. Data
presently available indicate a reduction of total blood mass and
mild hypovolemia. The significance of this finding or its extent
are not yet known. Clearly it is deserving of further study. It
was also noted in the initial studies with L-dopa by Cotzias
*et al (1967)* that a transient neutropenia occurred in the first
few weeks of treatment. This also occurs with pure L-dopa *(Yahr,
Duvoisin, Schear, et al., 1969)* and may still be observed in about
8-9% of patients. The significance of this phenomenon remains
uncertain, but so far serious neutropenias have been observed so
rarely that a casual relationship is uncertain. However, from 8
to 10% of patients develop a positive Coombs test, an incidence
similar to that occurring in hypertensive patients on chronic
methyldopa (Aldomet®) therapy *(Joseph, 1972; Henry et al., 1971)*.

There has also been some concern that chronic levodopa therapy
might be responsible for an apparent increase in the incidence of
dementia in our patients *(Wolf, Davis, 1973)*. The alternate
explanation favored by most clinicians is that the improvements in
motor function brought about by levodopa therapy and the prolongation of the patients' lives has brought into a relief a feature
of Parkinson's disease which was previously less apparent. That
diffuse cortical degeneration is part of the pathology of Parkinson's disease has been suggested both from pneumoencephalographic
studies *(Selby, 1968)* and post-mortem data *(Forno & Alvord, 1972)*.
The CT scan has made it possible to pursue this problem more
readily. Our preliminary experience would confirm the impression that significant cerebral atrophy is more frequent than would
normally be expected. An example may be seen in Figure 3.

It has been suggested that levodopa may stimulate the growth of
malignant melanomas and that Levodopa therapy should be withheld from
patients who have had a mole excised which proved to be malignant on
histological examination *(Skibba et al., 1972)*. The number of cases
described are too small to warrant a conclusion, but in view of this
possibility, it may be prudent to delay initiating levodopa therapy
until 1 or 2 years have elapsed.

The risks of levodopa therapy in patients with active cardiac
disease have not yet been fully explored. However, this is a complex problem. One would expect some risk for a patient with ischemic
heart disease on theoretical grounds. The occurrence of tachycardia
in Parkinson patients on L-dopa therapy and the lowering of blood
pressure naturally pose some risk. Also, improved motility resul-

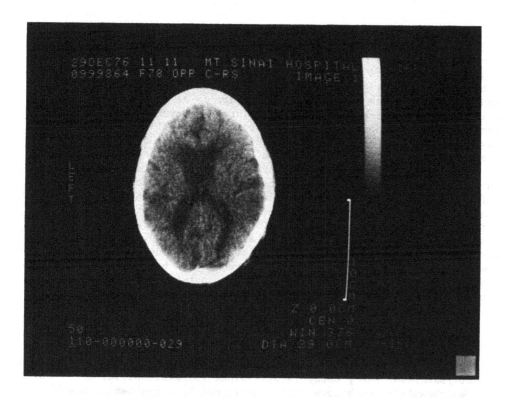

*Figure 3. CT scan in case of Parkinsonism with dementia and severe cerebral atrophy. Note large sulci and ventricles.*

ting from levodopa may make it possible for a previously akinetic patient to place more demands on his heart. The cardiac disease may thus be indirectly exacerbated. Consequently, levodopa should be used cautiously in the presence of ongoing heart disease. Patients subject to paroxysmal tachycardia may be placed on an anti-arrhythmic agent prior to beginning therapy.

LEVODOPA FAILURE

In view of the appreciable symptomatic relief provided by levodopa to most patients with Parkinson's disease, a failure of response is disappointing. A number of causes for such failure may be recognized. Leaving aside those patients in whom dose-related side effects have precluded an effective dosage there remains a small but significant group of patients who fail to respond at all to adequate dosage of levodopa alone or in combination with a peripheral decarboxylase inhibitor.

Complete failure of response to levodopa with no side effects
and no therapeutic benefit presents a serious challenge. The first
question is what is the diagnosis? Patients with striato-nigral
degeneration respond poorly if at all. If the incidence of this
entity is as high as 8-10% of patients classified as having Parkinson's disease as has been suggested (*Takei, 1973*) then this may
well be a major cause of treatment failure. However, it must be
admitted that some patients who fail to respond well to levodopa
have been found to have Parkinson's disease on post-mortem examination. Unfortunately, no alternative therapy appears to be available
in these cases. The diagnosis of striato-nigral degeneration can be
suspected on clinical grounds but cannot be made with certainty in
life. Some patients with progressive supranuclear palsy may initially respond well to levodopa; such a patient was included in
our original trial of levodopa in 1968 (*Yahr et al., 1969*). There
was a good initial response but a subsequent decline with the
development of other symptoms typical of that disorder. Similarly
some cases of olivo-ponto cerebellar degeneration have shown a good
response of their parkinsonian features but not of their ataxia or
other manifestations. The therapeutic benefit therefore is limited
in such cases. Patients with arteriosclerotic Parkinsonism usually
respond very poorly and as noted, cases of gait apraxia of whatever
etiology are also unresponsive.

Several iatrogenic causes of levodopa failure have been described. One of the first was the pyridoxine reversal of the L-dopa
effect (*Duvoisin, Yahr, Cote, 1970*). Since the availability of
the decarboxylase inhibitors, this should not be a problem although
the amount of carbidopa in the combination tablet presently available may not fully protect the patient from the pyridoxine reversal
especially when the dosage of the inhibitor is low and the pyridoxine is administered in large amounts. Dopamine receptor blocking
agents such as chlorpomazine, trifluoperazine, haloperidol, etc.
which may have been given to combat the emetic effect of levodopa has
also been responsible for some treatment failures. More recently,
papaverine (*Duvoisin, 1975*) has been identified as another commonly
used drug which can antagonize the levodopa effect.

A late failure of response to levodopa in a patient who had
previously done well may reflect the progression of the underlying
disease, especially cases of multiple system degeneration such as
olivo-ponto cerebellar degeneration or progressive supranuclear
palsy. These disorders generally progress more rapidly than
Parkinson's disease and the patients soon develop additional features such as ataxia, dystonia or dementia which are not responsive.
Late failure of response however, particularly if acute, should
suggest an intercurrent illness. An unexpectedly rapid decline in
the patient's status may be the first hint of a malignancy or of
other serious systemic disease. Thus a full evaluation of the
patient is indicated.

UNRESPONSIVE SYMPTOMS

There are a number of *bona fide* manifestations of Parkinson's disease which may not respond to levodopa therapy. Indeed, there are some which appear to be exacerbated, at least some of the time in some patients. One of the more common and distressing is the thermal paresthesia described above. It may be experienced as a coldness of a body part or a feeling of heat. Patients describe it as a "fire" when it is severe. The response to levodopa treatment is variable. In many cases it is reduced though usually not fully abolished. However in others, it is increased, diminishing when levodopa is withdrawn. In patients with the "on-off" effect, recurrent thermal paresthesia may herald the beginning of the "off" phase. No countermeasure appears to be consistently effective. Cyproheptadine, in doses of 2-4mg two or three times daily have relieved the symptoms in some patients. However, in the full dose of 4mg three or four times daily, this drug may mildly exacerbate the Parkinsonian state and thus care is required in titrating the dose.

Dysphagia is a frequent but usually manageable manifestation of Parkinson's disease. The pooling of saliva in the mouth and drooling reflects a disturbance in swallowing. Cinefluoroscopy regularly reveals cricopharyngeal achalasia *(Palmer, 1974)*. The patient reports that food simply won't go down. It seems to "get stuck" in the throat. The ultimate result is aspiration with chronic bronchitis and aspiration pneumonia. The patient eats slowly or not at all and begins to lose weight. There is some improvement on treatment with levodopa or with anticholinergic agents. The dysphagia is most severe in post-encephalitic patients and here, the response to anticholinergics can be dramatic. It is my impression that anticholinergics are more helpful than levodopa in controlling this symptom. However, the therapeutic response is insufficient in some patients and serious complications may ensue. Posterior cricopharyngeal sphincterotomy has been advocated by Palmer *(1974)* in this situation. If this cannot be done or fails to help, the patient may have to be fed by nasogastric tube or through a feeding gastrotomy.

Severe constipation is a very familiar complication of Parkinsonism. It is aggravated by anticholinergic drugs, amantadine and, to a lesser extent, by levodopa. Thus patients become regular users of various laxatives. Hydrophilic colloids and lubricants are preferable. Many patients, however, will require frequent enemas. When the dysfunction is severe, megacolon reminiscent of Hirschsprung's disease may develop. Volvulus and intestinal obstruction may develop and require appropriate surgery *(Caplan, Jacobson, & Rubinstein, et al., 1965)*.

Urinary tract dysfunctions are also a familiar problem in Parkinsonism. Urinary hesitancy, incomplete emptying and urge incontin-

ence are the usual manifestations. Cystometric studies may show a
hypotonic bladder or an uninhibited neurogenic bladder (Murnaghan,
1961). Prostatic obstruction in the male may complicate the situation. Again, the anticholinergic agents, amantadine and to a
lesser extent levodopa, may exacerbate the dysfunction. Occasional
individuals may require catheterization for transient episodes of
urinary retention. In more advanced stages of the disease, incon-
tinence may become a nursing problem particularly in those confined
to bed and chair.

INVOLUNTARY EYECLOSURE

A curious manifestation of Parkinson's disease and post-encephalitic parkinsonism which has not been extensively described is the
occurrence of involuntary eyeclosure. The patients may have to
manually lift their lids and in some extreme cases ophthalmic
surgeons have sutured the upper lids in an elevated position.
No drug therapy appears to benefit this unusual symptom. However,
it may be markedly exacerbated or appear for the first time after
evodopa therapy is begun. Several patients in my experience have
been unable to tolerate levodopa at all despite substantial benefit
in other respects because of continuous involuntary eyeclosure.

DEMENTIA AND PEDUNCULAR HALLUCINOSIS

James Parkinson had stated in his essay on the shaking palsy
(1817) that the intellect and senses were spared. It has generally
been held that intellectual decline is not an essential feature of
Parkinson's disease. It has become increasingly apparent with closer
study of large numbers of patients however that an organic dementia
is indeed a manifestation of Parkinson's disease as well as of
related multi-system degenerations with Parkinsonian features.
As noted above, it is becoming clear that a cortical degeneration
is a part of the pathology of these disorders. It is against this
background of an insidiously developing and progressive chronic
brain syndrome that drug psychotoxicity should be considered. The
first manifestation of this cortical deterioration may be an episode of confusion or visual hallucinations which disappear or markedly diminish when the drug dosage is reduced. There is a remarkable
consistency from patient to patient in the character of the visual
hallucinations. They are typical of peduncular hallucinosis, consisting of complex visual hallucinations which the patient may frequently recognize as unreal. A common hallucination is the vision
of numerous people milling about the house or room who appear to
the patient to be going about their business. They may seem to be
the same people day in and day out for long periods of time. The
patients can often describe in some detail entire families of such
imaginary persons. Sometimes they are confused with people on the

television screen.  The patient's family may first become aware of
this phenomenon when the patient reacts to these hallucinations.
Such reaction may often have a paranoid coloration which may produce
disputes with family members.

The anticholinergic agents are much more prone to precipitate
these phenomena.  In patients on multiple drug treatment, it is
best to begin by removing the adjunctive agents, continuing the levodopa as before pending further observation.  Other psychoactive
drugs including sleep medications, antihistiminic agents and tranquilizers should be avoided.  Neuroleptic agents such as chloroma-
zine are apt to exacerbate the hallucinations, probably due to
their central anticholinergic properties.  In more severe instances,
the hallucinations will continue after all other medications have
been discontinued.  It may then be necessary to reduce the dosage
of L-dopa.  It is possible to closely titrate the dosage of levodopa
in such cases against this toxic psychic manifestations.  Some degree of psychotoxicity may have to be accepted ultimately as the
unavoidable price for essential therapeutic benefit derived from
levodopa.

The progressive nature of the intellectual deterioration and
propensity to develop drug-induced psychotic manifestations is evident on following a given patient over a period of years.  For
example, a patient may develop psychotoxicity on therapeutic doses
of an anticholinergic agent which subsides on withdrawal of the
drug leaving him free of any mental manifestations for a period of
years.  The patient may then again develop psychotoxicity on levodopa therapy which again subsides when the dosage is diminished.
Then several years later, the toxicity will again become a problem
and persist even in the absence of any drug treatment whatever.  It
should be noted that hallucinations may require several weeks to
completely subside following withdrawal of the offending agent.

VISUAL DYSFUNCTIONS

The disturbances in vision and visual perception which occur in
Parkinson's disease are poorly understood.  Many patients complain of
difficulty reading or impairment of vision yet tests of visual acuity
appear to be normal and no visual field defects can be demonstrated.
One problem appears to be ocular latero-pulsion and festination.
Patients have difficulty tracking a line of print and finding the
beginning of the next line.  Paresis of accommodation by anticholinergic drugs is also a factor.  In this case blurring of vision
fluctuates during the day as the drug effect waxes and wanes.
Diplopia due to oculomotor disturbance is also not uncommon.  It
responds poorly to the use of prisms.  Finally, there appears to be
a disturbance of visual perception occurring centrally which has
still not been adequately studied to permit an understanding.

## INTERCURRENT ILLNESS

Levodopa therapy has had an impact on the occurrence and treatment of intercurrent illness among Parkinson patients. The increased mobility of the patients has rendered them subject to more injuries and accidents. Especially noteworthy has been an increased number of fractures, especially fractures of the femur, humerus and wrist. The management of these injuries has been greatly facilitated and orthopedic surgeons have been willing to treat them surgically whereas in the past they preferred to treat parkinsonian patients conservatively.

Levodopa therapy should be continued until the last dose before surgery. Usually, an operation is scheduled for the morning. Levodopa should be continued until the last dose of the evening before surgery. It should be resumed at a reduced dosage of 50-75% of the patients's customary dose on the first post-op day as soon as the patient can take fluids orally. No parenteral preparation of levodopa is currently available and rectal absorption appears to be unreliable. Generally, the post-operative course will be much better if levodopa is resumed promptly. Most patients will suffer only a partial recurrence of their parkinsonian state over a 24 hour period off their levodopa regimen.

These observations are also applicable to other surgical procedures such as prostatectomy and herniorrhaphy which the patients may require. Acute abdominal illness should be handled in as normal a manner as possible. Valuable time may be lost if one is diverted by the thought that the symptoms represent a drug reaction and the patient is observed for a time after withdrawal of levodopa. In fact, this usually only makes matters worse for recurrent tremor and rigidity will make evaluation and diagnositc studies more difficult to perform. Levodopa therapy should be continued, by nasogastric tube if necessary during whatever studies may be needed.

The cardiovascular action of levodopa may warrant withdrawing treatment in a patient who has a mycoardial infarction or other acute cardiac event or a cerebral vascular accident until the clinical status stabilizes. However, there may be cogent reason for not stopping treatment in some cases. Severe tremor and rigidity may itself represent a substantial stress and burden the patient's heart unnecessarily. In such a circumstance it is better to continue levodopa therapy, though the dose may be reduced to minimize the occurrence of dyskinesias and other levodopa side effects.

When very serious illness overshadows Parkinson's disease treatment of the latter may become superfluous. Levodopa may justifiably be gradually withdrawn, for example, in a terminal malignancy or in a patient in prolonged coma. In such cases, levodopa may no longer yield significant benefit.

In conclusion the proper treatment of parkinsonism requires the treatment of the whole patient. Our best treatment is only a

symptomatic remedy.  It must be given within the context of the
patient's pattern of life and with due regard to the patient's
overall state of health.  Thus it is most appropriate for parkinson patients to be cared for primarily by physicians willing and
able to assume a general responsibility for their care, i.e.,
the family physician or internist.

## REFERENCES

Caplan, L.H., Jacobson, H.G., Rubinstein, B.M. and Rotman, M.Z.
    (1965).  Megacolon and volvulus in Parkinson's disease.
    *Radiology 85:* 73-79.

Charcot, J.M. (1886) *Lecons sur les maladies du systeme nerveux.*
    Paris, Delahaye et Lecrosnier.

Cotzias, G., Van Woert, M. and Schieffer, L. (1976) *New Eng. J. Med.*
    *276:* 374-379.

Critchley, M. (1929).  Arterioschlerotic Parkinsonism.  *Brain 52:*
    23-83.

Denny-Brown, D. (1962).  *The Basal Ganglia.*  Oxford Univ. Press,
    London.  pp. 72-73 and Fig. 30.

Duvoisin, R.C. (1972).  Diphenidol for levodopa induced nausea and
    vomiting.  *J.A.M.A. 221:* 1408.

Duvoisin, R.C. Yahr, M.D. and Coté, L.J. (1969).  Pyridoxine reversal
    of L-dopa effects in Parkinsonism.  *Trans. Am. Neurol. Assoc.*
    *94:* 81-84.

Duvoisin, R.C. and Yahr, M.D. (1972).  In: *L-Dopa and Behavior* Ed. by
    S. Malitz, New York, Raven Press. pp. 57-72.

Duvoisin, R.C., Yahr, M.D., Lieberman, J., Antunes, J., and Rhee, S.
    (1972).  The striatal foot.  *Trans. Am. Med. Assoc. 97:* 267.

Duvoisin, R.C. (1975).  Antagonism of levodopa by papaverine.
    *J.A.M.A. 231 (8):* 845-846.

Duvoisin, R.C. (1975).  Alpha-methyldopa and Parkinsonism: Induction
    or Exacerbation.  *Neurology 25:* 376.

Duvoisin, R.C. and Marsden, C.D. (1975).  Note on the scoliosis of
    Parkinsonism.  *J. Neurol. Neurosurg, & Psychiat. 38:* 787-793.

Forno, L.S. and Alvorol, E.C. (1971).  In: *Recent Advances in Park-*
    *inson's Disease.*  Ed. by F.H. McDowell and C.H. Markham.
    pp. 119-162.

Gilbert, G.J. (1967).  *Lancet ii:* 442-443.

Henry, R.E., Goldberg, L.J., Sturgen, P. and Ansel, R.D. (1971).
    Serologic abnormalities associated with L-dopa therapy.  *Vox*
    *Sang. 20:* 306-316.

Joseph, C. (1972).  Occurrence of positive coombs test in patients
    treated with levodopa.  *New Eng. J. Med. 286:* 1401-1402.

Ratput, H., Kazi, K.G. and Rozdilski, B. (1972). Striatonigral
    degeneration response to levodopa therapy. *J. Neurol. Sci.*
    *16:* 331-341.
Selby, G. (1968). Cerebral atrophy in Parkinsonism. *J. Neurol. Sci.*
    *6:* 517-559.
Skibba, J.L., Pinckney, J., Gilbert, E.F. and Johnson, R.W. (1972).
    Multiple primary melanoma following administration of levodopa.
    *Arch. Pathol. 93:* 556-561.
Stadlan, E.M., Duvoisin, R.C. and Yahr, M.D. (1966) in *Proceedings*
    *of the Vth International Congress of Neuropathology.* Ed. by
    F. Luthy and A. Bischoff. Amsterdam, Excerpta Medica. pp.
    569-571.
Takei, Y. and Mirra, S.S. (1973) in *Progress in Neuropathology*, Vol. II
    Ed. by A.M. Zimmerman, New York, Grune and Stratton, pp.
    217-251.
Territo, M.C., Peters, R.W. and TAnaka, K.R., (1973) *J.A.M.A. 226:*
    347-348.
Wolf, S.M. and Davis, R.L., (1973). Permanent dementia in idiopathic
    Parkinsonism treated with levodopa. *Arch. Neurol. 29:* 276-278.
Yahr, M.D., Duvoisin, R.C., Schear, M.J., Barrett, R.E. and Hoehn,
    M.M. (1969). Treatment of Parkinsonism with levodopa. *Arch.*
    *Neurol. (Chicago) 21:* 343-345.

## DISCUSSION

*Dr. Fahn*
    Some personality change takes place in many of these patients.
They become indicisive; they lose their assertive drive, and if they
are an executive, they find they can't cope; they can't make a decision and pretty soon they are out of a job. This personality change
can be very disabling, and in my hands, anti-parkinson therapy has
not helped. I have a few other comments. Another form of pseudoparkinsonism that should be mentioned is normal pressure hydrocephalus,
another differential diagnosis in patients with parkinsonism and dementia. These patients have a freezing gait, trouble with their balance,
falling. This picture of parkinsonism can be corrected by surgical
means rather than by drug therapy. You showed a slide of correlating
clinical state and blood levels of levodopa in the rising and falling
states. I make a distinction between what I call "wearing off" and
what I call "on-off" phenomena. That slide is a very typical example
of "wearing off" phenomenon. There is a good correlation with blood
levels; the falling off phase is much slower than in the on-off and I
think the pharmacokinetics of levodopa is a much more important feature
in "wearing off" than in "on-off".

*Dr. Duvoisin*
    Yes, that's very true. I think the gait apraxia problem

includes low normal pressure hydrocephalus, and also is a feature
of patients with brain tumors in the striatum.  It has been described
on an arteriosclerotic basis by Barron & Meyers *(Brain, 1970)* and it
is probably the gait disturbance in the arteriosclerotic parkinson
patient.  It is not responsive to anything we do except in low
pressure hydrocephalus.

*Dr. Fahn*

Just in regards to normal pressure hydrocephalus, we have seen
two patients with typical normal pressure hydrocephalus and with
parkinson signs of a gait disorder.  But at postmortem, both of them
had lacunar states and hypertensive and arteriosclerotic disease.
This brings into relationship the three conditions; arteriosclerotic
parkinsonism, artesclerotic dementia and normal pressure hydrocephalus.

*Dr. Duvoisin*

I thought I knew what normal pressure hydrocephalus was three
or four years ago.  And now I am not so sure.  We have had so many
failures and late complications; almost a quarter of them have
developed subdural hematomas following surgery.  I sometimes regret
that we have undertaken the cysternograms to demonstrate the delayed
flow in cerebrospinal fluid.

*Dr. Fahn*

Someone had asked earlier that I make a comment about physical
therapy.  I didn't have a chance to.  I think physical therapy was
greatly emphasized in the pre-levodopa days; it has been less emphasized
in recent years.  I could only make a plea for some common sense in
its use.  I think all of us can benefit by some exercise, including
our parkinson patients, within reason.  The difficulty with physical
therapy for the more disabled patients is that it's good for the
duration of the therapy and the next twenty minutes, but it isn't
much good after that.  And to be ideal, it has to be given frequently.
In general, I do not like to see patients give up any activity,
because it then becomes very difficult to regain it.  I think it
becomes more important in the more advanced stages of the disease
to maintain independence.

*Dr. Mars*

I have recently reviewed the total number of patients that I
have seen over the years and once again recalculated the mean ages.
The mean ages are shifting; over the past 5 years they are shifting
towards an older age group by a couple of years.  I have no patients
in the 200 currently followed that are under 35 or 40.  I wonder
what your experience is.  I restrict this observation to primary
idiopathic Parkinson's disease individuals with no antecedent
history of clinically recognizable encephalitis nor any individuals

on any sort of drug therapy.

*Dr. Duvoisin*

Well, unfortunately, it's difficult to answer now by looking
at patient populations because the selective factors that determine
which patients come to teaching hospital clinics have changed.  We are
seeing a different population now.  Since levodopa therapy and Sinemet®
was developed internists and physicians in practice have been identi-
fying and treating these patients.  The patients that I see now,
include a high proportion of dopa-treatment failures, of people with
multiple system degenerations, and unusual features.  So I am not
seeing the same patients.  I would not know how to interpret your
observation.  I think it is true that we are not seeing quite so
many young ones but we never did see, in my lifetime, very many
young patients.  We are certainly following them a longer time
than formerly.  I haven't seen any without a real oculogyric crises,
but I have seen two or three persons who seem to have Parkinson's
disease and some dyskinesias before any treatment: I don't know
what that means.  You can think back and say, "Well, what could
have happened to the virus of encephalitis lethargica?  Is it really
possible that it totally disappeared, or is a modified virus
still around and is it still a factor?"  It is interesting to
speculate, but I have no further data.

*Dr. Calne*

I would just like to comment on Dr. Mars' inquiry about young
patients.  In the last two months, I have seen two patients under
40 years.  One of these patients was a most unusual case and in view
of your comments on the absence of post-encephalitic parkinsonism
since the pandemic, I wonder if you would like to offer a diagnosis.
This was a man of about 35 who developed over the course of five
years (without ever having had levodopa therapy or phenothiazine)
classical parkinsonism on one side and chorea on the other.  Now,
the only other situation where I have seen, patients who have both
chorea and parkinsonism, is in the postencephalitic colony in London.
This patient didn't have a history of encephalitis.

*Dr. Duvoisin*

Well, I have one, possibly two such patients now.  I don't know
what that means.

*Dr. Mars*

With respect to the question as to whether or not the von
Economo agent still remains in a viable pool, I don't think we can
answer that; but I think there have been cases sporadically reported
over the years since 1930 of individuals who do indeed meet the

clinical criteria for von Economo's encephalitis lethargica. I made
such a diagnosis in a patient approximately nine or ten months ago,
a young 25 year old girl who had presented with a profound personality
disturbance, increasing lethargy, somnolence, and sialorrhea; she then
went on to develop tremor and rigidity, with a very dramatic response
to Sinemet® therapy. She still remains with parkinsonian symptomotology eight months following the onset. The course of evolution of
the symptoms was approximately two or three months. We don't know
whether it's the same agent, but that's not to say that there are no
other agents with neuro toxicity.

*Dr. Duvoisin*

Yes, I agree with you. There are hints that there might be
some sort of phenomenon still continuing, but certainly nothing
comparable to the epidemics of the 1920's. It's very difficult to
really recognize what that was like. We have to go back and spend
some time looking at the old literature. There was a sizable number
of patients who really affected neurology very strongly; they grossly
outnumbered the Parkinson's disease population. A very large
proportion of them had oculogyric crises and I haven't seen that
in any of these somewhat unusual syndromes that I cannot classify.
It's too bad, because as Dr. Merrit once commented, when one faced
a difficult diagnostic problem in the 1930's or 40's or 50's, you
could always say it was encephalitis lethargica, but now you have
to admit honestly your ignorance. The last case that I know of is
a patient which Dr. Hoehn diagnosed, who probably had his encephalitis
in 1943 or '44 in an Army troop ship. So far as I know, he is one
of the last really classical cases who had the triad of ocular palsy,
bulbar palsy and somnolence. It's really a fascinating chapter of
neurological history; a disease which had such a profound impact and
then disappeared, before we could really establish its etiology.

*Dr. Messiha*

One question unrelated about the changes in the patients taste
with L-dopa therapy versus Sinemet® therapy, especially to coffee.
Do you notice the same complaint with Sinemet® therapy?

*Dr. Duvoisin*

I have not paid much attention to dysguesia. I think it
occurs; but it also occurred before L-dopa treatment. I think it's
part of the disease. I don't know its meaning. I think the pathology of the disease involves more than the striatum. Now that we
are aware of the mesolimbic dopamine system, it is perhaps possible
to suggest that some of the symptomotology and personality changes
that Dr. Fahn referred to might be related to limbic lobe involvement. There have been descriptions of patients who have loss of

smell, loss of interest in food, and in libido, all of which
returned towards normal on levodopa therapy.  This would imply
involvement of the dopaminergic limbic system in the disease.

*Dr. Pirch*

You made a comment about combined tricyclic antidepressant
and neuroleptic therapy which is used quite a bit today in psychiatry.  Could you further expound on your feelings about that?

*Dr. Duvoisin*

Well, I can understand the psychiatric reason for doing this
in the agitated, depressed patient.  I just see a small slice of
that population.  The patient whose depression is detected before
the onset of parkinsonism is treated and then the parkinsonism is
detected while the patient is still on a neuroleptic drug.  The
question then arises, is the parkinsonism iatrogenic?  You discontinue the neuroleptic and for a time the patient may seem to get
better, but six months or a year later, it's clear that Parkinson's disease is really present.  You know in your own mind that
the neuroleptic drug did not cause Parkinson's disease, but I have
run across a number of people who harbor a lingering doubt that
the neuroleptic drug may have caused the parkinsonism.

*Dr. Clark*

In that regard, would you comment on the role of depression
and disability in parkinson's disease?

*Dr. Duvoisin*

I do not share the popular opinion that depression is more
common in Parkinson's disease than in other chronic diseases.
The suicide rate amongst our patients has really not been any
higher than the suicide rate in other chronic conditions.  Psychia-
trists feel the situation is the other way around, that this is a
common association.  I frankly don't think we have good enough
data to be certain about this point.  The fact is, people get
depressed when they have a chronic disease.  It's something that
many practitioners overlook in their parkinsonian patients and treatment of the depression is something that we can do that may be
very helpful.  I have the impression that the dose of tricyclics
necessary is less in patients on levodopa or Sinemet® therapy
than in the average patient, that perhaps there is some synergistic
effect.  In fact, I would suggest that the use of tricyclics in a
single daily dose is probably the most common psychoactive drug
that I use in treating parkinsonian patients.  Now, Elavil® and
Tofranil® have some anti-parkinson activity which I think reflects
their anticholinergic properties.  You have to be careful; some

patients are so sensitive to the psychotoxic properties of the anticholinergics that they will get confusion and hallucinations even on
Elavil® or Benadryl®.  I have tried in such cases to go to some of
the tricyclics that are secondary amines and consequently have less
anticholinergic properties, such as protriptyline which is marketed
under the trademark name of Vivactil® in the United States.  I
think there is a little less psychotoxicity with it and I believe
that's a common experience among neurologists treating large numbers of parkinsonian patients.

# NEW APPROACHES IN THE MANAGEMENT OF HYPERKINETIC MOVEMENT DISORDERS

STANLEY FAHN, M.D.

Department of Neurology
Columbia University
College of Physicians and Surgeons
and
Neurological Institute of New York
New York, New York 10032

## ABSTRACT

This review covers recent advances in a variety of dyskinesias. Introduction of new drugs for the treatment of myoclonus and sensory biofeedback therapy for focal dystonia are expanding our concepts of these types of movement disorders. Progress in the treatment of action myoclonus is especially noteworthy and has led to the implication of serotonin deficit in the pathophysiology of this syndrome. Knowledge of the biochemical pathology of Huntington's chorea has outpaced therapy for this disorder, but new forms of therapy have been proposed based on the chemical findings. Basic pharmacologic studies suggest pathophysiologic mechanisms for the syndrome known as tardive dyskinesia, but treatment is still far from ideal for this disorder. Other movement disorders with recent therapeutic advances include essential tremor and hemiballism.

This review will cover only those dyskinesias in which new therapies have been advanced in the last few years. Aside from parkinsonism, which will not be discussed here, progress in the treatment of movement disorders has been slow, but steady. New drugs are being tested constantly, and the purpose of this review is to call attention to the ongoing evaluations in this field. Descriptions and etiologies for these dyskinesias are covered elsewhere (*Fahn, 1976a*) and therefore are not repeated here.

## ACTION MYOCLONUS

One of the major advances in movement disorder research in
recent years has been the verification that treatment with serotonin
precursors can significantly ameliorate the myoclonic jerks associated
with anoxic encephalopathy.  Lance and Adams described four patients
with this clinical syndrome in 1963 and established it as a separate
nosologic entity.  Action myoclonus is not a common sequela following
hypoxia; in fact, it is not mentioned in Courville's (1958) review
of cerebral anoxia.  Perhaps medical advances in recent years, allowing the hypoxic patient to survive, have contributed to the increasing
number of reported cases.  DeLean et al. (1976). found 20 reported
cases in the literature and described two additional patients.  Papers
not included in their review (Hirose et al., 1974) and subsequent
reports by Goldberg and Dorman (1976) and by Van Woert et al. (1976)
raise the total number of reported cases to 37 patients.  Commonly,
the anoxic state occurred during anesthesia, although other causes
of anoxia are occasionally responsible.  The duration of anoxia varies,
but longer than six minutes is usual.  Typically, the patient becomes
comatose, and remains in coma for a few days and has generalized
major motor seizures during this period, which can be controlled with
anticonvulsant medications such as phenytoin.  As the state of coma
lightens, myoclonic jerking develops, which becomes the major disability as the patient becomes fully conscious.  The myoclonic jerks
are not present at rest, except when startled.  The startle stimulus
can be mild and can be merely a visible gesture or the onset of
speech by someone nearby.  Use of the limbs brings out the myoclonus
(action myoclonus), and activities such as finger-to-nose testing,
handwriting, or walking exacerbate the involuntary movements.  It is
not known whether spontaneous cessation of this type of movement
disorder has ever occurred, and reported cases are those whose
symptoms have remained permanent, except with successful treatment.

Although moderate improvement of action myoclonus has occurred
with a variety of drugs (reviewed by DeLean et al., 1976), serotonin
precursors appear to be most effective.  Lhermitte and his colleagues
(1971, 1972) were the first to demonstrate that 5-hydroxytryptophan
(5-HTP), the immediate precursor of serotonin, can ameliorate action
myoclonus.  These workers used the racemic mixture of D,L-5-HTP.
Van Woert and Sethy (1975) refined this approach and utilized the
pure levorotatory isomer of 5-HTP plus carbidopa to inhibit peripheral L-aromatic amino acid decarboxylase.  These investigators
showed that this combination is effective in three patients.  More
recently, Van Woert et al. (1976) report continued improvement with
L-5-HTP/carbidopa therapy in a total of nine out of 12 patients
with action myoclonus secondary to anoxia.  Other causes of myoclonus
respond less well.  Gastrointestinal side effects of nausea, anorexia,
vomiting and diarrhea are troublesome, but these tend to disappear
with time and can be partly overcome by using phenothiazines and

diphenoxylate *(Lomotil) (Van Woert et al., 1976).*

DeLean *et al. (1976)* verified the beneficial effectiveness of
L-5-HTP/carbidopa in two patients with anoxia-induced action myoclonus.
Moreover, they also showed that L-tryptophan plus a monoamine oxidase
inhibitor can also reduce the myoclonus, but to a lesser degree. One
of their patients developed personality changes on L-5-HTP/carbidopa,
so the medications were discontinued. The other patient has been
maintained on L-5-HTP 1.8 g/d and carbidopa 150 mg/d for 6 months
with sustained improvement. Clearly, more patients with this syndrome need to be studied; but it would appear that serotonin precursors are worthy of continued investigation.

OTHER TYPES OF MYOCLONUS

Serotonin precursors have been administered to patients with
other causes of myoclonus with less benefit *(Van Woert et al., 1976).*
The myoclonus (tics) seen in the Gilles de la Tourette syndrome
commonly responds to haloperidol *(Shapiro et al., 1976).* I have
successfully employed haloperidol for segmental myoclonus secondary
to trauma. Steiner (personal communication) effectively treated
one patient with segmental myoclonus (presumably viral-induced)
with cyproheptidine, a serotonin antagonist. Hoehn and Cherington
(in press) found clonazepam and tetrabenazine to be effective in
controlling spinal myoclonus. From these individual reports it
seems that many different drugs can be effective in ameliorating
myoclonus, but possibly inconsistently. The causes of myoclonus
are varied *(see reviews in Charlton, 1975),* and the mechanisms of
this type of dyskinesia are also probably numerous, which may
account for the different therapeutic responses reported.

DYSTONIA

The dystonic states can be generalized or focal, hereditary or
sporadic, primary or secondary, and may be present at rest or only
with action *(Fahn and Eldridge, 1976).* I am impressed how frequently dystonia is misdiagnosed, either as a conversion reaction
or as some other type of involuntary movement disorder, particularly
if rapid, jerky spasms are present in addition to the sustained
dystonic movements. Dystonic postures are usually well recognized
and accepted, but this represents the full-blown, more advanced
stage. Commonly, dystonia begins with focal involvement and only
with action (i.e. use of a limb). It may remain limited or may
progress to become either multisegmental or generalized and eventually be present at rest.

An effective new approach in the treatment of focal dystonia
is the use of sensory biofeedback to train the patient to relax
the unwanted muscular contraction. Korein *et al. (1976)* introduced
this type of therapy and found it to be effective in 60% of patients

with torticollis. Spasmodic torticollis has otherwise been relatively
resistant to pharmacologic therapy, so that this new form of treatment
is most welcome. Sensory biofeedback therapy appears not to be effective for generalized dystonia because patients cannot concentrate on
relaxing more than one muscle at a time.

Drug therapy is worthy of extensive trial to control generalized
dystonia. Although a given patient may respond dramatically to a
specific drug, no drug has proven to be consistently effective in a
large number of patients with dystonia. Therefore, the clinician
should be prepared to test a series of drugs. Drugs that have been
occasionally successful include trihexyphenidyl, levodopa, haloperidol, diazepam, and carbamazepine (Eldridge and Fahn, 1976; Fahn,
1976a). Recently, Menkes (personal communication) has successfully
controlled the dystonic movements with L-tryptophan/tranylcypromine
combination in one patient whom I have personally seen. The response has been about 90% effective and has been maintained (approximately six months at present). It seems worthwhile to use the above
drugs first because of their proven usefulness in at least one patient, before testing other agents.

Unfortunately, whenever a specific drug is claimed to be effective in some patients, subsequent investigators find less benefit.
This has been the case with carbamazepine in dystonia (Geller et al.,
1976; Isgreen et al., 1976). Similar events were noted with levodopa in dystonia (Coleman, 1970; Chase et al., 1970; Barrett et al.,
1970; Fahn, personal observations), but occasional reports of
success are still reported with levodopa (Batshaw and Haslam, 1976;
Rajput, 1973). Apparently, those patients with some parkinson features in addition to dystonia respond favorably to levodopa (Allen
and Knopp, 1976). One note of caution should be given in regard to
levodopa therapy: Cooper (1972) feels that children treated with
this drug respond poorly to neurosurgical treatment for dystonia.
Since cryothalamotomy may be effective in some patients with dystonia
(Cooper, 1976), this procedure may need to be considered if the
dystonia is intractable to medical therapy and is disabling, painful, or intolerable to the patient. The patient should be willing
to accept speech deficit or worse neurologic damage as a possible
adverse effect of surgery before agreeing to this procedure.

In discussing dystonia it should always be remembered that
Wilson's disease can present with this type of movement disorder.
Since this is treatable with D-penicillamine, it should always be
searched for.

ESSENTIAL TREMOR

In recent years propranolol has been shown to be effective
in some patients in lessening the severity of essential tremor
(Winkler and Young, 1974; Tolosa and Loewenson, 1975), although
some investigators are less impressed (Sweet et al., 1974). Per-

sonal experience has shown that propranolol is clinically effective
only when the tremor is mild to moderate in amplitude.  The amount
of benefit is limited and never abolishes the tremor, but can allow
increased functional use of the affected arms, such as improving
handwriting, pouring liquids, and bringing liquids to the mouth.
Diazepam combined with propranolol can sometimes give additional
benefit *(Fahn, 1972a)*.

Ethyl alcohol remains the most effective agent in reducing the
tremor, but unfortunately chronic use of alcohol can lead to other
medical problems.  The benign nature of essential tremor, although
slowly progressive, may allow some elderly patients with mild tremor
to remain untreated.

## CHOREA, HEMICHOREA AND HEMIBALLISM

The most effective category of drugs for the choreic syndromes
remains the dopamine receptor blockers, namely the phenothiazines
and butyrophenones *(Fahn, 1976a)*, despite the recent biochemical
findings of reduced gamma-aminobutyric acid (GABA) *(Urquhart et al.,
1975)* and normal levels of dopamine *(Bernheimer et al., 1975)* in the
basal ganglia of patients with Huntington's disease.  The activities
of the enzymes catalyzing the synthesis of GABA and acetylcholine,
glutamic acid decarboxylase (GAD) and choline acetyltransferase
(CAT), respectively, are also reduced in the neostriatum *(McGeer
and McGeer, 1976)*.  These biochemical changes most likely reflect
neuronal loss in these structures and are therefore secondary effects,
much like dopamine loss in parkinsonism is secondary to loss of
nigral neurons.  This explanation fits well with the report of
Stahl and Swanson *(1975)* who showed that one patient with early
Huntington's disease who committed suicide had normal levels of
GAD and CAT activities.  Nevertheless, the choreic symptoms could
conceivably be secondary to deficient activity of GABA in the synapse.
The proof of such a hypothesis requires the demonstration that
replacement of GABA or GABA-mimetic agents can relieve the choreic
movements.  Attempts to treat with GABA have been unsuccessful, even
when GABA was combined with dipropylacetate, a GABA transaminase
inhibitor *(Shoulson et al., 1976)*.  This lack of efficacy may be
due to failure of GABA to enter the brain, rather than a failure
of cerebral GABA to relieve the symptoms, since a blood-brain
barrier to GABA exists *(Fahn, in press)*.  The GABA-mimetic drug,
muscimol *(Johnston, 1976)*, is currently being tested by Shoulson
to learn whether this approach is effective.

If basal ganglia deficiency of GABA in Huntington's disease
is responsible for chorea it would seem that the reduced number
of GABA-ergic striatopallidal neurons *(Fahn, in press)* plays a
key role in the sympatomatology.  The loss of these inhibitory
neurons would lead to a release of excitatory pallidothalamic
neuronal activity, resulting in chorea.  Why then should dopamine
antagonists be effective in reducing chorea?  A reasonable explana-

tion is that these drugs allow the disinhibition of residual cholinergic excitatory neurons in the neostriatum, which in turn activate
the residual GABA-containing neurons (see Figure 1 for proposed model
of connecting neurons in basal ganglia).

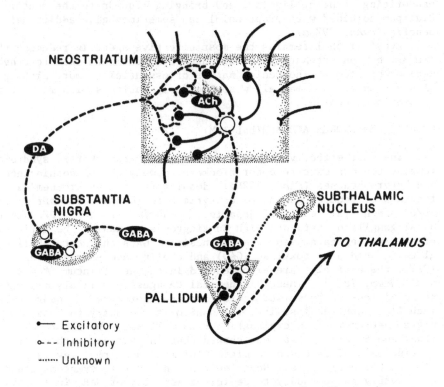

*Figure 1. A proposed model of some of the neuronal pathways in
basal ganglia, depicting their functions and suspected
neurotransmitters. Reproduced from Fahn (1976b), cour-
tesy of Raven Press.*

A similar explanation can account for the hemichoreic or hemiballism syndrome, which is most commonly caused by a lesion of the
contralateral subthalamic nucleus. The subthalamic nucleus sends
fibers (presumably inhibitory) to the globus pallidus, and a loss
of these fibers releases the pallidal efferent neurons. Drugs that
block dopamine receptors would increase GABA-ergic influence in the
pallidum by the mechanism described in the above paragraph. This
in turn inhibits the pallidal efferent neurons and controls the
hemichorea and hemiballism.

Probably any potent neuroleptic agent can be effective in
controlling chorea, hemichorea and hemiballism. My personal

experience has been primarily with perphenazine (Trilafon®) *(Fahn, 1972b; Johnson and Fahn, 1974)*. The details of perphenazine treatment have been presented elsewhere *(Fahn, 1976a)*.

## TARDIVE DYSKINESIA

The choreic-like movements of tardive dyskinesia (TD) are usually encountered in the elderly individual on long-term phenothiazine or butyrophenone therapy. Why some patients develop this complication of drug therapy, while others on the same medication dosage and duration do not, is not clear. There may be an analogy with the "on-off" phenomenon with chronic levodopa therapy. Both types of adverse effects develop after prolonged therapy with toxic dose levels. In TD, the patient had previously been parkinsonian from the neuroleptic drug according to Crane *(1972)*. With the "on-off" phenomenon, the patient had been choreic from levodopa, as has been discussed here *(see discussion after Klawans' paper, this volume)*. Both TD and the "off" phenomenon have been considered to be due to receptor mechanisms; TD due to supersensitivity after chronic receptor blockade *(Klawans, 1973)*, and the "off" phenomenon due to desensitization after chronic receptor stimulation *(Fahn, 1974)*. Neither of these proposed mechanisms are proven, and other possibilities should be considered. Prolongation of increased dopamine synthesis with neuroleptic therapy has been considered a possible contributing phenomenon in the pathophysiology of TD *(Fahn, 1976a)*.

The management of TD is complex. While higher doses of neuroleptic drug can suppress the involuntary movements, it seems contrary to medical principles to use even more of the offending agent in order to mask the symptoms. Rather, it would seem preferable to discontinue the drug and hope that the symptoms eventually subside, which may happen in perhaps one-third of the patients. Unfortunately, withdrawal of the neuroleptic agent usually augments the symptoms of TD, both the involuntary movements and the feelings of restlessness, which is most distressing to the patient. It is at this point that I treat with reserpine, which depletes the monoamines from their storage sites, beginning with small doses and slowly increasing it to avoid side effects *(Fahn, 1976a)*. If the dose of reserpine can be great enough, the TD will be suppressed, and occasionally reserpine can later be gradually withdrawn. Unfortunately, adverse effects of nasal stuffiness, depression, or hypotension interfere occasionally with this approach. Perhaps tetrabenazine could be used as a substitute for reserpine in this situation, but I have had no experience with this drug which is not commercially available in the U.S. Another difficulty in treatment is that many patients are unable to discontinue their neuroleptic drug due to persistence of the psychosis which continues to require medical treatment. These patients deserve a trial of reserpine combined with the dopamine receptor blocking drug that they have been receiving. I have not seen such a study carried out, but it seems a new approach worthy of study.

## CONCLUSION

A number of potent CNS-acting drugs are available today; it is likely that one or a combination of several may prove to be efficacious in a given patient with a dyskinesia. These drugs fall into two major classes: (1) those that act as neurotransmitter agonists or antagonists and (2) those that are neuron membrane suppressants, such as the anticonvulsants and the hypnotics. The clinician should be encouraged to test these agents systematically on the patient with an "intractable" dyskinesia, beginning with the drugs already reported to be effective. By sharing our experiences, we will learn a great deal about possible brain mechanisms contributing to specific dyskinesias and also how best to treat these disorders with the minimum side effects.

## REFERENCES

Allen, N. and Knopp, W. (1976). Hereditary parkinsonsim-dystonia with sustained control by L-dopa and anticholinergic medication. In: *Dystonia*. Advances in Neurology, Vol. 14. (Eldridge, R. and Fahn, S., Eds.) pp. 201-213. Raven Press, New York.

Barrett, R.E., Yahr, M.D. and Duvoisin, R.C. (1970). Torsion dystonia and spasmodic torticollis: results of treatment with L-dopa. *Neurology 20*, 107-113.

Batshaw, M.L. and Haslam, R.H.A. (1970). Multidisciplinary management of dystonia misdiagnosed as hysteria. In: *Dystonia*. Advances in Neurology, Vol. 14. (Eldridge, R. and Fahn, S., Eds.) pp. 367-373. Raven Press, New York.

Bernheimer, H., Birkmayer, W., Hornykiewicz, O., Jellinger, K. and Seitelberger, F. (1973). Brain dopamine and the syndromes of Parkinson and Huntington: Clinical, morphological and neurochemical correlations. *J. Neurol. Sci. 20*, 415-455.

Charlton, M.H., (Ed.) (1975), *Myoclonic Seizures*, Excerpta Medica, International Congress Series, No. 307, Amsterdam.

Chase, T.N. (1970). Biochemical and pharmacologic studies of dystonia. *Neurology 20*, 122-126.

Coleman, M. (1970). Preliminary remarks on the L-dopa therapy of dystonia. *Neurology 20*, 114-122.

Cooper, I.S. (1972). Levodopa-induced dystonia. *Lancet 2*, 1317-1318.

Cooper, I.S. (1976). Twenty-year followup study of the neurosurgical treatment of dystonia musculorum deformans. In: *Dystonia*. Advances in Neurology, Vol. 14. (Eldridge, R. and Fahn, S., Eds) pp. 423-452. Raven Press, New York.

Courville, C.B. (1953). Contributions to the Study of Cerebral
    Anoxia. Los Angeles, San Lucas Press.

Crane, G.E. (1972). Pseudoparkinsonism and tardive dyskinesia.
    *Arch. Neurol. 27,* 426-430.

DeLéan, J., Richardson, J.C. and Hornykiewicz, O. (1976). Benefi-
    cial effects of serotonin precursors in postanoxic action
    myoclonus. *Neurology 26,* 863-868.

Eldridge, R. and Fahn, S. (Eds.) (1976). *Dystonia.* Advances in
    Neurology, Vol. 14, Raven Press, New York.

Fahn, S. (1972a). Differential diagnosis of tremors. *Med. Clin.
    No. Am. 56,* 1363-1375.

Fahn, S. (1972b). Treatment of choreic movements with perphen-
    azine. *Dis. Nerv. Syst. 33,* 653-658.

Fahn, S. (1974). "On-off" phenomenon with levodopa therapy in
    parkinsonism: Clinical and pharmacologic correlations and the
    effect of intramuscular pyridoxine. *Neurology 24,* 431-441.

Fahn, S. (1976a). Medical treatment of movement disorders. In
    *Neurological Reviews* 1976. pp. 72-106. American Academy of
    Neurology, Minneapolis.

Fahn, S. (1976b). Biochemistry of the basal ganglia. In: *Dystonia.*
    Advances in Neurology, Vol. 14. (Eldridge, R. and Fahn, S.,
    Eds.) pp. 59-88. Raven Press, New York.

Fahn, S. (in press). Gamma-aminobutyric acid, glycine and other
    putative amino acid neurotransmitters. In: *Handbook of
    Clinical Neurology.*

Fahn, S. and Eldridge, R. (1976). Definition of dystonia and clas-
    sification of the dystonic states. In: *Dystonia.* Advances
    in Neurology, Vol. 14. (Eldridge, R. and Fahn, S., Eds.)
    pp. 1-5. Raven Press, New York.

Geller, M., Kaplan, B., and Christoff, N. (1976). Treatment of
    dystonic symptoms with carbamazepine. In: *Dystonia.* Advances
    in Neurology, Vol. 14. (Eldridge, R. and Fahn, S., Eds.)
    pp. 403-410. Raven Press, New York.

Goldberg, M.A. and Dorman, J.D. (1976). Intention myoclonus:
    Successful treatment with clonazepam. *Neurology 26,* 24-26.

Hirose, G., Singer, P., Bass, N.H. (1971). Successful treatment
    of posthypoxic action myoclonus with carbamazepine. *J.A.M.A.
    218,* 1432-1433.

Hoehn, M.M. and Cherington, M. (in press). Spinal myoclonus.
    *Neurology,* in press.

Isgreen, W.P., Fahn, S., Barrett, R.E., Snider, S.R. and Chutorian,
    A.M. (1976). Carbamazepine in torsion dystonia. In: *Dysto-
    nia.* Advances in Neurology, Vol. 14. (Eldridge, R. and
    Fahn, S., Eds.) pp. 411-416. Raven Press, New York.

Johnson, W.G. and Fahn, S. (1974). Treatment of vascular hemi-
    chorea and hemiballismus with perphenazine. *Trans. Am.
    Neurol. Assoc. 99,* 22-224.

Johnston, G.A.R. (1976).  Physiologic pharmacology of GABA and its
    antagonists in the vertebrate nervous system.  In: *GABA in
    Nervous System Function* (Roberts, E., Chase, T.N., and Tower,
    D.B., Eds) pp. 395-411.  Raven Press, New York.
Klawans, H.L. (1973).  The pharmacology of tardive dyskinesias.
    *Am. J. Psychiat. 130*, 82-86.
Korein, J., Brudney, J., Grynbaum, B., Sachs-Frankel, G., Weisinger,
    M., and Levidow, L. (1976).  Sensory feedback therapy of
    spasmodic torticollis and dystonia: Results in treatment of
    55 patients.  In: *Dystonia*.  Advances in Neurology, Vol. 14.
    (Eldridge, R. and Fahn, S., Eds.) pp. 375-402.  Raven Press,
    New York.
Lance, J.W. and Adams, R.D. (1963).  The syndrome of intention or
    action myoclonus as a sequel to hypoxic encephalopathy.
    *Brain 86*, 111-136.
Lhermitte, F., Marteau, R. and Degos, L.-F. (1972).  Analyse pharma-
    cologique d'un nouveau cas de myoclonies d'intention et
    d'action post-anoxiques.  *Rev. Neurol. Paris 126*, 107-114.
Lhermitte, F., Peterflavi, M., Marteau, R., Gazengel, J. and Serdaru,
    M. (1971).  Analyse pharmacologique d'un cas de myoclonies
    d'intention et d'action post-anoxiques.  *Rev. Neurol. Paris.
    124*, 23-31.
McGeer, P.L. and McGeer, E.G. (1976).  The GABA system and function
    of the basal ganglia: Huntington's disease.  In: *GABA in
    Nervous System Function*.  (Roberts, E., Chase, T.N., and Tower,
    D.B., Eds.) pp. 487-495.  Raven Press, New York.
Rajput, A.H. (1973).  Levodopa in dystonia musculorum deformans.
    *Lancet 1*, 432.
Shapiro, A.K., Shapiro, E.S., Bruun, R.D., Sweet, R., Wayne, H. and
    Solomon, G. (1976).  Gilles de la Tourette's syndrome:
    Summary of clinical experience with 250 patients and suggested
    nomenclature for tic syndromes.  In: *Dystonia*.  Advances in
    Neurology, Vol. 14. (Eldridge, R. and Fahn, S., Eds.) pp.
    277-283.  Raven Press, New York.
Shoulson, I., Kartzinel, R., and Chase, T.N. (1976).  Huntington's
    disease: Treatment with dipropylacetic acid and gamma-amino-
    butyric acid.  *Neurology 26*, 61-63.
Stahl, W.L. and Swanson, P.D. (1974).  Biochemical abnormalities in
    Huntington's chorea brains.  *Neurology 24*, 813-819.
Sweet, R.D., Blumberg, J., Lee, J.E., and McDowell, F.H. (1974).
    Propranolol treatment of essential tremor.  *Neurology 24*,
    64-67.
Tolosa, E.S. and Loewenson, R.B. (1975).  Essential tremor: treatment
    with propranolol.  *Neurology 25*, 1041-1044.
Urquhart, N., Perry, T.L., Hansen, S. and Kennedy, J. (1975).  GABA
    content and glutamic acid decarboxylase activity in brain of
    Huntington's chorea patients and control subjects.  *J. Neuro-
    chem. 24*, 1071-1075.

Van Woert, M.H., Jutkowitz, R., Rosenbaum, P. and Bowers, M.B., Jr. (1976). Serotonin and myoclonus. *Monagr. Neural Sci.* *3*, 71-80.
Van Woert, M.H. and Sethy, V.H. (1975). Therapy of intention myoclonus with L-5-hydroxytryptophan and a peripheral decarboxylase inhibitor, MK 486. *Neurology 25*, 135-140.
Winkler, G.F. and Young, R.R. (1974). Efficacy of chronic propranolol therapy in action tremors of the familial, senile or essential varieties. *N. Engl. J. Med. 290*, 984-988.

*DISCUSSION*

*Dr. de la Torre*
About six years ago, we successfully used the dopa decarboxylase inhibitor with 5-HTP for seizures induced by drugs, and I was wondering if you have tried this treatment for convulsive seizures in epilepsy? My second question is, doesn't it seem like a contradiction that you can find beneficial effects using reserpine as well as with the combination decarboxylase inhibitor and 5-HTP?

*Dr. Fahn*
Regarding the first part of your question, I have no experience using these drugs in treating epilepsy and I'm not aware of such reports. In regards to your second question, treatment of action myoclonus with serotonin precursors, has been effective in the majority of cases reported. These patients don't respond to reserpine. Reserpine has been helpful in other types of myoclonus such as spinal myoclonus present at rest and not with action. I think one of the main points I wanted to make about action myoclonus and serotonin is that there may well be a deficiency of some of the serotonin neurons; 5-HIAA has been reported to be low in spinal fluid, either before or after probenecid in these patients. Whether one should be using combination 5-HTP with carbidopa, which is quite toxic compared to L-tryptophan, or use L-typtophan plus a monoamine oxidase inhibitor is a question that needs to be resolved. There are probably different mechanisms of action between 5-HTP and tryptophan. Tryptophan is eventually converted to serotonin specifically in serotonin containing neurons. 5-HTP will form serotonin wherever there is aromatic L-amino acid decarboxylase. So it will form 5-HT not only in serotonin-containing neurons, but also in other monoamine-containing neurons. Whether this difference is important for their effectiveness in action myoclonus is not clear. This difference might also explain why 5-HTP exacerbates parkinsonism, whereas tryptophan does not.

*Dr. Mars*
I want to talk a bit about torsion dystonia, dystonia musculorum deformans. As you pointed out, the therapy we have for that

disease is abysmal. There have been reports that a definite percentage of those patients with torsion dystonia, have an alteration in dopamine β-hydroxylase in plasma with an elevation in quantity of that particular enzyme. If DBH in plasma is indeed an indicator of overall sympathetic activity, then what compounds could one use that might be centrally effective in inhibition of DBH; we tried giving a patient large doses of Antabuse®, hoping that some of it would get in. It obviously did; she became quite confused, delirious and quite frankly, acted intoxicated for a couple of days, without the benefit of any alcohol. The drug had to be discontinued. It also showed some signs of hepatic toxicity with alterations in her liver enzymes. That didn't turn out to be effective, and I wondered if you had tried it or if anybody else in this room has tried anything like that. Also, I wonder if anyone has had the opportunity of employing lithium in that disease state?

*Dr. Fahn*

Let me just make a comment about the DBH studies and dystonia before talking about these specific drugs you mentioned. First of all, plasma DBH was reported to be elevated in the autosomal dominant rather than in the recessive form. There is considerable debate about the significance of elevated DBH level in plasma in patients with dystonia. Some workers believe that plasma DBH levels is a familial characteristic and more studies on unaffected family members are required before coming to any conclusions. As far as using Antabuse® or lithium, I have no experience with either of these drugs, in the treatment of dystonia. But I agree that it would be worthwhile testing them and reporting their effects.

*Dr. Mars*

Let me point out that the patient who had the Antabuse® did show some definite clinical improvement before she got toxic. She is now having some benefit from very small doses of clonopin and that's a drug also that we might consider.

*Dr. Fahn*

I will add another drug that I have only tried on one patient that seems to be effective: methaqualone. Unfortunately, this drug can be easily abused, and one must be very cautious before prescribing it.

*Dr. de la Torre*

I wanted to ask you a philosophical question regarding one of your subjects with dystonia that you reported was extremely scholarly in school, because I have several friends who are dystonic and are quite intelligent. I was wondering if you think whether that is a coincidence or if you think that maybe the catecholamines in the brain somehow are in a state of disarray and are conducive to this?

*Dr. Fahn*
     The observation of intellectual achievement being greater in
Ashkenazie patients with the autosomal recessive dystonia is reasonably
ably well documented.  In my personal experience, these patients
do very well in school and they impress me as having superb perception and comprehension.  The other types of dystonia don't seem
to show this, by the way; just this particular form.  Why is there
this association?  It has been suggested that superior intelligence
has provided them with a positive survival benefit, allowing for
some type of environmental selection, even though they have a
physical disability.  In this manner, the particular gene was selected out.  What is the relationship of amines in the brain and dystonia?  I am not convinced that amines are involved in dystonia
whatsoever.  One patient we have studied biochemically, who had
a postencephalitic type of dystonia, showed low levels of GABA
in two regions of the brain.  We need many more cases; one case
by itself is not significant.

*Dr. Duvoisin*
     First, let me compliment you on the beautiful presentation.
Two questions: one, regarding reserpine.  The original rationale
for using this drug in tardive dyskinesia was that being the only
powerful neuroleptic available to use that was totally different
from all the other neuroleptics in having a presynaptic site of
action, that we didn't run the risk of exacerbating or causing
more tardive dyskinesia.  There seems to be a little uncertainty
about that point.  In a paper by Christianson decribing changes in
the substantia nigra in tardive dyskinesia, two patients were said
to have been on reserpine.  And Sheldon Wolfe described a case,
published in the Bulletin of the Los Angeles Neurological Association, of a man who, while on reserpine treatment, had a vascular
accident and an episode of dysmnesis which appeared to be short
lived.  Do you know of any other reports; or does anyone here know
of a case, of tardive dyskinesia that is certainly related to reserpine?  And the second question is: in the treatment of some dysmne-
sias we use drugs that can cause tardive dyskinesia; have we yet
seen patients to whom we have added tardive dyskinesia to their
previous movement disorder.

*Dr. Fahn*
     I must announce to everybody here that I believe you were one of
of the first ones to point out that tardive dyskinesia is a rare,
if ever, occurrance in patients on reserpine, whereas it does occur
on the other drugs.  I think at the time I was reviewing this literature four years ago, I found only one isolated case in a large series
from Denmark, and in the tables I found somebody had received reser-

pine.  So it is quite rare compared to the other neuroleptics.
Whether it's rare because it's used less than the other neuroleptics
is not clear.  Certainly the mechanism of action is different from
other neuroleptics and this may be the crucial point.  Other than
the reports you have mentioned, I am not aware of other studies on
this particular point.  The pathophysiology of tardive dyskinesia
is unknown.  It may be related to chemical denervation with supersensitivity of the dopamine receptors or it may be due to sub-
stained increased synthesis of dopamine, or a combination of both
factors.  Because the mechanism of action of reserpine differs from
that of other neuroleptics, it is possible that its effectiveness
depends on its ability to deplete storage levels of dopamine and
thereby permanently alters the pathophysiologic abnormality.  I
would even speculate that perhaps reserpine can be used in conjunction with other neuroleptics to control tardive dyskinesia particularly in patients who need these other drugs to control psychosis.
I should mention that there was a recent report about the relief
of tardive dyskinesia in three patients using cyproheptadine which is
a serotonin antagonist.  The total number of patients tested with
this drug was not given.  We have tried cyproheptadine on one
patient so far and it was ineffective.  As far as the pathology
of the substantia nigra, as reported in the Swedish paper, we have
studied one patient with tardive dyskinesia postmortem and we
found the substantia nigra to be normal.

*Dr. Duvoisin*
     What about the risk of creating tardive dyskinesia in patients
with movement disorders?

*Dr. Fahn*
     This is a good question, and the answer is not yet available.
In the movie I showed of a woman with tardive dyskinesia, she was
given a neuroleptic drug not because of psychosis, but because she
was grieving over the sudden death of her husband.  After eight
weeks, she developed the syndrome.  Fortunately, this was reversed
with reserpine and she was able to eventually come off the drug.  But
this is the risk with neuroleptics.  Tardive dyskinesia can occur
in all kinds of patients, I think.  We use neuroleptics to control
choreic movements.  Will they eventually develop tardive dyskinesia
on top of their chorea?  How about the dystonic patients that
take these drugs?  In these other neurologic disorders, I have
yet to see tardive dyskinesia.  One might legitimately question the
ability to differentiate the involuntary movements between tardive
dyskinesia from Huntington's chorea.  This is not easy, but I
think it's possbile, even on the clinical level.  I believe that we
can distinguish the two syndromes clinically, when an experienced
clinician has seen a number of patients with both syndromes.

*Dr. Calne*

I wonder if I could ask you about the natural history of some
of these spontaneous focal dyskinesias. It seems that the common
denominator in your very last review of therapy is that some drugs
seem to help some patients, but there is an inadequacy of controlled
observation for various good reasons. Now obviously, with the development of pharmacology, everybody is looking at these patients
much more carefully than even before; one does wonder how much
fluctuation do these diseases go through, spontaneously? How
much remission may you expect to see with the passage of time,
without any interference from drugs?

*Dr. Fahn*

That is a very good question. There are clearly going to be
some patients who do have some spontaneous improvement; I don't see
many of those, but I believe they do occur. For example, some
patients with torticoll could improve spontaneously, and they may
be the ones who respond to whatever drug you are using. So there
are probably some people who do have some spontaneous improvement
and certainly in the generalized form of the progressive dystonia
such as the Ashkenazi Jewish form of torsion dystonia, many of them
do have fluctuations in severity, regardless of what drug they are
on; so one must be cautious. As a general rule, the patients that
I see usually have it for life; for example writer's cramp persists
as does generalized dystonia, there are times when the symptoms will
temporarily disappear, such as under hypnosis and during sleep. The
severity of dystonia can fluctuate a little bit, but the disease
tends to persist. The natural history of dystonia reported by Cooper
and by Marsden is one of progression with time, particularly if the
age of onset is during childhood.

*Dr. Potter*

I would like to ask a question about your tryptophan treatment. When you give dietary tryptophan to a normal individual,
perhaps one percent would be converted to serotonin; a considerable
quantity may go to niacin. I was just wondering has anybody looked
at these individuals who have various types of dystonia that respond
to tryptophan and can these individuals perhaps be shown to be
niacin deficient?

*Dr. Fahn*

I can't answer about the niacin deficiency at the moment.
Dietary tryptophan is well utilized in the body, tryptophan pyrrolase
in the liver metabolizes ninety percent of it, at least; but if you
give exogenous levels of tryptophan orally, you can get elevated
levels of serotonin in the brain and increased turnover of serotonin with elevation of 5-HIAA. In experiments done in Glowinski's

laboratory, intraperitoneal injections of tryptophan would result
in the release of serotonin into the ventricular fluid.  I think
many biochemical studies have shown that the brain level of serotonin is controlled by the plasma level of tryptophan.  Other
neutral amino acids that compete with the transport of tryptophan
into brain are also important factors.  It turns out that the controlling mechanism for serotonin is tryptophan conversion to 5-HTP
because the enzyme tryptophan hydroxylase has a very high Km and
the enzyme is not saturated in normal conditions; only when you
give exogenous levels of tryptophan can you saturate the enzyme
and give rise to increased synthesis of serotonin.  One way we
try to augment the beneficial effects of tryptophan is to give a
a monoamine oxidase inhibitor along with it.  A patient will first
be placed on parnate ten milligrams three times a day, and then
start adding tryptophan gradually and increasing it.  This is what
we are doing with out patient with action myoclonus; we have also
tried it on three patients with dystonia.  One patient couldn't
tolerate the parnate, and tryptophan alone did nothing.  Another
patient, whether on parnate or off had improvement of speech from
tryptophan.  He has been on it for at least four years now.  We
might want to mention the surgical therapy of dystonia.  This
can be quite effective in controlling dystonia, but one really
wants to make sure that the patient has intractable and unacceptable
dystonia.  The family should be well aware of the risk of surgery
before we attempt this form of treatment.

*Dr. Messiha*
     On the question of tardive dyskinesia, your experience with
reserpine, which is a biogenic amine depleter, and the other experience of Cole *et al.* in Boston on tetrabenazine, which is a cerebral
catecholamine depleter, are all based on the hypothesis of negative
feedback and excessive formation of dopamine.  However, you have
probably noted the use of lithium therapy in tardive dyskinesia in
the Scandinavian literature, which has not been confirmed by the
reports from the Mt. Sinai group.  I wonder if you have any comments
in this regard.

*Dr. Fahn*
     I personally have had no experience with lithium.  In the
anecdotal reports that I have read, one person said that lithium
seemed to help, when I asked for a reprint, he wrote on the reprint
that when the patient went off the drug, he was still benefitted and
the physician no longer feels that lithium was effective in his patient.
I am not sure where lithium stands today, and I would have strong
doubts about it.  Certainly it does nothing for Huntington's chorea
in our experience.  It does not appear to be terribly effective for
that.  Deanol has been tried with mixed results.

*Dr. Messiha*

The question is really to Dr. Mars, and is related to his experience with Antabuse®. As you know, Antabuse® is an enzyme inhibitor of dopamine β-hydroxylase, the enzyme converting dopamine to norepinephrine. I wonder what is the reaction you have seen and its relationship to alcoholic-like reaction? Can you comment, if there were any psychological manifestations or any psychiatric manifestations with it?

*Dr. Mars*

I don't use Antabuse®. This was a patient with classical torsion dystonia. We had a large body of laboratory and clinical observations on her. Her urinary profiles had been repeatedly studied; we have measured the DBH levels and found them to be very significantly increased in plasma, but we could not identify the cerebrospinal fluid. Magnesium levels were also elevated in the blood. Because of the known effect of Antabuse® on DBH, we wondered whether it would be worth a trial. She was given very small doses of Antabuse® and, on one gram a day, she began to show very definite improvement clinically. She was able to walk independently, without assistance or having to hold on to a wall or using furniture for support. But as the dose was increased up to two grams a day, we were extremely careful to make sure that she received no alcohol sponges, no food that conceivably could have alcohol or wine mixed in it or added to some of the sauces. She became disoriented, giggly, had flightive ideas, and acted as if she was in the early stage of alcohol intoxication. This necessitated the immediate discontinuance of the drug, and it took another few days for the effects to wear off entirely. I am not sure whether this was a direct effect of the Antabuse® or whether perhaps there was some sort of an abnormal reaction between the Antabuse® and metabolic alcohols. This is one of the things that had gone through our mind: whether in fact she did have something akin to an acetaldehyde reaction, because of endogenous alcohol and metabolite formation.

# THE ON-OFF EFFECT IN PARKINSON'S DISEASE TREATED WITH LEVODOPA WITH REMARKS CONCERNING THE EFFECT OF SLEEP

EDWARD C. CLARK and BERTRAM FEINSTEIN

Department of Neurosciences
Mount Zion Hospital and Medical Center
San Francisco, California 94101

## ABSTRACT

The "On-Off Effect" in levodopa treated Parkinson's disease began in a few patients during the first year of treatment. The number of patients suffering from this phenomenon increased rapidly the first three or four years with some continuing increase throughout the six years of the study. Even those whose disease had worsened would become even more incapacitated during parts of each day.

One group of patients experienced their initial "On" effect upon arising at their usual hour of awakening. This would last for 1 to 3 hours and was their best time of day.

## INTRODUCTION

One of the unexpected complications of levodopa in Parkinson's disease was the "On-Off Effect". Patients manifesting this phenomenon may swing from almost complete "normality", at times complicated by involuntary movements (the "On" Effect) to complete parkinsonian immobility with tremor (the "Off" Effect) within a short period of time.

Finding the cause of this complication is an important key to the mystery of how to treat Parkinson's disease. Consequently, this investigation was made to study the natural history of the "On-Off Effect" over a 6 year period as well as the effect of sleep on this phenomenon.

175

## METHODS

The "On-Off Effect" was studied in 138 patients with Parkinson's disease treated with levodopa. The initial group started the medication in 1969. By 1975, 128 patients had begun the drug 5 or 6 years before and 10 had started levodopa 1 to 4 years before. At the end of the study 14 patients were no longer being followed. Thirty-three patients had died. Seventy-two patients had previous thalamotomies and 66 were unoperated. The largest number of patients were in the 6th decade of life. Men numbered 86, and women 52. One-hundred-and-thirty-five patients were classified as suffering from Parkinson's disease of unknown cause.

In sharp contrast to other studies, levodopa was begun at low doses and increased slowly in this group. No standard levodopa dosage schedule was used in the treatment of these individuals. Most patients were begun at 0.5 gram or 1 gram of the medication a day. Although not always successful, every effort was made to find a plateau where the patient would have a few or no symptoms of Parkinson's disease and no toxic side effects. If side effects occurred, the amount of medication given was either decreased or divided into smaller and more frequent doses. Consequently, the levodopa might be given four, six or eight times a day, after food. Other modifications were made, as necessary.

During the 6 years of treatment the amount of levodopa given daily to these patients ranged from 0.5 gram to 9 grams a day, varying from year to year. Almost all patients were continued on their pre-levodopa medication.

The "On-Off Effect" was evaluated at each patient visit by questioning the patient and any accompanying person. When any question arose the patient was asked to keep a diary which could be later constructed into a graph. In addition, in one group the patient and his bed-partner were questioned about the patient's Parkinson's symptoms during sleep and upon awakening.

## RESULTS

In 138 patients, 81 of whom were followed for 6 years (Table 1), the "On-Off" phenomenon rose rapidly in the third year to 22% of the entire group. It reached 35% by the end of the sixth year. By the third year, 26% of the "50% to 100% improved" group suffered from the "On-Off" phenomenon, and for parts of each day might be immobile or nearly so. By the end of the 6th year, 32% experienced the swings of this effect. At the end of the 3rd year, 7% of the "0% to 49% improved" group improved and worsened during the "On-Off Effect". At the end of the 6th year, 485 fluctuated "on and off". The "worse" group also fluctuated, in part. By the end of the 6th year, 26% would become even worse during parts of the day.

TABLE 1.   NUMBER AND PERCENTAGE OF CASES EXPERIENCING THE "ON-OFF EFFECT"

| Year | GRAND TOTAL Total # of cases | Total # On-Off | % On-Off | 50% to 100% IMPROVED Total # of cases | Total # On-Off | % On-Off | 0% to 49% IMPROVED Total # of cases | Total # On-Off | % On-Off | WORSE Total # of cases | Total # On-Off | % On-Off |
|---|---|---|---|---|---|---|---|---|---|---|---|---|
| 1 | 123 | 3 | 2% | 53 | 2 | 4% | 70 | 1 | 1% | 0 | 0 | 0% |
| 2 | 119 | 9 | 8% | 81 | 9 | 11% | 37 | 0 | 0% | 1 | 0 | 0% |
| 3 | 104 | 23 | 22% | 72 | 19 | 26% | 2 | 2 | 7% | 3 | 2 | 67% |
| 4 | 97 | 29 | 30% | 64 | 21 | 33% | 23 | 7 | 30% | 10 | 1 | 10% |
| 5 | 89 | 24 | 26% | 52 | 15 | 29% | 23 | 5 | 22% | 14 | 4 | 29% |
| 6 | 81 | 28 | 35% | 41 | 13 | 32% | 21 | 10 | 48% | 19 | 5 | 26% |

The "On-Off Effect" presented itself as a fairly consistent rhythm
in some patients, but not all.  At times this was associated with the
taking of the levodopa.  As the years passed, the "On" portion of the
rhythm tended to shorten.

Thus, finding the cause of this phenomenon is a very important
key to the mystery of how to treat Parkinson's disease.  But the
elusiveness of this mystery lies in the apparent lack of consistency
of the response of many patients to a given dose of levodopa or
blood level.  Because of this each unusual response to levodopa
should be evaluated in hope of contributing to the solution of this
problem.

Barbeau (Barbeau, 1974) and Marsden (Marsden and Parkes, 1976)
have made separate classifications of various types of "On-Off
Effect" that they have observed.  These illustrate that on the one
hand there is the "On-Off Effect" with a fairly predictably rhythm.
This is often but not always associated with the time of taking the
levodopa.

A half-hour or so after taking the medication, the Parkinson's
symptoms may disappear.  Somewhere along the way, involuntary movements or dyskinesias may develop.  After another hour or two, or
more, the dyskinesias disappear and the Parkinson's symptoms re-
appear, and for a time the patient may become literally immobile.

As example of this fairly predictable phenomenon is a patient
who by spacing his doses can walk into the theater, sit through the
play more or less immobile, with tremor, and then walk out of the
theater at the end of the play, a half-an-hour after taking a dose
of levodopa.  Another example is a man with Parkinson's disease who
delivers laundry for a living.  He can space his medication so that
he has an hour-and-a-half or two hours in the morning and a similar
period in the afternoon of usuable mobility.  His improvement,
although not perfect, is predictable enough that he manages to make
morning and afternoon deliveries of laundry and thus continues to
make a living.

On the other hand, there are patients whose "On-Off" pattern
of behavior does not seem necessarily to be related to the timing
of the dosage, nor to the levodopa blood level.  The behavior of
one of this group is charted here in Figures 1, 2 and 3, to illustrate both the unpredictability of the "on-Off Effect" as well as
the effect of sleep.

It has long been known that most of the symptoms of Parkinson's
disease disappear in the majority of patients during sleep (Bailey,
1906; April, 1966).  In fact, sleep is often an excellent means of
temporarily suppressing the symptoms of Parkinson's disease, as the
tremor is often absent for varying periods of time after awakening
(McDowell & Lee, 1976).

In order to evaluate the effect of sleep, a group of patients
whose initial improvement each day seemed to be related to sleep
and their usual awakening in the morning was studied.

Figure 1 is a graph of a patient's Parkinson's symptoms and levodopa dyskinesias as evaluated hourly by the patient and her daughter during one day from 6 a.m. until 11 p.m.  At that time the patient had taken levodopa for four months and was receiving 4 grams a day in four divided doses.

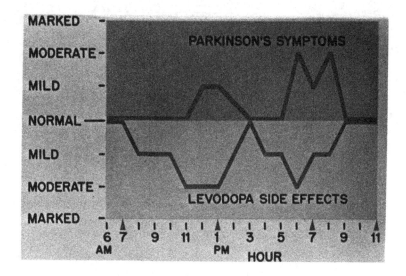

*Figure 1. Graph of a patient's Parkinson's symptoms and levodopa dyskinesias (side effects) as evaluated hourly for one day by the patient and her daughter.  The patient had been taking levodopa for 4 months and was receiving 4 grams a day in divided doses.*

In viewing this graph as a whole, it is obvious that there is a lack of correlation between the dosage, parkinson's symptoms and levodopa side effects.  However, limiting ourselves to the early morning hours, it is apparent that the patient had no symptoms of Parkinson's disease when she got out of bed at 6 a.m., some seven hours after her last gram of levodopa and one hour before the next dose of levodopa.

Figure 2 shows a composite of the patient's response to levodopa for all seven days of  this same week.  Here one sees that much of the time the patient was "normal" by her estimation. However, there is no constant rhythm and no consistent response to a given dose of levodopa.  Here in each of the seven days, the patient awakened from sleep "normal", and continued that way for at least an hour or more before developing any difficulties.

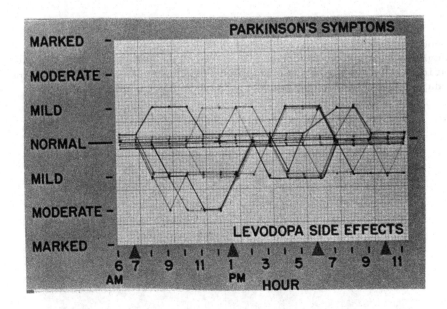

*Figure 2. Composite of patient's response to levodopa hourly for seven days of same week as Fig. 1. The levodopa "side effects" were dyskinesias (involuntary movements).*

Figure 3 is a year later, and shows a seven day composite of the day to day curves of the same patient, who was now taking 2.5 grams of levodopa in five divided doses. Here it is apparent that the patient awakened at 6 a.m. and took here levodopa half-an-hour later. On all seven days she was able to get out of bed with no discernible Parkinson's symptoms and had none for the first two hours of each day. However, the graph of Figure 3 reveals that she had immediate evidence of involuntary movements on awakening on two days, before taking her morning dose of levodopa. This may indicate a higher brain level of dopamine than expected for that hour of the day. Why this might be so is not clear. This is being emphasized, as one would expect the dopa blood level to be low at this time, and it has been so reported (*Muenter and Tyce, 1971*).

In addition to this patient, five other patients whose best time of day was upon awakening, were studied. These patients showed continuing improvement from the time of their usual awakening for one to three hours, even though one arose at 4:30 a.m. and the others from 6 to 8 a.m., on a regular basis.

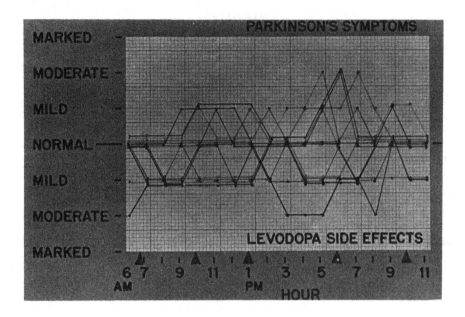

*Figure 3. Composite of patient's response to levodopa for seven
days one year after Fig. 2. The patient was now receiving
2.5 grams of levodopa in five divided doses. The patient
took her first dose of levodopa 15 min to 30 min after
arising. The levodopa "side effects" were dyskinesias
(involuntary movements).*

Thus sleep would appear to play a role in their improvement
at this time. However, the matter is complicated by the fact that
four of these patients had a great deal of parkinsonian difficulty
in the middle of the night when getting out of bed to go to the
bathroom. In addition, one patient felt "normal" on awakening.
She stated that on occasions she would then take her levodopa and
go back to sleep. When she awakened an hour or so later, she would
be much more rigid and have tremor.

While there are other possible explanations, it would appear
probable that the improvement these patients showed on awakening
was not directly related to sleep alone, but, more importantly, to
the usual time of awakening in the morning.

## ACKNOWLEDGEMENTS

Gratitude is expressed to Robert E. Cook, M.D. for his profes-
sional assistance, Anna S. Vikart, Ruby Silverstone, Mary Lewis and
Beth Robles for the technical help.

## REFERENCES

April, R.S. (1966). Observations on parkinsonian tremor in all
    night sleep. *Neurology 16*, 720-724.
Bailey, P. (1906). Diseases of the Nervous System Resulting From
    Accident and Injury. P. 332. D. Appleton & Co., New York.
Barbeau, A. (1974). The clinical physiology of side effects in
    long term L-DOPA therapy. In: *Advances in Neurology*, Vol. 5,
    Fletcher H. McDowell & André Barbeau. Raven Press,
    New York, pp. 347-365.
Marsden, C.D., and Parkes, J.D. (1976). "On-Off" effects in pat-
    ients with Parkinson's disease on chronic levodopa therapy.
    *Lancet i*, 292-296.
McDowell, F.H., and Lee, J.E. (1976). Extrapyramidal diseases.
    In: *Clinical Neurology*. Baker, A.E., and Baker, L.H., eds.
    Harper and Row, Haggerstown, Md, Chapter 26, p. 19.
Muenter, M.D., and Tyce, G.M. (1971). L-DOPA therapy in Parkinson's
    disease: Plasma L-DOPA concentrations, therapeutic response,
    and side effects. *Mayo Clinic Proc. 46*, 231-239.

# ADENYLATE CYCLASE FROM VARIOUS DOPAMINERGIC
# AREAS OF THE BRAIN AND THE ACTION OF LOXAPINE

YVONNE C. CLEMENT-CORMIER

Department of Pharmacology
The University of Texas Medical School at Houston
Houston, Texas 77025

## ABSTRACT

The present report is a comparative study of adenylate cyclase
activity in various areas of the brain identified as dopaminergic.
Low levels of dopamine were found to stimulate adenylate cyclase
from the striatum, median eminence, olfactory tubercle, nucleus
accumbens and amygdala. Apomorphine, known to mimic the pharmacological and physiological effects of dopamine, stimulated adenylate cyclase from these areas. Several different classes of drugs
effective in the treatment of schizophrenia were potent inhibitors
of the stimulation by dopamine of the enzyme from these various regions. The drugs studied included representatives of the phenothiazine, butyrophenone, dibenzodiazepine and dibenzoxazepine classes.
The inhibition by the dibenzoxazepine, loxapine, which is structurally very similar to the dibenzodiazepine, clozapine, was competitive
with respect to dopamine. The calculated inhibition constant (Ki)
for loxapine of about 15 nM was similar to that observed for some of
the more potent phenothiazines. The results, considered together
with previously published data, support the possibility that the
therapeutic effects as well as the extrapyramidal and endocrinological
side effects, of these antipsychotic agents may be attributable to
their ability to block the activation of adenylate cyclase in various
select areas of the brain.

183

# INTRODUCTION

It is well known that many antipsychotic drugs produce an extra-pyramidal syndrome indistinguishable from Parkinson's disease (Holli-ster, 1972; Hornykiewicz, 1971). These extrapyramidal side effects may arise from the ability of these drugs to block the dopamine receptor of the caudate nucleus (Carlsson, 1963; Nybäck 1968). Many investigators have indirectly characterized the dopamine receptor in physiological, pharmacological and biochemical studies. Most re-cently, a dopamine-sensitive adenylate cyclase was demonstrated in homogenates of the caudate nucleus, olfactory tubercle, and nucleus accumbens (Kebabian, 1972; Clement-Cormier, 1974, 1975; Karobath, 1974). These studies have suggested that an intimate association exists between this dopamine-sensitive adenylate cyclase and the "dopamine receptor" of these areas since the biochemical and pharma-cological properties of this enzyme were similar to the reported properties of the dopamine receptor.

Dopamine has been implicated as a neurotransmitter in several other regions of the mammalian central nervous system in addition to those areas mentioned above. Recently, the amygdala, cerebral cortex and median eminence have been identified as regions receiving dopaminergic innervation (Hornykiewicz, 1966; Ungerstedt, 1970; Björklund, 1973; Thierry, 1973; Kavanagh, 1973). Previous studies have supported the correlation between dopaminergic innervation of limbic system and the extrapyramidal motor system and the occurrence of dopamine-sensitive adenylate cyclase in these two areas (Clement-Cormier, 1974). Thus, it was of interest to verify the presence of a dopamine-sensitive adenylate cyclase in the amygdala and median eminence.

It has been proposed that the extrapyramidal side effects of the antipsychotic drugs may be related to their ability to block stimulation by dopamine of adenylate cyclase activity in the caudate nucleus and that therapeutic effects of the antipsychotic drugs may be related to a similar action on a dopamine-sensitive adenylate cyclase in the limbic system (Clement-Cormier, 1974). Furthermore, it has been suggested that the endocrinological side effects of the antipsychotic drugs may result from a blockade of dopamine receptors in the median eminence (Martin, 1973). The results presented in this communication are consistent with a model in which the dopamine receptor of neural tissue is intimately associated with a dopamine-sensitive adenylate cyclase. The results are also compatible with the possibility that inhibition of this enzyme may provide an explanation, at the molecular level, for the therapeutic effects, as well as for the side effects, of some widely used antipsychotic agents.

## METHODS

ATP (adenosine $-5^1$- triphosphate), cyclic AMP (cyclic adenosine $-3^1,5^1$- monophosphate), and EGTA (ethylene glycol-bis[β-amino ethy-lether]-N,N$^1$- tetraacetic acid) were purchased from Sigma; 3-hydroxy-tyramine (dopamine) was from CalBiochem; inorganic salts were all reagent grade; loxapine was a gift from Lederle Laboratories. All phenothiazines and related compounds were obtained, in high purity, from their commercial distributor.

The procedure for the dissection of the rat caudate nucleus [the nucleus caudate putamen *(Konig, 1970)*] olfactory tubercle and nucleus accumbens have been described *(Clement-Cormier, 1974)*. The amygdala was dissected according to the guidelines in Knippel and König for the rat brain and the median eminence as published by Kavanagh and Weisz *(1973)*.

After the tissues were obtained, they were pooled and were homogenized in 50 volumes (w/v) of 2mM tris-(hydroxymethyl) amino-methane-maleate buffer (pH 7.4)-2mM EGTA. The standard assay system (final volume 0.25ml for the median eminence and 0.5 ml for all other areas) contained (in mmol/liter): tris-(hydroxymethyl) aminomethane-maleate, 80.2; ATP, 0.3; MgSO$_4$, 1.2; theophylline 10; EGTA 0.6 (in-cluding the amount introduced with the tissue homogenate); tissue homogenate (0.025 ml for the median eminence and 0.050 ml for other areas) and test substances as indicated. Incubation was 2.5 min for all areas except the median eminence which was for 5 min at 30$^o$C. The reaction was terminated by boiling and cyclic AMP measure as described by Clement-Cormier *et al. (1975)*. Under the experimental conditions enzyme activity was proportional to time and enzyme con-centration. Protein was determined essentially by the method of Lowry *et al.(1951)*.

## RESULTS

The effects of various concentrations of dopamine and norepine-phrine on the adenylate cyclase of a homogenate of the median eminence is shown in Table 1. Adenylate cyclase activity was stimulated by low concentrations of dopamine; half maximal increase in enzyme activity was observed with 5 μM dopamine. In contrast, the β-adren-ergic agonists L-isoproterenol had no significant effect on adenylate cyclase activity with concentrations as high as 1000 μM. L-norepine-phrine stimulated adenylate cyclase activity of the median eminence to the same maximal level as did dopamine. Greater concentrations of L-norepinephrine than of dopamine were required to achieve a given increase in enzyme activity. Half-maximal stimulation of the enzyme was obtained with 30 μM L-norepinephrine and maximal stimulation was obtained with 300 μM L-norepinephrine. Similar to results ob-served in the olfactory tubercle and caudate nucleus, the increase

TABLE 1.   *EFFECT OF DOPAMINE AND NOREPINEPHRINE ON ADENYLATE CYCLASE*
*ACTIVITY IN A HOMOGENATE OF THE RAT MEDIAN EMINENCE*

| Addition | | Enzyme Activity picomoles $mg^{-1}$ $min^{-1}$ |
|---|---|---|
| None | | 78.4 |
| Dopamine | 1.0 µM | 93.4 |
| | 10.0 µM | 121.5 |
| | 100.0 µM | 136.6 |
| | 1000.0 µM | 134.5 |
| Norepinephrine | 1.0 µM | 83.4 |
| | 10.0 µM | 92.6 |
| | 100.0 µM | 118.4 |
| | 1000.0 µM | 133.0 |

*Data are expressed as the mean ± S.E.M. (N=4)*

in enzyme activity in the presence of a combination of dopamine and
L-norepinephrine interacts with the same receptor as does dopamine.
  Fluphenazine, one of the most potent phenothiazine compounds
both as an antipsychotic agent as well as in producing extrapyramidal side effects in patients, has been shown to be a potent competitive antagonist of dopamine-sensitive adenylate cyclase in the olfactory tubercle and caudate nucleus *(Clement-Cormier, 1974)*.  It was
of interest to test fluphenazine in the median eminence in addition
to the dibenzodiazepine clozapine, a potent antipsychotic with low
extrapyramidal side effects, the butyrophenone, haloperidol and
loxapine, a dibenzoxazepine whose chemical structure is very similar
to clozapine.  Table 2 shows the calculated inhibition constants
($K_i$) for these agents on several dopaminergic areas.  In all areas

TABLE 2.    *CALCULATED INHIBITION CONSTANTS (Ki) FROM SEVERAL DOPAMINERGIC AREAS OF THE BRAIN FOR REPRESENTATIVES OF THE PHENOTHIAZINE, BUTYROPHENONE, DIBENZODIAZEPINE AND DIBENZOXAZEPINE CLASSES.*

| Source of Enzyme | Enzyme Activity picomoles $mg^{-1}$ $min^{-1}$ | | $K_i$ | | | | |
|---|---|---|---|---|---|---|---|
| | Control | + Dopamine (40 μM) | Chloro-promazine | Fluphen-azine | Halo-peridol | Cloza-pine | Loxa-pine |
| Caudate nucleus | 105.1 | 280.0 | 90 nM | 8.0 nM | 32 nM | 60 nM | 15 nM |
| Olfactory tubercle | 50.9 | 109.8 | 60 nM | 7.0 nM | 30 nM | 60 nM | 14 nM |
| Nucleus accumbens | 80.0 | 120.2 | 75 nM | 7.5 nM | -. | 59 nM | 10 nM |
| Median eminence | 83.2 | 126.6 | 70 nM | 7.5 nM | 38 nM | 61 nM | 13 nM |
| Amygdala | 103.8 | 180.6 | 80 nM | - | - | - | - |

*The $K_i$ value was calculated either from relationship $Km' / Km = 1 + \frac{I}{K}$, where $Km'$ and $Km$ are the concentrations of dopamine required to give half-maximal activation of the enzyme, in the presence and absence of test substance respectively, and I is the concentration of the inhibitor from the relationship $I_{50} = K_i ( 1 + \frac{S}{Km} )$, where $I_{50}$ is the concentration of drug required to give 50% inhibition of the enzyme activity, and S is the concentration (40 μM) of dopamine.*

studied, including the amygdala, these agents inhibited dopamine stimulation of adenylate cyclase. Loxapine was found to be a rather potent inhibitor of adenylate cyclase in both the olfactory tubercle and the caudate nucleus. Further studies with loxapine in the olfactory tubercle (Figure 1) and the striatum (data not shown) indicate that this compound is a competitive inhibitor of adenylate cyclase activity.

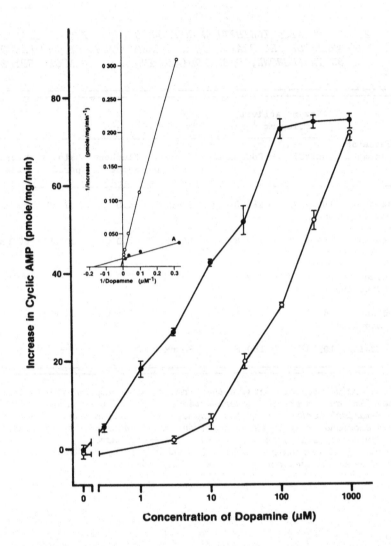

Figure 1.    Effect of various concentrations of dopamine, alone (•)
             or in combination with 0.25 μM loxapine (o), on adenylate
             cyclase activity in a homogenate of the olfactory tuber-
             cle of the rat.  In the absence of added dopamine and
             loxapine 70.0 ± 1.8 pmole of cyclic AMP mg protein$^{-1}$
             min$^{-1}$ was formed.  The increase in cyclic AMP above basal
             level (i.e., the level in the absense of both dopamine
             and loxapine) is plotted as a function of dopamine con-
             centration form 3 μM to 300 μM.  (A) control; (b) 2.5 x
             10$^{-7}$M loxapine.

## DISCUSSION

Results herein show that the dibenzoxazepine, loxapine, is a
potent inhibitor of adenylate cyclase in various dopaminergic areas
of the brain. The demonstration that loxapine is a potent competitive inhibitor of adenylate cyclase in the olfactory tubercle pre-
dicts that it is a good antipsychotic agent. However, the fact
that it is also a potent inhibitor of the caudate enzyme suggests
that its high extrapyramidal side effects may be due to its ability
to antagonize the stimulation by dopamine of the caudate enzyme.
7-OH loxapine, a natural metabolite of loxapine has recently been
shown to be a potent inhibitor of the caudate enzyme *(Coupet and
Szues, 1976).* Based on these experiments, we would predict that this
metabolite which is thought to potentially be a good antipsychotic
would also be a potent inhibitor of the olfactory tubercle enzyme.
Finally, the evidence presented here that a dopamine-sensitive
adenylate cyclase occurs in the median eminence and that antipsychotic drugs are potent antagonists of this enzyme is compatible with
with idea that the endocrinological side effects of the antipsychotic
drugs may result from a blockade of dopamine receptors in this area.

## ACKNOWLEDGEMENTS

This work was supported by NIH Grant 5 F 22 AM-01482-02.

## REFERENCES

Bjorklund, A. Moore, R.Y. Norbin, A. and Stenevi, U. (1974). The
    organization of Tubero-hypophyseal and reticulo-infundibular
    catecholamine neuron systems in the rat brain. *Brain Research
    51,* 171-191.
Carlsson, A. and Lindquist, M. (1963). Effect of chlorpromazine or
    haloperidol on formation of 3-methoxytyramine and normetane-
    phrine in mouse brain. *Acta Pharmacol. et Toxicol. 20,* 140-144.
Chen, Y.-C. and Prusoff, W.H. (1973). Relationship between the
    inhibition constant (Ki) and the concentration of inhibitor
    which causes 50 per cent inhibition ($I_{50}$) of an enzymatic re-
    action. *Biochem. Pharmacol. 22,* 3099-3108.
Clement-Cormier, Y.C., Kebabian, J.W., Petzold, G.L. and Greengard,
    P. (1974). Dopamine-sensitive adenylate cyclase in mammalian
    brain: 2 possible site of action of antipsychotic drugs. *Proc.
    Nat. Acad. Sci. 71,* 1113-1117.
Clement-Cormier, Y.C., Parrish, R.G., Petzold, G.L., Kebabian, J.W.
    and Greengard, P. (1975). Characterization of a dopamine-
    sensitive adenylate cyclase in the rat caudate nucleous.
    *J. Neurochem. 25,* 143-149.

Coupet, J. and Szucs, V.A.   (1976).   The effects of loxapine and its
       metabolites on the dopamine-sensitive adenyl cyclase of rat
       striatal homogenates.  *Fed. Proc. 35,*  456.
Hollister, L.E.   (1973).   Clinical Use of Psychotherapeutic Drugs.
       C.C. Thomas, Springfield, Illinois.
Hornykiewicz, O.   (1971).   Neurochemical pathology and pharmacology
       of brain dopamine and acetylcholine: Rational basis for the
       current drug treatment of parkinsonism.  *Contemp. Neurol. Series.*
       *8,* 34-65.
Hornykiewicz, O.   (1966).   Dopamine (3-hydroxytyramine) and brain
       function.  *Pharmacol. Rev. 18,* 925-964.
Karobath, M. and Leitich, H.   (1974).   Antipsychotic drugs and dopa-
       mine-stimulated adenylate cyclase prepared from corpus stria-
       tum of rat brain.  *Proc. Nat. Acad. Sci. USA 71,* 2915-2918.
Kavanagh, A. and Weisz, J.   (1973).   Localization of dopamine and
       norepinephrine in the medial basal hypothalamus in the rat.
       *Neuroendocrinology 13,* 201-212.
Kebabian, J.W., Petzold, G.L. and Greengard, P.   (1972).   Dopamine-
       sensitive adenylate cyclase in caudate nucleos of rat brain,
       and its similarity to the "dopamine receptor".  *Proc. Nat.*
       *Acad. Sci. USA 69,* 2145-2149.
Konig, J. and Knippel, R.   (1970).   The Rat Brain, A Stereotoxic
       Atlas of the Forebrain and Lower Parts of the Brainstem.
       Krieger, New York.
Lowry, O.H., Rosebrough, N.J., Farr, A.L. and Randall. R.J.   (1951).
       Protein measurement with the folin phenol reagent.  *J. Biol.*
       *Chem. 193,* 265-275.
Martin, J.B.   (1973).   *New Engl. J. Med.* (1973).   Neural regulation
       of growth hormone secretion.  *288,* 1384-1393.
Miller, R.J., Horn. A.S. and Iverson. L.L.,   (1974).   The action of
       neuroleptic drugs on dopamine-stimulated adenosine cyclic
       $3^1,5^1$- monophosphate production in rat striatum and limbic
       forebrain.  *Mol. Pharmacol. 10,* 759-766.
Nyback, H. and Sedvall, G.   (1968).   Effect of chlorpromazine on
       accumulation and disappearance of catecholamines formed from
       tyrosine -[14]C in the brain.  *J. Pharmacol. Exp. Ther. 162,*
       294-301.
Thierry, A.M., Blanc, G. Sabel, A., Stinus, L. and Glowinski, J.
       (1973).   Dopamine terminals in the rat cortex.  *Science 182,*
       499-501.
Ungerstedt, U.1971).   Postsynaptic supersensitivity after 6-hydroxy-
       dopamine induced degeneration of the nigro-striatal dopamine
       system.  *Acta Physiol. Scand. 367* (1): 69-94.

# PHARMACOPSYCHIATRY AND IATROGENIC PARKINSONISM

CÉSAR PÉREZ DE FRANCISCO AND RODRIGO GARNICA PORTILLO

National Institute of Neurology
México 22, D.F. México

## ABSTRACT

Through the study of the pharmacological and clinical actions of chlozapine, a new drug used in psychiatry, we are questioning one of the traditional statements on the therapeutic action of antipsychotics: the affirmation that those must have, concomitantly, antipsychotic action and intense extrapyramidal effects (drug-induced parkinsonism).

Combining our own investigations and those of other authors, the generally accepted concepts on the possible biochemical mechanisms involved in the etiology of endogenous psychosis are criticized. Although there is evidence of alterations of the dopaminergic system in schizophrenia and also changes due to the action of neuroleptics, we cannot reject, given the dissociation of effects obtained with chlozapine, the possibility that the repercussion on the nigrostriatal dopaminergic system be only one of the many probably mechanisms of action of psychotropic drugs. Thus, such anatomical and neurochemical systems could be involved only in a secondary manner in the biochemical alterations typical of schizophrenia.

## INTRODUCTION

Psychopharmacological tradition states that the incisiveness of a neuroleptic runs parallel to its capacity for unleashing drug-induced parkinsonism. In all departments of psychiatry, this positive correlation is accepted as a truth, without exception. Although the mechanism of action is not yet completely understood, it was accepted that the antipsychotic effect, that is the curative effect, of the drugs was due to the modification of the dopaminergic system.  This led to a tremendous impulse in the study of the nigro-striatal system in a great many neurochemical and neurophysiological laboratories all over the world.  But the other two systems, the mesolimbic and the tuberoinfundibular, are probably more important from the psychiatric point of view (Nieto, 1976).

During this decade, new neuroleptics have sprung up, the actions of which are more complex, and, above all, as in the case of chlo-zapine, which achieve a complete dissociation between their thera-peutic effects and their parkinsonian capacity.  So much so, that some investigators have proposed the use of that dibenzodiazepine in dyskinesias of varied etiologies.

At the Psychiatric Department of the National Institute of Neurology in Mexico, we have diagnosed post-encephalitic parkinsonian syndromes, genetic ones, as well as those produced by a great vari-ety of neuroleptics.  The experience which we have acquired with chlozapine during the past two years, revealed to us its desirable effects, but above all stimulated us to try to reason out the almost complete absence of neuroleptic impregnation with this drug.

THE NEUROLEPTIC RANGE

Our experience encompasses clinical investigations with seda-tives, polyvalent, incisive and long-acting neuroleptics.  This has allowed us to locate chlozapine reasonably well amongst them (Pérez de Francisco, Dureau, and Bury, 1965; Pérez de Francisco, 1975; Riquelme García, Pérez de Francisco, and Nieto Gómez, 1973; Pérez de Francisco, Riquelme García, and Nieto Gómez, 1972; Pérez de Francisco, and Nieto Gómez, 1966; Pérez de Francisco, 1975; Pérez de Francisco, 1970; Pérez de Francisco, Riquelme García, and Nieto Gómez, 1972; Nieto, Krassowsky; Pérez de Francisco, Dávila, Ortíz, and Reséndiz, 1964; Pérez de Francisco, 1972; Pérez de Francisco and Lecona Desmond, 1973; Pérez de Francisco, 1972; Pérez de Francisco, 1972; Pérez de Francisco and Gómez, 1971; Pérez de Francisco and Riquelme García, 1971).

In a recent investigation with pipothiazine, we analyzed the undesirable effects in a population of 25 studied patients.  There was tremor, akathisia, different levels and distributions of mus-cular hypertonia, and a few cases with difficulty in visual accomo-dation.  Such symptoms and signs are not rare findings in any anti-psychotic treatment (Pérez de Francisco, in press).

With the same therapeutic intentions and in a population of 38 patients with similar psychopathological profiles, we have used chlozapine in doses of up to 500 mg per day.  In this group, there were also collateral and/or undesirable effects, but within the spectrum of mental confusion and psychomotor excitation, or that of orthostatic hypotension.  Only four patients developed sialorrhea, one had a slight rigidity of the lower jaw, and another discrete tremor and barely perceptible muscular rigidity (Perez de Francisco

*and Garnica Portillo).*  Given our medical philosophy on the use of
antiparkinsonian drugs in antipsychotic treatments, that is jointly
with the neuroleptics used, we cannot attribute the absence of drug-
induced parkinsonism to their effect.

It may be important to clarify this criterion on the use of
antiparkinsonians.  We never use them routinely, and do so only in
emergency situations such as in a dystonis with torticollis.  And
the reasons for not using them routinely are: if antiparkinsonian
drugs reduce the intensity of the collateral effects, it is logical
to think that they also diminish the antipsychotic potency of the
neuroleptic being used.  The optimal therapeutic dosage of neuroleptics is located at the subparkinsonian level.  The isolated
effect of the antiparkinsonian medicine influences the evolution
of the sickness as it produces discrete excitation which clearly
opposes the main intention of the majority of neuroleptic cures.
And, finally, the addiction to antiparkinsonians which we observe
more frequently among today's youth, has allowed us to see toxic
psychoses due to such drugs, which definitely proves that the
active principles with antiparkinsonian effects are also psycho-
tomimetics *(Pérez de Francisco, Nieto Gómez and Castilla, 1970).*
We insist that their use is indicated only in cases of extreme
impregnation or in acute emergency situations.

## COMMENTARY

Already in 1969, Stille and Hippius noted how ignorant we are
of the mechanisms of action of psychopharmacological drugs in
general.  In that Symposium which was held in Liege, all partici-
pants generally agreed that the therapeutic action of a neuroleptic
is indefectibly tied to the extrapyramidal effects it produces.
Also, some laboratory experiments with animals allow the definition
of the neuroleptic profile of an active principle:
    1) cataleptogenic or catatonigenic action,
    2) action antagonistic to the stereotyped reactions produced
       by apomorphine and by amphatamines,
    3) the inhibitory action of the conditioned reflex of escape.
On that occasion they should also have questioned such statements
when dealing with chlozapine which is a drug with antipsychotic
action but without parkinsonizing effects.

We would not like to dwell upon the chemical synthesis and
characteristics of chlozapine, but to recall the work of Gerlach et al.
*(1975).*    They compared the antipsychotic actions of chlozapine
and haloperidol, finding them similar, although chlozapine was
more effective in certain symptoms such as anxiety, sleep induction,
as well as in conceptual disorganization and mannerisms *(Gerlach,
Koppelhus, Helweg and Monrad, 1975).*

At the Psychiatric Department of the National Institute of
Neurology, we have also studied chlozapine in relation with what
we have called ranges of action.  In about half of over 50 patients,

we used doses which varied from 95 to 500 mg (antipsychotic range),
while in the others we used only an evening doses of 25 to 50 mg,
with the induction of sleep as our only goal.  We were able to
observe the antipsychotic effects when we used high doses, with
minimal or nonexistant extrapyramidal collateral effects, and the
easy induction of sleep in the cases which received low doses.
Of course, we did observe collateral effects not related at all to
extrapyramidal action (Pérez de Francisco and Garnica Portillo,
in press).

Some authors have attributed the absence of extrapyramidal
effects with chlozapine to the fact that it would affect the dopaminergic system very little.  For example, the transformation of
dopamine to its immediate metabolite, homovanillic acid (HVA) was
investigated in 2 patients treated with chlozapine and compared
with three who received haloperidol.  The authors themselves admit
in the small sample involved, but they recognize that there seems
to exist a tendency to less conversion of dopamine to HVA with
chlozapine as compared with haloperidol.

The physiopathogenesis could be outlined in the following manner.
Chlozapine would block the dopaminergic receptors, but its anticholinergic properties would counterarrest the clinical and experimental effects due to the diminution of dopamine in the corpus
striatum.  Chlozapine, as opposed to haloperidol, would show little
affinity for the dopaminergic receptors of the striated body, and
on the other hand, would have a greater affinity for the receptors
located in the limbic system, which would be very important in
explaining and producing its antipsychotic effect.

In general, it is accepted that the antipsychotic action of
neuroleptics is due to their antidopaminergic capacity, which is
the basis for the positive correlation between antipsychotic action
and extrapyramidal effects.  However, it seems that chlozapine
possesses a slight antidopaminergic effect but an intense antinoradrenergic action.  It is possible that this antinoradrenergic
effect be involved in the antipsychotic mechanism of action
(Boissier, Hippius and Pichot, 1974).

Due to its minimal extrapyramidal effects, and its possible
action on the cholinergic system, we are working on the possibility
that chlozapine functions on that cholinergic system in one way or
the other, depending upon the patient.  In some patients with
clinical manifestations of psychomotor excitation and mental confusion, chlozapine would exert an anticholinergic effect, and the
toxic results would be comparable to those caused by the atropinics.
In exchange, there would be the opposite effect in patients where
sialorrhea and enuresis would suggest clear cholinomimetic actions.
We cannot deny how disconcerting have been these findings which we
have not been able to correlate positively to any kind of a variable.  We are starting to suspect in our patients genetic differences
which would set a different metabolic pathway for cholozapine to
follow.

# REFERENCES

Nieto, G.D. (1976). Psicosis anfetamínicas. In: *Editores Jorge Maisterrena y Carlos Valverde R. Las anfetaminas.* Publicación de trabajos de investigacion. Cuadernos cientificos CEMEF Vol. 6. México.

Perez de Francisco, C., Dureau, F. and Bury, A.J. (1965). Un neurolentico mayor: el haloperidol. *Neurología, Neurocirugía, Psiquiatría.* 6, 55-61.

Pérez de Francisco, C. (1975). Tratamientos biológicos de las psicosis. *La Prensa Médica Mexicana.* Vol. XI Números 7-8, 221-232.

Riquelme García, E., Pérez de Francisco, C., and Nieto Gómez, D. (1973). Tratamiento de sostén y resocialización de pacientes psicóticos cróni cos con penfluridol, un neuroléptico de accion prolongada. *Psiquia tría. 3.* 47-51.

Pérez de Francisco, C., Riquelme García, E. and Nieto Gómez, D. (1972). Tratamiento de sostén en pacientes psicóticos con pimozide. Reporte de 50 casos. *Revista Psiquiátrica Gharma. 52.* 27-33.

Pérez de Francisco, C.,, Nieto Gómez, D. (1966). Tratamiento de las psicosis con tioridazina. *Neurología, Neurocirugía, Psiquiatría 7,* 225-230.

Pérez de Francisco, C. (1975). Three long-acting neuroleptic drugs. Comparative study. *International Journal of Neurology 10,* 41-45.

Pérez de Francisco, C. (1970). Nuevos tratamientos en la psicosis maniacodepresive. *Revista del Instituto Nacional de Neurología 4,* 48-57.

Pérez de Francisco, C., Riquelme García, E., and Nieto Gomez, D. (1972). Investigación clínica del pimozide, un neuroléptico de acción prolongada. *Revista APAL 2,* 115-120.

Nisto, D.;, Krassowsky;, J., Pérez de Francisco, C., Dávila, J., Ortíz, R. and Reséndiz, J. (1964). Ensayos terapeuticos con un nueva derivado de la tioridazina. *Neurología, Neurocirugía, Psiquiatris 5,* 165-166.

Pérez de Francisco, C. (1972). Ensayo clinica de un neuroléptico de acción prolongada (Fluspirilene). *Actas Luson Espanolas de Neurología y Psiquiatria 30.*

Pérez de Francisco, C. and Lecona Desmond, R. (1973). El sulpiride en neurosis y trastornos de personalidad. *Revista médica del Hospital General de México, 36,* 575-586.

Pérez de Francisco, C. (1972). Butirofenonas y difenilbutilpiperidinas. Coloquio interdisciplinario sobre los neurolépticos. Hospital psiquiátrico Fray Bernardino Alvarez, S.S.A. Sandoz de México, S.A. México, D.F., 29 de septiembre pp. 23-31.

Pérez de Francisco, C. and Gómez, S. (1971). Utilización del sulpiride en psicocardiología. *Revista de la Facultad de Medicina.* Vol. XIV Num. 6. México, noviembre-diciembre. pp. 447-451.

Pérez de Francisco, C. and Riquelme García, E. (1971). Una butirofenona
    acción prolongada. Evaluación clínica del pimozida. V
    Congreso Mundial de Psiquiatría. *La Prensa Médica Mexicana*.
    México, p. 464.
Pérez de Francisco, C.; Gaxiola Rodriguez, B.E.; Velez M.: Pipo-
    tiacina y farmacoterapia de large accion. *Revista del
    Instituto Nacional de Neurologia*. (En prensa).
Perez de Francisco, C. and Garnica Portillo, R.: Clozapina en farma-
    copsiquiatría clínica. Utilización de la franja antipsicótica
    en un estudio abierto de 38 cases. *Medicina. Revista Mexi-
    cana. in press.*
Pérez de Francisco, C.: Nisto Gómez, D.; Castilla, J. (1970). Psicosis
    tóxicas. *Revista El Médico*. Año 20 No. 7. México, pp. 50-51.
Gerlach, J., P. Koppelhus, E. Helweg and A. Monra (1975). Clozapine and
    Haloperidol in a Single-Blind Cross-Over Trial: Therapeutic
    and Biochemical Aspects in the Treatment of Schizophrenia.
    En: On the methodology of the pharmacological and clinical
    trials of psychotropic drugs. Simposic llevado a cabo en
    Moscú.
Boissier, J.R., Hippius, H. and Pichot, P. (1975). Neuropsychopharma-
    cology Proceedings of the IX Congress of the Collegium Inter-
    nationale Neuropsuchopharmacologicum. Paris, 7-12,
    July, 1974. Excerpta Medica, Amsterdam.

# COMPARISON OF LITHIUM AND HALOPERIDOL THERAPY IN GILLES DE LA TOURETTE SYNDROME

H.M. ERICKSON, JR., J.E. GOGGIN AND F.S. MESSIHA

Departments of Psychiatry, Pharmacology and Therapeutics
and Pediatrics
Texas Tech University School of Medicine
Lubbock, Texas 79409

## ABSTRACT

Three patients suffering from Gilles de la Tourette Syndrome were initially treated with haloperidol. Depressive side effects and symptom breakthrough necessitated the search for another agent. The efficacy of lithium carbonate in treating stereotyped hyperkinetic behavior (such as is seen in Gilles de la Tourette syndrome) prompted the evaluation of lithium carbonate. An objective behavioral observation technique, clinical ratings and the patient's subjective reports were used to systematically record the response to treatment during the entire course of the study. Initially blood plasma $Li^+$ levels in the 0.5 to 0.6 mEq/L range were obtained and these correlated with reduced frequency, as well as intensity, of involuntary motor acts (tics) and sounds. When the $Li^+$ blood levels had stabilized at 0.8 to 0.9 mEq/L the major tics and involuntary sounds cleared dramatically.. The patients experienced no side effects and have been followed for several months without recurrence of the original symptoms.

## INTRODUCTION

Gilles de la Tourette *(1885)*, a student of Charcot at the Salpetriere in Paris  has described a syndrome characterized by the onset of involuntary tics in late childhood which progressively increased after puberty and were often associated with coughing, jumping and other motor outbursts.  The most distinctive feature of the syndrome is the coprolalia, or profanity, that accompanies these tics.  In many cases involuntary guttural or barking sounds may preceed and/or accompany the coprolalia.  Echolalia may also be present.  The incidence of Gilles de la Tourette syndrome (T.S.) is unknown, however Woodrow *(1974)* suggests a prevalence of 4 cases per 100,000.  Woodrow *(1974)* also reports that T.S. is more common in males than females (3:1).  Indirect evidence suggests dopaminergic dysfunction in T.S. as indicated by increased dopamine (DA) excretion *(Messiha et al., 1971; Messiha and Knopp, 1976)*.  Increased DA excretion has also been observed in manic states and tends to decrease towards normal levels with subsequent stabilization on lithium carbonate ($Li_2CO_3$) *(Messiha et al., 1970; Messiha et al., 1974)*.  The management of stereotyped hyperkinetic behavior, as seen in T.S. by a DA-receptor blocker such as haloperidol (HAL), coupled with the favorable response of dyskinesias, i.e. chorea *(Dalen, 1973)*, to lithium therapy prompted the evaluation of $Li_2CO_3$ in T.S. and its comparison to HAL.

## METHOD

Case 1 is a 15 year old boy of superior intelligence.  At age 10 years facial tics and involuntary "hissing" sounds were noted. Two years later these symptoms were replaced with bilateral, major tics involving the shoulders and by coprolalia, associated at times with copropraxia.  By age 13 these symptoms were so severe that they almost precluded his attending school in spite of high scholastic ability.  Following 18 months of unsuccessful psychotherapy the patient was admitted to our clinic and the diagnosis of Gilles de la Tourette syndrome was made.  Classical treatment with HAL 1.0 mg. t.i.d resulted in complete remission of symptoms.  However, a personality change involving excessive dependence and dullness with loss of spontaneity, prompted us to treat the patient with $Li_2CO_3$.

To obtain an objective analysis of lithium's effectiveness in ameliorating the target symptoms of T.S. a behavioral observation technique was used.  The observation technique was a modified version of the time-sampling method described by Goggin *(1975)*.  The patient's symptoms were systematically recorded for 10 minutes during every office visit in an experimental room setting through an observation mirror.  The patients were aware they were being observed for purposes of the study.  The behavioral observation

TABLE 1.  BEHAVIOR RATING FORM (PARENT RATING)

Patient Name_____

DIRECTIONS: Please circle number alongside the term that most appro-
            priately applies to your child now:

| MY CHILD | NOT AT ALL | JUST A LITTLE | QUITE A BIT | VERY MUCH |
|---|---|---|---|---|
| 1. Is slow, lethargic, passive, dependent | 0 | 1 | 2 | 3 |
| 2. Hands in pockets | 0 | 1 | 2 | 3 |
| 3. Obscene gestures | 0 | 1 | 2 | 3 |
| 4. Is excitable, impulsive | 0 | 1 | 2 | 3 |
| 5. Unusual movements | 0 | 1 | 2 | 3 |
| 6. Is easily frustrated, demands must be met immediately | 0 | 1 | 2 | 3 |
| 7. Profane language | 0 | 1 | 2 | 3 |
| 8. Tics | 0 | 1 | 2 | 3 |
| 9. Noises | 0 | 1 | 2 | 3 |
| 10. Explodes when he does not get his way (temper tantrum) | 0 | 1 | 2 | 3 |

COMMENT: In your judgment, is your child
         since your first rating
         (Circle One)        Worse=0  Same=1  Improved=2  Improved=3

How serious a problem do you
think your child has at this
time?  (Circle One)          None=0 Minor=1  Moderate=2     Severe=3

categories included individually designated target symptoms of T.S.
Each specified behavior was scored immediately after it occurred.
The target symptoms measured included involuntary sounds, coprolalia
and involuntary motor acts (tics).  Involuntary sounds included all
inarticulate utterances (barks, grunts and helps, et cetera) and

verbalizations which were phonetically similar to obscenities but are disguised by the patient. Involuntary motor acts included all facial grimaces as well as bodily tics. Ratings were independently made by the physician and the parents at the time of $Li^+$ blood determinations. The rating scale is shown in Table 1. Numbers 0 to 3 on the clinical response ordinates represent a clinical rating scale that ranges from 0, reflecting no symptoms at all, to 3, indicating severe symptoms.

HAL was decreased from a daily dosage of 3.0 mg to 1.5 mg prior to discontinuing all medication for seven days. This was followed by increasing dosages of $Li_2CO_3$. HAL was co-administered with $Li_2CO_3$ therapy to minimize the reoccurrence of symptoms. Blood samples were obtained for the quantitative determination of plasma $Li^+$ concentration by atomic absorption spectroscopy through-out the study.

## RESULTS

Figure 2 depicts the effect of HAL and $Li_2CO_3$ on the patient's involuntary sounds. While he was receiving HAL 3 mg/day he had no involuntary sounds or involuntary motor acts. When HAL was decreased to 1.5 mg/day a mild exacerbation of target symptoms was evident. During the drug-free period the symptoms reoccurred to the very severe level. The behavioral assessment of the involuntary sounds shown in Figure 1 is inconsistent with the clinical ratings. An initial clinical response with institution of lithium carbonate occurred and this correlated with the plasma $Li^+$ level as seen in Figure 3. This initial response to lithium did not completely clear the involuntary sounds, and because the patient had enrolled in a summer school class it was decided to reinstitute a very small amount (0.25 mg/day) of HAL. This brought about further ameliora-tion of the involuntary sounds. Discontinuation of HAL and con-tinued build-up of $Li_2CO_3$ to a maintenance dosage of 1,800 mg/day resulted in complete remission of symptoms at plasma $Li^+$ of 0.8 to 0.9 mEq/L. Late in the course of the study the patient's daily dose of lithium was increased to 2,100 mg/day for the purpose of deter-mining the effect of this higher dosage on blood level.

The patient's coprolalia responded well to lithium therapy as seen in Figure 2. The coprolalia responded to lithium in a manner comparable to the involuntary sounds. The patient has not exper-ienced the depressed, dependent behavior on $Li_2CO_3$ that occurred during HAL therapy. On the behavioral observation technique the patient showed a greater frequency of coprolalia while on HAL therapy compared to his later response to lithium.

Figure 3 shows blood plasma $Li^+$ concentration and the response of involuntary motor acts (tics) to drug therapy. The frequency and intensity of tics respond initially to lithium treatment at a

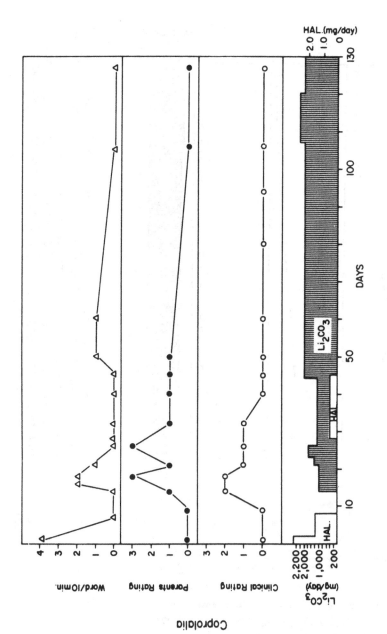

*Figure 1.* Response of coprolalia to treatment with haloperidol (HAL) and lithium carbonate (Li₂CO₃) alone and combined. Drug dosages expressed as mg/day. Coprolalia evaluated by three raters on a scale of 0 to 3 with 0 indicating the absence of symptoms and 3 reflecting severe symptoms.

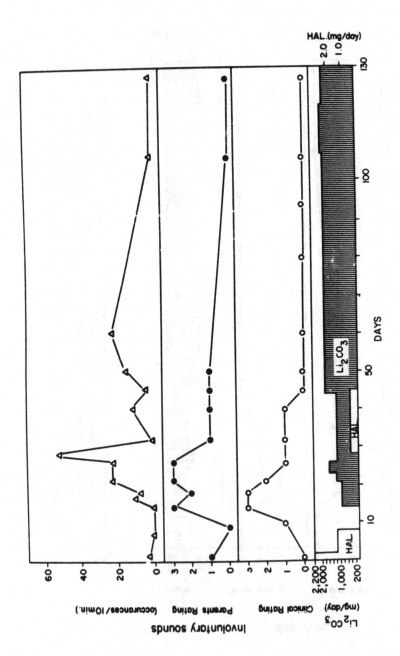

Figure 2. Response of involuntary sounds to treatment with haloperidol (HAL) and lithium carbonate (Li₂CO₃) alone and combined. Drug dosages expressed as mg/day. Involuntary sounds evaluated by two raters on a scale of 0 to 3 with 0 indicating absence of symptoms and 3 reflecting severe symptoms. The upper graph represents frequency of involuntary sounds expressed as occurrences/10 minutes.

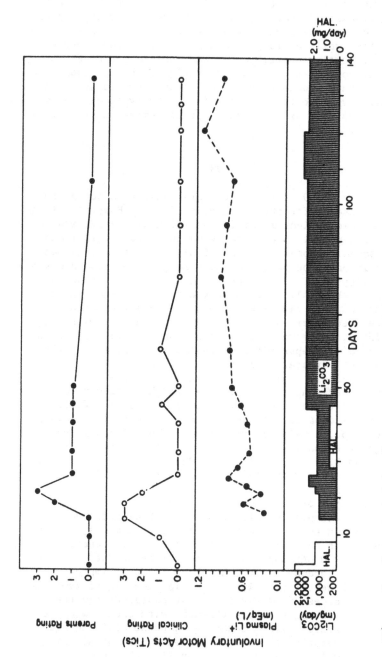

*Figure 3.* Response of involuntary motor acts (tics) to treatment with haloperidol (HAL) and lithium carbonate (Li₂CO₃) alone and combined. Drug dosages expressed as mg/day. Tics evaluated by three raters on a sclae of 0 to 3 with 0 indicating absence of symptoms and 3 reflecting severe symptoms.

blood lithium level of 0.5 to 0.6 mEq/L.  This was followed by a complete remission of tics at a blood level of 0.8 to 1.0 mEq/L.

Two additional T.S. patients are being successfully treated with $Li_2CO_3$.  One of these was suffering from severe depression with suicidal ideation while on long term HAL therapy.  The other experienced severe depression shortly after the institution of HAL necessitating its discontinuation.  The patient's disabling major motor tics and involuntary sounds were dramatically improved as reflected in their subjective reports, the behavioral observations and clinical ratings.  Both have experienced a marked remission of symptoms at plasma $Li^+$ levels of 0.8 to 1.0 mEq/L.

## DISCUSSION

In this study $Li_2CO_3$ therapy strongly suggests a new pharmacotherapeutic approach for the management of T.S.  However, little is known of the biochemical mechanism by which $Li^+$ exerts its pharmacological and behavioral effects on this neurological disorder. One of us *(Messiha)* proposed the use of $Li_2CO_3$ in the management of T.S.  This is based on the reported relationship between dopaminergic overactivity and T.S. *(Messiha et al., 1971)*.  Furthermore, abnormalities in the small cells of the corpus striatum, an area of high DA content which is involved in the regulation of motor activity, have been observed in the brain of a patient with T.S. *(Balthazar, 1956)*.  Moreover, brain DA has been implicated in the pathophysiology of extrapyramidal disorders as indicated by the reduced content of striatal DA in Parkinson's disease *(Ehringer and Hornykiewic, 1960)*.  This suggests an inverse relationship in the mechanisms underlying the akinetic and dyskinetic movement disorders relative to functional amounts of DA and/or an altered sensitivity of the dopaminergic receptors.  For example, administration of levodopa, a DA precursor, improves Parkinson's symptoms, while prolonged treatment may induce dyskinesia.  Hyperkinetic disorders such as T.S. and Huntington's Chorea are aggravated by levodopa but successfully treated with a central dopamine receptor-blocker such as HAL.

Other modalities of treatment have been utilized in the management of T.S.  For example, barbituates, phenothiazines, sympathomimetics, insulin shock, electroconvulsive treatments, psychotherapy and hypnosis have all been tried with little benefit to T.S. patients.  Since 1960 HAL has been considered treatment of choice for these patients because it brought about dramatic improvement of symptomatology.  However, this initial rapid clearing of symptoms at relatively low doses of HAL is often not sustained and the symptoms tend to eventually "break through" with each new higher dosage level.  Fernando, *(1976)* describes a personality change including loss of spontaneity which occurred in two of his six T.S. patients.  Similarly, a marked personality change as a consequence of HAL therapy was noted in our first T.S. patient from

being a spontaneous, gregarious teenager to being dependent and
insecure. The fact that the patient's coprolalia on the behavioral
assessment reached its highest peak during the initial stage of
HAL therapy was inconsistent with the clinical ratings. Perhaps
the patient's high level of copropalia was related to anxiety about
being observed for the first time. Our successful use of $Li_2CO_3$
in this T.S. patient has been supported by the marked improvement
of two other cases being treated with $Li_2CO_3$ alone. This suggests
the use of $Li_2CO_3$ in Gilles de la Tourette disease and other
tic-like syndromes. A search of the literature revealed no other
studies on the efficacy of $Li_2CO_3$ in the treatment of Gilles de la
Tourette syndrome *(Dalen, 1973)*. Our findings suggest that hypersensitivity and/or hyperactivity of the dopaminergic system may
be an important mechanism closely linked to the etiology of T.S.

## REFERENCES

Balthazar, K. (1956). Ueber das anatomische Substrat der general-
        isierten Tic-krankheit (maldie des tics, Gilles de la Tour-
        ette): Entwicklungshemmung des Corpus Striatum. *Arch.
        psychiat. Nervekr. 195,* 531-549.
Dalen, P. (1973). Lithium therapy in Huntington's Chorea and
        tardive dyskenesia. *Lancet i,* 107-108.
Ehringer, H. and Hornykiewicz, O. (1960). Verteilungvon Noradrena-
        lin und Dopamine im Gehirn des Menschen und ihr verhalten be:
        Erkrankungen des extrapyramidalen systems. *Klin. Wsch. 38,*
        1236-1239.
Fernando, S.J.M. (1976). Six cases of Gilles de la Tourette's
        Syndrome. *Brit. J. Psychiat. 128,* 436-441.
Gilles de la Tourette, (1885). Etude sur une affection nerveuse
        caracterisee par de l'incordination motorice accompagnee
        d'echolalie et de coprolali. *Arch. Peurol. (Paris) 9,* 158-200.
Goggin, J.E. (1975). Sex differences in theactivity level of pre-
        school children as a possible precursor of hyperactivity.
        *J. Genet. Psychol. 127,* 75-81.
Messiha, F.S., Agallianos, D. and Clower, C. (1970). Dopamine
        excretion in affective states and following lithium carbonate
        therapy. *Nature 225,* 868-869.
Messiha, F.S., Knopp, W., Vanecko, S., O'Brien, J., Corson, S.
        (1971). Haloperidol therapy in Tourette's syndrome: Neuro-
        logical, biochemical and behavioral correlates. *Life Science
        10 (1),* 449-457.
Messiha, F.S., Savage, C., Turek, I. and Hanlon, T. (1974). A
        psychopharmacological study of catecholamines in affective
        disorders. *J. Nerv. Ment. Dis. 158,* 338-347.
Messiha, F. and Knopp, W. (1976). A study of endogenous dopamine
        metabolism in Gilles de la Tourette's disease. *Dis. Nerv.
        Syst. 37,* 470-473.
Woodrow, K.M. (1974). Gilles de la Tourette's disease - A review.
        *Amer. J. Psychiatry. 131,* 1000-1003.

# DOPAMINE RECEPTORS HYPERSENSITIVITY: FURTHER CONFIRMATION FOLLOWING DRUG ABUSE MODEL

ABRAHAM FLEMENBAUM

Department of Psychiatry
Texas Tech University School of Medicine
Lubbock, Texas 79409

## ABSTRACT

Controversial multiple investigations have reported that chronic administration of amphetamine or similar drugs in different animals produces a reverse tolerance or a receptor hypersensitivity. However, most studies utilized large doses given chronically and for lengthy periods of time.

Real life drug abusers tend to utilize drugs in a cyclic pattern of intermittently increasing doses and then "crashing off" depending on the availability of drugs and psychiatric treatment.

In this experiment I intended to demonstrate receptor hypersensitivity with less chronic administration of drugs (in this case only six dosages) given in about two weeks, intermittently, and in increasing dosages to simulate somewhat closer a drug abuse model. I also utilized a lengthier period of time of waiting in-between the pretreatment and post-treatment evaluation (eight weeks). The subjects were 16 Sprague-Dawley rats of initial weight of 150 – 200 grams, acclimated to photoelectric cell cages. They were given either D- or L-amphetamine in alternating days for two weeks and in increasing dosages. Both activity and stereotype behavior (SB) were measured. The animals were given eight weeks of rest and then retested with a subthreshold dose of the same drug previously utilized and two days later with the smallest dose of the same medication again. The results showed that the latency and the

threshold was decreased and the response was maximized but this was
statistically true only for SB, as it did not reach statistical
significance for hyperactivity.

The relationship of this phenomenon of dopamine receptor hypersensitivity and the clinical findings in dyskinetic disorders, is
discussed; also some ideas for further research in this area are
brought to light.

## INTRODUCTION

While many studies have shown no change in behavior or tolerance
with repetitive administration of amphetamine, or similar drugs, a
number of papers have reported progressive changes ("reverse tolerance") associated with repetitive and continuous administration of
amphetamine-like substances to different species of animals.  The
administration of cocaine to dogs and rats has been associated
with increasing susceptibility to cocaine-induced convulsions and
for amphetamine-increased effects on activity and SB.  (Mago, 1969;
Segal and Mandell, 1974; Ellinwood and Kilbey, 1975; Klawans and
Margolin, 1975; Post and Kopanda, 1976).

Post and co-workers demonstrated a progression of severity of
cocaine-induced dyskinesia in animals treated for more than ten
weeks.  By comparing this with Lidocaine, a compound with local
anesthetic potency equal to cocaine but with no known amine potentiation, they discounted amine effects and found a similarity in
the quality and course of the effects of both drugs to the phenomenon of electrical kindling.  They observed that a repetitive but
intermittent stimulation is critical for the development of electrical kindling, but that chronic non-intermittent stimulation will
retard the kindling phenomenon.  (Post and Kopanda, 1976).

Onthe other hand, Klawans and Margolin, (1975b) demonstrated
amphetamine induced dopaminergic hypersensitivity in guinea pigs
treated non-intermittently (daily) for three weeks, and re-evalu-
ated repeatedly after several days to a one month interval (see
Discussion).  I found that non-intermittent pharmacological stimulation of up to ten weeks is the norm for most of the previous
reports while intermittent stimulation methodology has been applied
mainly in electrical stimulation studies.

Further demonstration of receptor hypersensitivity is important
to the understanding of the pathoneurophysiology of not only some
psychoses, but also on L-dopa-induced dyskinesia and other dyskinetic disorders.  Because of reported species and strain differences
in dopamine receptor sensitivity (Segal et al., 1975), it is
important to duplicate the above experiments with the following
differences: 1. Use a different species of research animal.  2.
Perform intermittent pharmacological stimulation of the receptors.
3. Expose the animals to relatively short drug periods.  4. Allow
long "off" drugs period of time before retesting.

## METHOD

The subjects of this study were 16 male Sprague-Dawley rats of 150 to 200 grams of initial weight. Housed in groups of four, the rats were given one week of acclimation to photoelectric cell cages, and one week of observation of activity and SB after saline injections. The animals were divided in two groups of eight and given six doses each of either D- or L-amphetamine on alternating days with weekends off and at increasing dosages (See Figures 1 and 2) up to 3.5 mg/kg of d-amphetamine and 12.5 mg/kg of l-amphetamine.

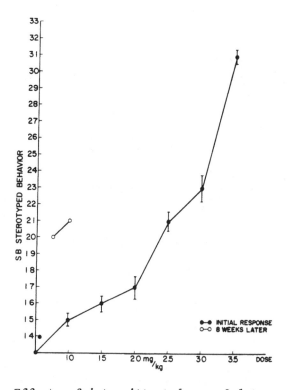

*Figure 1. Effects of intermittent doses of d-Amp on S.B.*

All injections were given IP at 1ml/kg. Both hyperactivity and SB were measured at the same time every day for two hours, beginning 5-10 minutes after medication. The animals were then given eight weeks of rest before a subthreshold, and two days later the smallest test dose of the same drug was tried again. The data were analyzed with the t-test utilizing pooled variances (Table I).

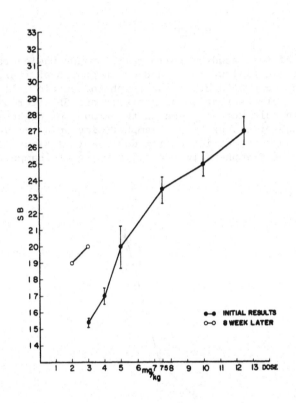

*Figure 2. Effects of intermittent dose of L-Amp on S.B.*

## RESULTS

### A. INITIAL RESPONSE

Figures 1 and 2 demonstrate statistically significant increases of SB with each increase of the dose of both D- and L-amphetamine. Figures 3 and 4 are the same except that they measure activity. The activity increases with the dose up to a point at which time it decreases. We have observed this phenomenon before as related with the animals presenting such high levels of SB that the general activity measured by the counter decreases. Also and probably because of large variance the increases in activity are not always statistically significant when increasing the dose.

### B. RESPONSE AFTER EIGHT WEEKS

All the figures also show the results of the measurements of SB and activity eight weeks after termination of the first series

TABLE 1.   EXPERIMENT ONE. D-AMPHETAMINE COMPARISON OF SUBTHRESHOLD
           + SMALLEST DOSE AFTER EIGHT WEEKS TO SMALLEST INITIAL DOSE

|       | $\bar{X}$ | SD | t | P |
|-------|------|-----|------|-------|
| SB 1  | 15.0 | 0.7 | - | - |
| SB 2  | 20.7 | 1.1 | 18.2 | 0.000 |
| Act 1 | 903  | 275 | - | - |
| Act 2 | 1555.7 | 455 | 3.4 | 0.01 |

TABLE 1.   EXPERIMENT TWO.   L-AMPHETAMINE COMPARISON OF SUBTHRESHOLD
           + SMALLEST DOSE AFTER EIGHT WEEKS TO SMALLEST INITIAL DOSE.

|       | $\bar{X}$ | SD | t | P |
|-------|------|-----|------|-------|
| SB 1  | 15.4 | 0.5 | - | - |
| SB 2  | 19.9 | 0.6 | 15.7 | 0.000 |
| Act 1 | 976  | 421 | - | - |
| Act 2 | 1182.7 | 173 | 1.32 | NS (0.11) |

NOTE: SB 1 = Stereotyped behavior on first trial on 1.0 mg/kg.
      SB 2 = Average obtained ten weeks later on D-amphetamine 0.5
             and then 1.0 mg/kg.
      Act 1 = Same as SB 1 but measuring activity.
      Act 2 = Same as SB 2.

of six shots.  Both activity and SB were measured at subthreshold
doses of .5 mg of D-amphetamine, and two days later at the minimum
dose of 1.0 mg/kg of the same drug in the same eight animals, or
the subthreshold dose of 2 mg/kg of L-amphetamine and two days
later at the minimum dose previously utilized of 3.0 mg/kg.  Here
again there is a statistically significant increase of SB and an
increase of activity which was not statistically significant (See
all Figures and Table I).
     Briefly, for both D- and L-amphetamine there was an increase
of SB in direct correlation with increases of the dose and this
was always significant.  There was also a decrease of latency and
threshold to the SB effectiveness of the drugs in the sense that
subthreshold doses produced significantly higher levels of SB that

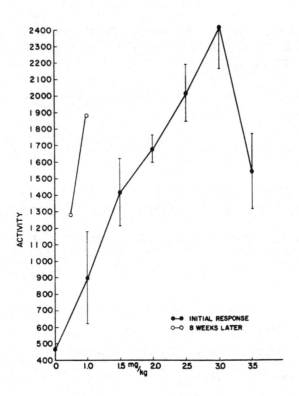

*Figure 3. Effects of intermittent doses of D-Amphetamine on activity.*

started earlier in the experimental session. Although the same can
be said for the measurements of hyperactivity, the measurements
did not always reach significance, thus showed only a trend in the
same direction.

## DISCUSSION

The duplication of the work reported above again suggests the
formation of a type of "reverse tolerance", or what Klawans called
agonist-induced hypersensitivity. However, this was done with some
differences from previous studies, i.e., most previous studies
reviewed utilized continuous (non-intermittent) administration of
amphetamine, or amphetamine-like substances. Klawans administered
daily doses of amphetamine for three weeks. His animals were tested
again for SB on days 3,7,10,20 and 34. This readministration of
the drugs for testing and retesting may have helped to maintain a
receptor state compatible with high SB response. Also, in human
life situations, amphetamine or similar drug abusers tend to
utilize them on an "on" and "off" basis, with periods of "highs"

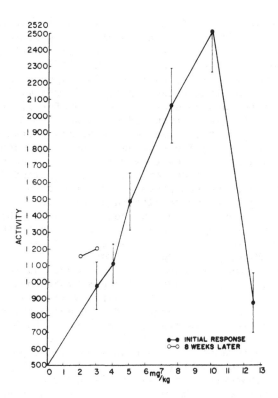

*Figure 4. Effects of intermittent doses of L-Amphetamine on activity.*

and increasing doses, and then "crashes" with no drug use.  Abusers
also undergo long periods without drugs for varied reasons.  To
follow the drug abuse model more closely, it was determined to give
the drugs intermittently and in increasing doses.  The drugs were
used for a short period of time:  six doses within less than three
weeks.  Then the rats were completely unexposed to drugs for eight
weeks before retesting for SB and hyperactivity.  Test results
showed a statistically significant increase of SB and a tendency
(but it did not reach statistical significance) for an increase of
hyperactivity.  These results are compatible with *intermittent*
agonist-induced receptor hypersensitivity at the DA level as SB
has been clearly related with DA receptors while hyperactivity may
relate to NE and other receptors *(Creese and Iversen, 1974; Creese
and Iversen, 1975; Costall and Naylor, 1973)*.

Although the pathophysiological mechanisms of L-dopa and
amphetamine-induced dyskinesias and psychoses are poorly understood, the amphetamine-induced SB (a widely used animal model for
psychoses and dyskinesias) has been solidly associated to its

action on DA receptors sites of the corpus striatum. It has been
repeatedly demonstrated that both the locomotor and stereotyped
responses induced by amphetamine are dependent on functional
integrity of the nigrostriatal dopamine pathway (*Creese and Iversen,*
*1974; Creese and Iversen, 1975),* as is the SB response of apomorphine stimulation of dopamine receptors (*Costall and Naylor, 1973*).
A widely accepted pathophysiological explanation for dyskinetic
movements is the one initially proposed by Klawans *et al, (1974,*
*1975),* among others, that the prolonged use of major tranquilizers,
with their longstanding dopamine blockade, results in mechanical
dennervation of the dopamine receptors which then become hypersensitive. Upon reduction of dopamine blockade on withdrawal of
the major tranquilizer, the receptors hyper-respond to the dopamine
available. This over-response results in dyskinesia.

     Contrary to the dennervation hypersensitivity hypothesis,
multiple reports have shown an increased sensitivity to the effects
of drugs - the so-called "reverse tolerance" - induced by chronic
agonist treatment (*Mago, 1969; Segal and Mandell, 1974; Ellinwood*
*and Kilbey, 1975; Klawans and Margolin, 1975; Post and Kopanda,*
*1976),* which Klawans called "agonist"-induced hypersensitivity
(*Klawans and Margolin, 1975*). In this overview Klawans mentions
that hypersensitivity can be demonstrated with apomorphine, a
direct dopamine agonist. This suggests that the pathophysiology
of this mechanism is not related to the distribution, storage, or
release of monoamines; rather, it is post-synaptic or pharmacologically located at the receptor site.

     Because the pathogenesis of Parkinson's disease involves a
degeneration of dopamine containing neurons in the substantia nigra,
with depletion of this neurotransmitter in the striatum, it is
intuitive to conclude that L-dopa induced dyskinesias are caused
by a dennervation hypersensitivity of the striatum dopamine receptor sites.

     The concept of dennervation hypersensitivity explains the fact
that normal persons who recieve L-dopa rarely develop dyskinetic
movements, while parkinson patients do. It does not explain other
observations: (1) Although initially the dyskinesias are present
about the same time as maximal dopa effect on parkinsonian symptoms, later in the course of therapy dyskinesia begins within minutes of L-dopa ingestion; (2) There is a direct relationship between
duration of L-dopa therapy and level of dyskinesia in which more
than 70% of the patients have dyskinetic movements by the end of
two years of therapy while very few have it during the first few
weeks of treatment; (3) In many patients there is a direct relationship between the duration of dyskinesia and its severity with the
dyskinesia becoming more severe while on treatment with L-dopa;
(4) Therapists have found a reverse relationship between the duration of dyskinesia and the dosage of L-dopa necessary to elicit
dyskinesias. This is further evidenced by recurrance of abnormal
movement a few weeks or months after dosage of L-dopa had been

further reduced and abnormal movements had disappeared. The above mentioned difficulties with L-dopa therapy are better explained by a chronic agonist-induced hypersensitivity than by the dennervation hypersensitivity (Klawans and Margolin, 1975). It may well be that these two mechanisms coincide.

To further support a theory of agonist-induced hypersensitivity, other studies should be mentioned: in humans, Kramer (1972) suggested that amphetamine addicts may experience an almost immediate reactivation of the paranoid ideation when they take amphetamine, even after prolonged periods of abstinence; monkeys that had been exposed to methadone, but were drug free when given methamphetamine at low doses, immediately developed pronounced oral dyskinesias (Eibergen and Carlson, 1975). Methadone, the reverse of apomorphine, is known to block dopamine receptors. Moreover, a supersensitivity to apomorphine develops following sesation of long term neuroleptic treatment (Tarsy and Baldessarini, 1974).

Although these phenomenona follow closely the dennervation hypersensitivity theory, they were demonstrated *after* prolonged periods of lack or absence of blocking or "dennervation", so that, to some extent, they conform to the pattern of receptor-agonist-hypersensitivity.

Similarly, a study (Klawans and Wiener, 1974) disclosed that in disorders believed to involve physiological alteration within the basal ganglia with increased sensitivity to DA, i.e., Huntington's and Sydenham's chorea, chorea associated with SLE, etc., a single IV dose of 10 mgs/kg of amphetamine was sufficient to exacerbate or uncover the chorea.

Dyskinesias produced by amphetamine apparently occur only after chronic abuse, not initially. This again suggests an altering of the physiology of the receptors by chronic exposure to an agonist. Even paranoia produced by chronic doses of amphetamine is initially mild and easily controlled. But, with continued administration, it begins earlier, becomes more severe and lasts longer. Increased sensitivity is maintained even after prolonged abstinence of the drug (Kramer, 1972).

Several areas still are unexplored, i.e., sex; effect of benzodiazepines; cholinergic drugs and clozapine. Also the question remains, if there is a real difference between this phenomenon and the better known "dennervation hypersensitivity".

It has been shown that chronic administration of ethynylestradiol significantly prolongs amphetamine SB (Lal and Sourkes, 1972), hence, it is important to re-evaluate all the results using female animals. Also, chlordiazepoxide and other minor tranquilizers in high doses prolong amphetamine SB (Lal and Sourkes, 1972), and hyperactivity (Cox et al., 1971; Davies et al., 1974). It would be of significance to determine if this relation can be supported in animals and by clinical observations of patients on large doses of benzodiazepines while on L-dopa or neuroleptics, showing them to have a higher incidence of L-dopa-induced dyskinesias. Secondly,

cholinomimetics are clearly involved in the physiology of DA
receptor response (Wolfarth et al., 1974), and their relationship
to L-dopa dyskinesias needs further evaluation.

Dopamine receptor hypersensitivity (as measured by apomorphine
response) produced by withdrawal of neuroleptics have been demonstrated in all antipsychotics with the exception of clozapine (Sayers,
et al., 1975). It would be worthwhile to explore the effects of
clozapine on receptor hypersensitivity, and how this particular dopamine blocker's different response relates to Creese and Snyder's DA
agonist-antagonist receptor state (Creese et al., 1975 and 1976).

In our work, as in Klawan's, amphetamine pretreatment produced
a decreased latency and threshold, while increasing intensity of
amphetamine-induced stereotyped behavior. After his extensive
review of the literature on psychosis, dyskinesias and stereotyped
movement associated with amphetamine and amphetamine-like drugs, we
concur with him that "the evidence strongly suggests that these
phenomenona share a common pathophysiology of increased dopamine
activity (hypersensitivity) and that agonist-induced supersensitivity may serve as a useful model for these disorders".

## REFERENCES

Costall, B. and Naylor, R.J. (1973). The role of telencephalic
    dopaminergic systems in the mediation of apomorphine-stereo-
    types behaviour. *Euro. J. Pharm. 24*, 8-24.
Cox, C., Harrison-Read, P.E., Steinberg, H. *et al*: (1971). Lithium
    attenuates drug-induced hyperactivity in rats. *Nature 232*,
    336-337.
Creese, I. and Iversen, S.D. (1974). The role of forebrain dopamine
    systems in amphetamine induced stereotyped behavior in the
    rat. *Psychopharmacologia (Berl.) 39*, 345-357.
Creese, I. and Iversen, S.D. (1975). The pharmacological and ana-
    tomical substrates of the amphetamine response in the rat.
    *Brain Res. 83*, 419-436.
Creese, I., Burt, D.R. and Snyder, S.H. (1975). Dopamine receptor
    binding: Differentiation of agonist and antagonist states.
    *Life Sci. 17*, 993-1002.
Creese, I., Burt, D.R. and Snyder, S.H. (1976). DA receptor binding
    predicts clinical and pharmacological potencies of antischizo-
    phrenic drugs. *Science 192*, 481-483.
Davies, C., Sanger, D.J., Steinberg, H., *et. al*. (1974). Lithium
    and alpha-Methyl-p-Tyrosine prevent "manic" activity in
    rodents. *Psychopharmacologia (Berl) 36*, 263-274.
Eibergen, R.D. and Carlson, K.R. (November 7, 1975). Dyskinesias
    elicited by Methamphetamine:Susceptibility of former Methadone-
    consuming monkeys. *Science 192*, 588-590.
Ellinwood, E.H. and Kilbey, M.M. (1975). Amphetamine stereotypy;
    the influence of environmental factors and prepotent behavioral
    patterns on its topography and development. *Biol. Psychiatry.
    10*, 3-16.

Iversen, S.D. and Creese, I. (1975).  Behavioral correlates of dopa-
     minergic supersensitivity.  In *Advances in Neurology*.
     (Caine, D.B., Chase, T.N. and Barbeau, A., Eds.) *9*, 81-92.
     Raven Press, N.Y.

Klawans, H.L. and Weiner, W.J. (1974).  The effect of d-amphetamine
     on choreiform movement disorders.  *Neurology 24*, 312-318.

Klawans, H.L. Crosset, P. and Dana, N. (1975).  Effect of chronic
     amphetamine exposure on stereotyped behavior: Implications
     for pathogenesis of L-DOPA-Induced dyskinesias.  In *Advances
     in Neurology*.  (Caine, D.B., Chase, T.N. and Barbeau, A.,
     Eds.) *9*, 105-112.  Raven Press, N.Y.

Klawans, H.L. and Margolin, D.I. (1975).  Amphetamine-induced dopa-
     minergic hypersensitivity in guinea pigs.  *Arch. Gen. Psychiat.
     32*, 725-732.

Kramer, J.C. (1972).  Introduction to amphetamine abuse.  In Current
     Concepts on Amphetamine Abuse.  *National Institute of Mental
     Health Publication* 72-9085 (Ellinwood, E.H. and Cohen, S.,
     Eds.) pp. 177-184.  Washington, D.C., U.S. Government Printing
     Office.

Lal, S. and Sourkes, T.L. (1972).  Potentiation and inhibition of
     the amphetamine stereotype in rats by neuroleptics and other
     agents.  *Arch. Int. Pharmacodyn. 199*, 289-301.

Mago, L. (1969).  Persistence of the effect of amphetamine on
     stereotyped activity in rats.  *Eur. J. Pharmacol. 6*, 200-201.

Post, R.M. and Kopanda, R.T. (June 1976).  Cocaine, Kindling and
     Psychosis.  *Am. J. Psychiat. 133*, 627-632.

Sayers, A.C., Bürki, H.R. , Ruch, W. and Asper, H. (1975).  Neuro-
     leptic-induced hypersensitivity of striatal dopamine receptors
     in the rat as a model of tardive dyskinesias.  Effects of
     Clozapine, Haloperidol, Loxapine and Chlorpromazine.  *Psycho-
     pharmacologia 41*, 97-104.

Segal, D.S. and Mandell, A.J. (1974).  Long-term administration of
     d-amphetamine: Progressive augmentation of motor activity
     and stereotypy.  *Pharmacol. Biochem. Behav. 2*, 249-255.

Segal, D.S. Geyer, M.A. and Wiener, B.E. (25 July 1975).  Strain
     differences during intra-ventricular infusion of norepin-
     phrine: Possible role of receptor sensitivity.  *Science 189*,
     301-303.

Tarsy, D. and Baldessarini, R.J. (1974).  Behaviour super-sensitivity
     to apomorphine following chronic treatment with drugs which
     interfere with the synaptic function of catecholamines.
     *Neuropharmacology 13*, 927-940.

Wolfarth, S., Dulska, E. and Lacki, M. (1974).  Comparison of the
     effects of the intranigral injections of cholinomimetics
     with systemic injections of the dopamine receptor stimulating
     and blocking agents in the rabbit.  *Neuropharmacology 13*,
     867-875.

# L-DOPA-INDUCED HYPOTENSION: DEPRESSION OF SPINAL SYMPATHETIC NEURONS BY RELEASE OF 5-HYDROXYTRYPTAMINE

DONALD N. FRANZ, ROBERT J. NEUMAYR, AND BRADFORD D. HARE

Department of Pharmacology
University of Utah College of Medicine
Salt Lake City, Utah 84132

## ABSTRACT

In studies designed to determine the respective functional roles of two bulbospinal monoaminergic pathways to sympathetic preganglionic neurons, both L-dopa and precursors of 5-HT depressed transmission through excitatory spinal reflex and bulbospinal sympathetic pathways. Transmission through spinal reflex pathways was secondarily enhanced after L-dopa. Pharmacological tests indicated mediation of these effects by monoamines. After antagonism or depletion of central 5-HT, L-dopa only enhanced transmission through both pathways. The results indicate that hypotension and other sympathoinhibitory effects of L-dopa are produced at the spinal level by release of 5-HT from terminals of bulbospinal 5-HT pathways that are inhibitory to sympathetic preganglionic neurons. The excitatory effects of L-dopa are apparently mediated by release of catecholamines from bulbospinal noradrenergic pathways that are excitatory.

## INTRODUCTION

Although the ability of L-dopa to produce hypotension in man and in experimental animals is well known, the predominant mechanism and site of this action have not been resolved. Experimentally, L-dopa has been shown to impair transmission at both peripheral adrenergic synapses and sympathetic ganglia (*Whitsett, Halushka and Goldberg, 1970; Antonaccio and Robson, 1974b*). However, the marked depression of preganglionic, sympathetic nervous activity produced by L-dopa and the failure of peripheral decarboxylase inhibitors to modify the sympathoinhibitory effects of L-dopa point to a predominant action at sites in the central nervous system *(Watanabe, Chase and Cardon, 1970; Henning, Rubenson and Trolin, 1972; Baum and Shropshire, 1973, 1974; Schmitt, Schmitt and Fenard, 1973; Antonaccio and Robson, 1974a; Coote and MacLeod, 1974; Watanabe, Judy and Cardon, 1974).*

Since L-dopa reaching the central nervous system is converted to catecholamines and since the brainstem contains major sites for central sympathetic integration, the hypotensive effect of L-dopa has been attributed to stimulation of adrenergic receptors that presumably function to inhibit medullary vasomotor centers *(Van Zwieten, 1973).* However, recent studies in our laboratory, designed to assess the respective functional roles of two bulbospinal, monoaminergic pathways to spinal sympathetic centers *(Dahlström and Fuxe, 1965),* indicate that depression of sympathetic preganglionic nerve activity by L-dopa is mediated by release of 5-hydroxytryptamine (5-HT) from inhibitory 5-HT bulbospinal pathways to sympathetic preganglionic neurons in the spinal cord rather than by direct effects of synthesized catecholamines on higher centers *(Hare, Neumayr and Franz, 1972; Neumayr, Hare and Franz, 1974).* Furthermore, the inhibitory 5-HT pathways appear to act reciprocally with excitatory noradrenergic (NE) bulbospinal pathways to regulate the sympathetic outflow at the spinal level.

## METHODS

In order to assess the sensitivity of sympathetic preganglionic neurons to the putative transmitters, NE and 5-HT, the effects of their precursors were tested on transmission through two, separate spinal sympathetic pathways in cats made spinal at C-1 under ether anesthesia. Carotid and vertebral arteries were occluded to render the brain ischemic. Animals were paralyzed with Flaxedil® and artificially respired. Upper thoracic, preganglionic white rami were exposed retropleurally and prepared for recording of evoked sympathetic discharges. Spinal preparations were preferred for these studies to confine the test systems to the spinal cord.

The diagrams in Figure 1 depict the two different pathways upon which paramacological tests were performed. The cross section of the thoracic spinal cord on the left illustrates the polysynaptic, spinal sympathetic reflex pathway. Sympathetic discharges recorded from preganglionic rami were evoked by stimulation of small myelinated afferent fibers in adjacent intercostal nerves at 15/min *(Beachem and Perl, 1964; Franz, Evans and Perl, 1966).* This spinal pathway contains no monoaminergic neurons *(Dahlström and Fuxe, 1965).* The other spinal sympathetic pathway is illustrated on the right; preganglionic discharges were evoked at 6/min by intraspinal micro-

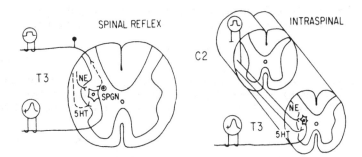

*Figure 1.*    *Schematic representation of pathways for spinal sympathetic*
             *reflexes (left) and for intraspinally evoked sympathetic*
             *discharges (right) recorded from T3 preganglionic rami.*
             *Approximate locations of bulbospinal, monoaminergic path-*
             *ways and their terminations at sympathetic preganglionic*
             *neurons (SPGN) are also shown.  NE, norepinephrine; 5-HT,*
             *5-hydroxytryptamine.*

electrode stimulation of a descending excitatory pathway in the
dorsolateral funiculus at C2-3.  This pathway is continuous with
medullary vasomotor centers and appears to utilize NE as a transmitter *(Neumayr, Hare and Franz, 1974)*.  The preganglionic neurons
are presumably the only neural elements common to both pathways.

The diagrams also show terminations of the two bulbospinal,
monoaminergic pathways at sympathetic preganglionic neurons *(Dahlström and Fuxe, 1965)*.  If these pathways do influence the preganglionic neurons, selective release of their respective transmitters,
either spontaneously or by activation, would be expected to exert
their characteristic effects on the excitability of these neurons.
Monoamine precursors were administered to induce selective release,
and other drugs affecting monoaminergic transmission were also tested
alone or in conjunction with the precursors.

In addition to recording individual responses on film during
each experiment, the sizes of evoked sympathetic discharges were
measured on-line by integrating the analog sum of 16 or 32 conse-
cutive responses with a signal averaging computer (Nicolet 1072).
After establishing that average responses were stable during a 1-2
hr control period, they were sampled every 5 or 10 minutes after
precursor or drug treatment.  In the absence of such treatment, the
evoked responses remained stable for many hours (2 S.D. $\leq \pm$ 10%).
The effects of each precursor or drug treatment were observed in
3-12 cats with only minor quantitative variations among the results.

All drugs and precursors were administered as solutions through
an indwelling catheter in a cephalic vein except parachlorophenylalanine (PCPA) which was injected intraperitoneally as a suspension.
Arterial blood pressure, body temperature, and end-tidal $CO_2$ concen-

tration were monitored throughout surgical and experimental procedures
and were maintained for optimal physiological conditions.

## RESULTS

Intravenous administration of 50 mg/kg of the 5-HT precursor,
D,L-5-HTP, severely depressed preganglionic discharges for prolonged
periods regardless of whether they were evoked by spinal reflex

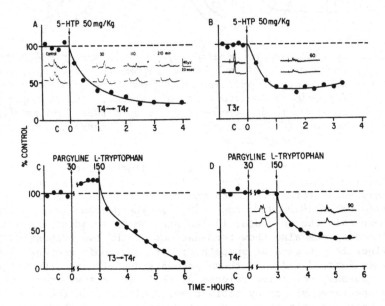

*Figure 2.   Effects of 5-HT precursors on spinal sympathetic reflexes
(A and C) and on intraspinally evoked discharges (B and D)
in four separate experiments.   A and B, effects of 50 mg/kg
of 5-HTP on reflexly and intraspinally evoked responses.
C and D, effects of 150 mg/kg of L-tryptophan on each type
of response after 30 mg/kg of pargyline.   Upper traces in
A, B and D are single responses; lower traces are averages of 16 responses which were integrated to determine the
size of responses throughout all experiments.   Post-drug
responses are plotted as percentages of control responses.
Numbers above traces designate time after drug injection,
in minutes.   Control data (C on abcissa) were collected
for at least one hour prior to drug administration.   Spinal reflex pathways in A and C indicate spinal nerve stimulated (T4 and T3) and preganglionic ramus from which
response was recorded (T4 in each).   Responses in B and
D were recorded from T3 and T4 preganglionic rami, respectively.*

pathways (Figure 2A) or by intraspinal pathways (Figure 2B). The depression induced by a dose of 25 mg/kg was minimal and recovered to control levels by about 1 hr. Two kinds of evidence indicated that the depression was mediated by intraneuronal conversion to and release of 5-HT. Inhibiting central decarboxylation of 5-HTP by pretreatment with 500-600 mg/kg of Ro 4-4602 completely prevented the depression by 5-HTP. Inhibition of monoamine oxidase by pargyline (30 mg/kg) markedly increased the potency of 5-HTP so that equivalent depression could be produced by only 5-10 mg/kg, doses that were only a fraction of the minimally effective dose of 5-HTP alone. L-tryptophan was also modestly depressant, but after pre-treatment with pargyline, this natural 5-HT precursor produced marked depression of both spinal sympathetic reflexes (Figure 2C) and intraspinally evoked sympathetic discharges (Figure 2D).

Further evidence that the depressant effect of the precursors was due to release of 5-HT was provided by experiments in which the typically modest depression produced by 30 mg/kg of 5-HTP was markedly potentiated by 5 mg/kg of imipramine or chlorimipramine administered either before the precursor of afterward during partial recovery. Such potentiation is consistent with the ability of these drugs to block reuptake of released 5-HT.

The inhibitory responses to 5-HTP were not blocked by methysergide; instead, methysergide also depressed sympathetic responses. The failure of classical 5-HT antagonists to block inhibitory effects of 5-HT on central neurons has been confirmed by iontophoretic studies (Haigler and Aghajanian, 1974). However, tolazoline was found to antagonize the depression by 5-HTP in both systems (Figure 3A and B). Tolazoline was more effective when given prior to 5-HTP as shown in Figure 3C and D; it also appeared to be more effective in antagonizing the effect of 5-HTP on the intraspinal than on the spinal reflex pathway. Possible reasons for these differences have not been determined.

The depressant effect of 5-HT on sympathetic discharges is consistent with the vasodepressor and sympathoinhibitory effects of stimulation within the raphe region of the medulla which contains the bulbospinal 5-HT cell bodies (Dahlström and Fuxe, 1965; Neumayr, Hare and Franz, 1974) and indicates that these bulbospinal 5-HT pathways to sympathetic preganglionic neurons are inhibitory.

The effects of L-dopa were somewhat more complicated than those of the 5-HT precursors. On spinal sympathetic reflexes (Figure 4A), L-dopa routinely produced a biphasic effect, first a prominent, transient depression, then a prolonged enhancement of reflex responses to 125-225% of control values. On intraspinally evoked discharges, L-dopa produced only depression which recovered within about 3 hours (Figure 4B) The degree and duration of both depression and enhancement were approximately dose-related between doses of 15 and 50 mg/kg. Both effects were prevented by inhibiting central decarboxylase with a large dose of Ro 4-4602, and the potency of L-dopa was increased 5-10 times by inhibiting monoamine oxidase

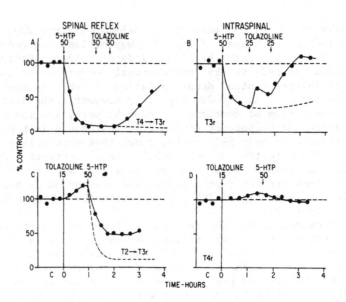

Figure 3.   *Antagonism of 5-HTP-induced depression of spinal sympathe-*
            *tic reflexes (A and C) and of intraspinally evoked sympa-*
            *thetic discharges (B and D) by tolazoline.  Dashed curves*
            *in A, B and C approximate the usual effects of 5-HTP alone.*
            *Drug doses are in mg/kg.  Graphs are constructed as in*
            *Figure 2.*

with pargyline.  Therefore, the effects of L-dopa were attributed to
intraneuronal synthesis of catecholamines and release of active monoamines rather than to direct effects of the precursor.

Although the enhancement of sympathetic reflexes by L-dopa was
consistent with an excitatory role for the NE pathway, the depressant activity was not.  However, other investigators have shown that
dopamine synthesized from L-dopa within 5-HT terminals can induce
a transient release of 5-HT by displacement *(Ng et al., 1970; Ng,*
*Colburn and Kopin, 1972).*  Since this mechanism could account for
the depressant activity, the effects of L-dopa were tested in cats
depleted of 5-HT stores by a 3-day pretreatment with parachlorophenylalanine (PCPA, 100 mg/kg/day) prior to the day of experiments.
In these animals the depression of sympathetic preganglionic neurons
after L-dopa was almost or completely eliminated, so that spinal
sympathetic reflexes were only enhanced (Figure 4C) and transmission through the intraspinal pathway was also enhanced instead of
depressed (Figure 4D).

Elimination of the depressant effects of L-dopa by depleting
central stores of 5-HT suggested that those effects were actually
induced by release of 5-HT from the inhibitory bulbospinal 5-HT

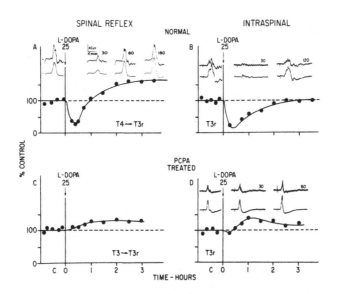

Figure 4. *Respective effects of 25 mg/kg of L-dopa on spinal sympathetic reflexes (A) and on intraspinally evoked discharges
(B) in normal cats. In cats depleted of central 5-HT
by pretreatment with parachlorophenylalanine (PCPA), both
types of response (C and D) were only enhanced after
L-dopa. Figures are constructed as in Figure 2.*

terminals. The experiments depicted in Figures 5 and 6 provided further support for this proposal. After depletion of both NE and 5-HT
by a large dose of reserpine (Figure 5A), the depressant effect of
L-dopa on sympathetic reflexes was much smaller than normal, but the
phase of enhancement was still apparent. Presumably, the modest
depression reflected release of a small amount of residual 5-HT
whereas replenishment and release of depleted catecholamines by
L-dopa accounted for further enhancement. As shown in Figure 5B in
which L-dopa produced the typical enhancement of intraspinally evoked
discharges in a PCPA-pretreated cat, partial replenishment of central
5-HT stores by a slow infusion of 5-HTP restored the ability of
L-dopa to produce a transient depression. Likewise, a prior loading
dose of 5-HTP in a normal cat (Figure 5C) markedly augmented the
depressant effect of L-dopa on spinal sympathetic reflexes.
     Since tolazoline was found to antagonize the depressant effect
of 5-HTP, it was also tested against the depressant effect of L-dopa.
As shown in Figure 6A and B, small doses of tolazoline almost immediately blocked the typical depression of both spinal sympathetic
reflexes and intraspinally evoked discharges after L-dopa and rapidly replaced the depression with enhancement. Given prior to L-dopa,

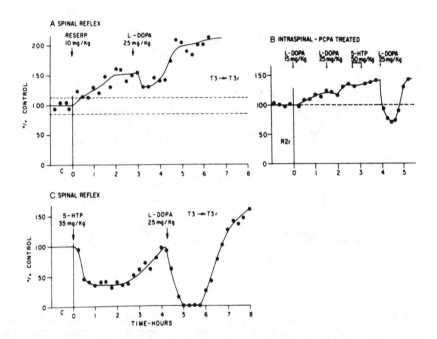

*Figure 5.*   *Experiments showing the relationship between the depres-*
           *sant effect of L-dopa on spinal sympathetic pathways and*
           *central levels of 5-HT.   A. Reduction of the depressant*
           *effect of L-dopa on spinal sympathetic reflexes after*
           *acute depletion of central monoamines by reserpine.*
           *B. Reestablishment of the ability of L-dopa to depress*
           *intraspinally evoked discharges by infusion of 5-HTP*
           *in a cat depleted of central 5-HT by pretreatment with*
           *PCPA.   C. Enhancement of the depressant effect of L-dopa*
           *on spinal sympathetic reflexes following recovery from*
           *5-HTP.*

tolazoline, like PCPA-pretreatment, prevented the depression so that
transmission through both pathways was only enhanced (Figure 6C and
D).

     At any stage during enhancement of spinal sympathetic reflexes
by L-dopa, the enhancement could be blocked by 3 mg/kg of chlorpromazine without affecting normal transmission through the reflex
pathway.  However, transmission through the intraspinal (presumably
NE) pathway was rapidly blocked by chlorpromazine.  On the other
hand, desipramine (2-5 mg/kg) further enhanced the excitatory effect
of L-dopa on either pathway and greatly increased transmission
through the intraspinal pathway when given alone.  The respective
effects of chlorpromazine and desipramine were not modified by
pretreatment with tolazoline.

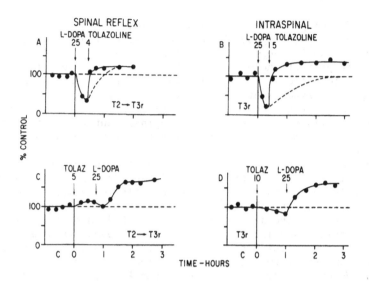

*Figure 6.    Reversal (A and B) or prevention (C and D) of the depres-
sant effects of L-dopa (25 mg/kg) on spinal sympathetic
reflexes and on intraspinally evoked discharges by tolazoline (mg/kg).   Dashed curves in A and B indicate usual
effects of L-dopa alone.   Graphs are constructed as in
Figure 2.*

## DISCUSSION

The systematic effects of monoamine precursors and of other
drugs affecting central monoamines on transmission through the two
spinal sympathetic pathways add considerable support to anatomical
(*Dahlström and Fuxe, 1965; Réthelyi, 1972*) and functional (*Neumayr,
Hare and Franz, 1974*) evidence that sympathetic preganglionic neurons are innervated by two monoaminergic pathways arising in the
medulla.   These pathways appear to act reciprocally on the sympathetic neurons, the bulbospinal NE pathways being exicitatory and
the bulbospinal 5-HT pathways being inhibitory.   The concept of
reciprocal innervation is well established in the periphery and has
been increasingly advanced for monoaminergic pathways in the CNS
(*Viala and Buser, 1969; Birkmayr et al., 1972; Flórez, Delgado and
Armijo, 1972; Jovet, 1973; Wise, Berger and Stein, 1973*).
The present results with 5-HT precursors confirm and extend
previous studies on spinal sympathetic reflexes (*Hare, Neumayr and
Franz, 1972; Coote and MacLeod, 1974*).   Their inhibitory effect on
transmission through sympathetic preganglionic neurons appears to
be mediated by release of 5-HT from bulbospinal and 5-HT terminals.
This mechanism may account for the dose-related sympathoinhibitory

effects of 5-HT precursors in intact animals which were also determined to be mediated by synthesis and release of 5-HT within the CNS
*(Antonaccio and Robson, 1975; Baum and Shropshire, 1975)*.  The possibility that part of the effects of 5-HT precursors in intact animals
may be due to actions of 5-HT on higher centers cannot be excluded
by the present experiments.  However, the close correspondence among
effective doses required to depress sympathetic activity in intact
vs. spinal animals suggests that the spinal centers of sympathetic
integration are the primary sites of action for the sympathoinhibitory
effects of 5-HT.

Considering the excitatory nature of the bulbospinal NE pathways,
L-dopa would be expected to raise the level of catecholamines in the
NE terminals and to increase the excitability of sympathetic preganglionic neurons as was observed secondarily in the spinal reflex studies.  Therefore, the depressant effect of L-dopa on responses evoked
by both pathways was initially puzzling.  However, reports that
L-dopa, after conversion to dopamine, could induce transient release
of 5-HT from 5-HT terminals in brain slices or from isolated synap-
tosomes *(Ng et al., 1970; Nf, Colburn and Kopin, 1972)* suggested a
similar mechanism in our studies.  This possibility was verified by
altering the central levels or effects of 5-HT.  Reducing 5-HT stores
by pretreatment with PCPA or reserpine or blocking the effect of
5-HT by tolazoline eliminates or markedly reduces the depressant
effect of L-dopa and discloses its excitatory effect mediated by
catecholamines released from NE terminals.  On the other hand, the
depressant effect is intensified or reestablished by increasing 5-HT
levels with 5-HTP.  The relationship between the degree of depression
produced by L-dopa and the central levels of 5-HT indicates that
5-HT release is responsible for the deprkssion.  Furthermore, the
lack of L-dopa-induced deprewsion when central decarboxylase activity
is inhibited signifies nhat dopamine formation is necessary for
release of 5-HT.

Since monoaminergic neurons are generally considered to be
selective for uptake of their respective precursors, the uptake of
L-dopa by 5-HT neurons may appear inconsistent.  However, L-dopa is
normally synthesized only within catecholamine neurons after selective
uptake of L-tyrosine.  Apparently, exogenously administered L-dopa, as
an abnormal extraneuronal metabolite, is taken up by both catecholamine
and 6-HT neurons and converted to dopamine.  The 5-HT-releasing
effect of L-dopa has also been invoked by other investigators to
account for its effects on other centrally mediated phenomena
*(Freidman and Gershon, 1972; Da Prada et al., 1973; Gaillard et al.,
1974; Jacobs, 1974)*.

The inhibitory effect produced by 5-HT release from 5-HT terminals after L-dopa predominates over the excitatory effect of L-dopa
produced by catecholamine release from NE terminals.  This imbalance
could be due either to greater release of 5-HT or to its higher

synaptic efficacy. The more efficient regulation of transmitter synthesis in catecholamine than in 5-HT neurons *(Costa and Meek, 1974)* may contribute to a greater release of 5-HT. Elimination of the depressant effect of 5-HT reveals the excitatory effects of L-dopa operating through the NE terminals. The failure of L-dopa alone to enhance transmission through intraspinal NE pathways appears to be related to periodic activation of those pathways; the ability of L-dopa to enhance transmission through spinal reflex pathways is lost when tested alternately with intraspinal pathways in the same experiment *(Neumayr and Franz, unpublished observations)*.

The present evidence that L-dopa, in doses equivalent to those used clinically, can markedly depress sympathetic preganglionic neurons by releasing 5-HT can at least partially account for the postural hypotension encountered during chronic therapy of Parkinson's disease. The transient nature of this side effect in some patients may reflect partial depletion of central 5-HT or changes in its metabolism *(Birkmayr et al., 1972; Goodwin et al., 1973)*. Furthermore, hypotension, bradycardia and reduced sympathetic nerve activity induced by similar doses of L-dopa in intact animals *(Henning, Rubenson and Trolin, 1972; Baum and Shropshire, 1973, 1974; Schmitt, Schmitt and Fenard, 1973; Coote and MacLeod, 1974; Watanabe, Judy and Cardon, 1974)* are also apparently mediated by central 5-HT release *(Antonaccio and Robson, 1974a)*. Although the sympathoinhibitory effects of L-dopa are generally ascribed to stimulation of adrenergic receptors at supraspinal sites, the present results suggest that release of 5-HT from bulbospinal 5-HT neurons at sympathetic preganglionic neurons in the spinal cord is the primary mechanism and site of action.

It seem very unlikely that 5-HT release by L-dopa is confined to the spinal cord, but the possible influence of this action in higher centers on the therapeutic or other side effects of L-dopa defies speculation. The functional roles of 5-HT pathways to the striatum and to the rest of the brain are almost completely obscure, and their probable interactions with other monoaminergic neurons remain largely unexplored. However, the proposal that L-dopa may be converted to dopamine and released by striatal 5-HT terminals of parkinsonian patients *(Ng et al., 1972)* offers an intriguing possibility.

## ACKNOWLEDGEMENTS

This research was supported by U.S. Public Health Service Grants FR-05428, NS-04553, and GM-00153. For generous supplies of drugs we are indebted to the following companies: Abbott Laboratories (pargyline), Ciba Pharmaceutical Co. (chlorimipramine), Hoffman-LaRoche Inc. (RO 4-4602), Pfizer Inc. (PCPA); and USV Pharmaceutical Corp. (desipramine).

## REFERENCES

Antonaccio, M.J. and Robson, R.D.   (1974a).   L-dopa hypotension in
     dogs: Evidence for mediation through 5-HT release.  *Archs int.*
     *Pharmacodyn. Thér. 212*, 89-102.
Antonaccio, M.F. and Robson, R.D.   (1974b).   An analysis of the peri-
     pheral effects of L-dopa on autonomic nerve function.  *Br. J.*
     *Pharmac. 52*, 41-50.
Antonaccio, M.J. and Robson, R.D.   (1975).   Centrally-mediated
     cardiovascular effects of 5-hydroxytryptophan in MAO-inhibited
     dogs: modification by autonomic antagonists.  *Archs int. Pharma-*
     *cody. Thér. 213*, 200-210.
Baum, T. and Shropshire, A.T.   (1973).   Reduction of sympathetic out-
     flow by central administration of L-dopa, dopamine and norepine-
     phrine.  *Neuropharmacology 12*, 49-56.
Baum, T. and Shropshire, A.T.   (1974).   Influence of heart rate on
     the reduction of sympathetic outflow produced by L-dopa.  *Am.*
     *J. Physiol. 226*, 1276-1280.
Baum, T. and Shropshire, A.T.   (1975).   Inhibition of efferent sympa-
     thetic nerve activity by 5-hydroxytryptophan and centrally
     administered 5-hydroxytryptamine.  *Neuropharmacology 14*, 227-233.
Beacham, W.S. and Perl, E.R.   (1964).   Background and reflex dis-
     charge of sympathetic preganglionic neurons in the spinal cat.
     *J. Physio. (Lond.) 172*, 400-416.
Birkmayr, W., Danielczyk, W., Neumayer, E. and Riederer, P.   (1972).
     The balance of biogenic amines as a condition for normal behav-
     ior.  *J. Neural Transm. 33*, 163-178.
Coote, J.H. and MacLeod, V.H.   (1974).   The influence of bulbospinal
     monoaminergic pathways on sympathetic nerve activity.  *J.*
     *Physio. (Lond.) 241*, 453-475.
Costa, E. and Meek, J.L.   (1974).   Regulation of biosynthesis of
     catecholamines and serotonin in the CNS.  *Ann. Rev. Pharmac.*
     *14*, 491-511.
Dahlström, A. and Fuxe, K.   (1965).   Evidence for the existence of
     monoamine neurons in the central nervous system.  II. Experi-
     mentally induced changes in intraneuronal amine levels of
     bulbospinal neuron systems.  *Acta physiol. scand. 64*, Suppl.
     247, 1-36.
Da Prada, M., Carruba, M., Saner, A., O'Brien, R.A. and Pletscher,
     A.   (1973).   The action of L-dopa on sexual behavior of male
     rats.  *Brain Res. 55*, 383-389.
Flórez, J., Delgado, G. and Armijo, J.A.   (1972).   Adrenergic and
     serotonergic mechanisms in morphine-induced respiratory de-
     pression.  *Psychopharmacologia 24*, 258-274.
Franz, D.N., Evans, M.H. and Perl, E.R.   (1966).   Characteristics
     of viscerosympathetic reflexes in the spinal cat.  *Am. J.*
     *Physiol. 211*, 1292-1298.
Friedman, E. and Gershon, S.   (1972).   L-dopa: centrally mediated
     emmission of seminal fluid in male rats.  *Life Sci. 11*, 435-440.

Gaillard, J.M., Bartholini, G., Herkert, B. and Tissot, R.  (1974).
    Involvement of 5-hydroxytryptamine in the cortical synchroni-
    zation induced by L-dopa in the rabbit. *Brain Res. 68*, 344-350.
Goodwin, F.K., Post, R.M., Dunner, D.L. and Gordon, E.K.  (1973).
    Cerebrospinal fluid amine metabolites in affective illness:
    The probenecid technique. *Am. J. Psychiat. 130*, 73-79.
Haigler, H.J. and Aghajanian, G.K.  (1974).  Peripheral serotonin
    antagonists: Failure to antagonize serotonin in brain areas re-
    ceiving a prominent serotonergic input.  *J. Neural Transm. 35*,
    257-273.
Hare, B.D., Neumayr, R.J. and Franz, D.M.  (1972).  Opposite effects
    of L-dopa and 5-HTP on spinal sympathetic reflexes.  *Nature
    (Lond.) 239*, 336-337.
Henning, M., Rubenson, A. and Trolin, G.  (1972).  On the localization
    of the hypotensive effect of L-dopa.  *J. Pharm. Pharmac. 24*,
    447-451.
Jacobs, B.L.  (1974).  Evidence for the functional interaction of
    two central neurotransmitters. *Psychopharmacologia 39*, 81-86.
Jouvet, M.  (1973).  Serotonin and sleep in the cat.  *In Serotonin
    and Behavior* (Barchas, J. and Usdin, E., Eds.) pp. 385-400.
    Academic Press, New York.
Neumayr, R.J., Hare, B.D. and Franz, D.N.  (1974).  Evidence for
    bulbospinal control of sympathetic preganglionic neurons by
    monoaminergic pathways. *Life Sci. 14*, 793-806.
Ng, L.K.Y., Chase, T.N., Colburn, R.W. and Kopin, I.J.  (1970).
    L-dopa-induced release of cerebral monoamines. *Science (Wash.)
    170*, 76-77.
Ng, L.K.Y., Chase, T.N., Colburn, R.W. and Kopin, I.J.  (1972).
    L-dopa in parkinsonism: A possible mechanism of action. *Neuro-
    logy (Minneap.) 22*, 688-696.
Ng, L.K.Y., Colburn, R.W. and Kopin, I.J.  (1972).  Effects of L-dopa
    on accumulation and efflux of monoamines in particles of rat
    brain homogenates. *J. Pharmac. exp. Ther. 183*, 316-325.
Réthelyi, M.  (1972).  Cell and neuropil architecture of the inter-
    mediolateral (sympathetic) nucleus of cat spinal cord. *Brain
    Res. 46*, 203-213.
Schmitt, H., Schmitt, H. and Fenard, S.  (1973).  Localization of
    the site of the central sympatho-inhibitory action of L-dopa
    in dogs and cats. *Eur. J. Pharmac. 22*, 211-216.
Van Zwieten, P.A.  (1973).  The central action of antihypertensive
    drugs mediated via central $\alpha$-receptors.  *J. Pharm. Pharmac.
    25*, 89-95.
Viala, D. and Buser, P.  (1969).  The effects of DOPA and 5-HTP on
    rhythmic efferent discharges in hind limb nerves in the rabbit.
    *Brain Res. 12*, 437-443.
Watanabe, A.M., Chase, T.N. and Cardon, P.V.  (1970).  Effect of
    L-dopa alone and in combination with extracerebral decarboxy-
    lase inhibitor on blood pressure and some cardiovascular
    reflexes. *Clin. Pharmac. Ther. 11*, 740-746.

Watanabe, A.M., Judy. W.V. and Cardon, P.V. (1974). Effect of
    L-dopa on blood pressure and sympathetic nerve activity after
    decarboxylase inhibiton in cats. *J. Pharmac. exp. Ther. 188*,
    107-113.
Whitsett, T.L., Halushka, P.V. and Goldberg, L.I. (1970). Attenua-
    tion of postganglionic sympathetic nerve activity by L-dopa.
    *Circulat. Res. 27*, 561-570.
Wise, C.D., Berger, B.D. and Stein, L. (1973). Evidence of α-norad-
    renergic reward receptors and serotonergic punishment receptors
    in the rat brain. *Biol. Psychiat. 6*, 3-21.

# ANTINOCICEPTIVE EFFECT OF DOPAMINERGIC NEUROTRANSMISSION EVOKED BY MESENCEPHALIC STIMULATION ON SPINAL INTERNEURONAL ACTIVITY IN CATS

SIMON J. FUNG AND CHARLES D. BARNES

Department of Physiology
Texas Tech University School of Medicine
Lubbock, Texas 79409

## ABSTRACT

Adult cats, precollicularly decerebrated and immobilized with Flaxedil® (2 mg/kg, i.v.), were used in the study. Recordings of laminae IV and V cell activity elicited by natural stimulation to the left hind limb or electrical stimulation to the left sural nerve exposed in the popliteal fossa was made at the level of $L_6$ and $L_7$. Brain stimulation consisting of 100 msec trains of rectangular pulses (0.1 msec, 100 Hz, 3/sec for 1 min, 5-10 V intensity) was delivered to substantia nigra, periaqueductal gray and raphe nucleus in the midbrain via concentric bipolar electrodes. Noxious peripheral input evoked activity ranging from a few spikes to long duration repetitive discharges. Stimulating the three brain sites individually resulted in inhibitory, facilitatory or no effect on the firing pattern of laminae IV and V cells. Cells responded to non-noxious activation, however, were without change following central stimulation. The inhibitory effect on the dorsal horn cells was abolished by injecting bulbocapnine (20 mg/kg, i.v.) or tetrabenazine (40 mg/kg, i.v.), suggesting a role of dopaminergic control of the midbrain on laminae IV and V cells. This was further substantiated by the finding that administration of L-dopa (20 mg/kg, i.v.) or apomorphine (20 mg/kg, i.v.) reversed the previous drugs effect and reestablished the brain stem inhibition on the spinal transmission of noxious impulses.

# INTRODUCTION

Based on the contention that parkinsonism is associated with pain of a central origin (*Snider et al., 1975*) and that L-dopa treatment can also decrease pain in Parkinsonian patients who also had breast cancer and bone pain (*Minton, 1975; Nixon, 1975; Tolis, 1975*), one could be led to suspect that a dopamine pathway has access to the central mechanism for pain.

Mayer and Hayes (*1975*) have demonstrated that morphine and electrical stimulation of the periaqueductal gray (PAG) produced analgesia by a common mechanism. Moreover, Verri et al. (*1967*) inferred that the analgesic action of morphine is closely related with cerebral catecholamines. It is proposed that electrical stimulation produced analgesia be utilized to test whether it also has common elements with dopamine's association with pain.

The present experiments were undertaken to investigate the neural inhibition produced by focal electrical brain stimulation of mesencephalic sites on laminae IV and V cells which are responsible for the spinal transmission of pain impulses (*Besson et al., 1972; Wagmann and Price, 1969; Pomeranz et al., 1968*). The role of dopaminergic neurotransmission in the brain stimulation produced analgesia is further delineated by using a number of dopaminergic modifying drugs.

# METHODS

Observations were made on thirty-one adult cats weighing 1.9 to 3.8 kg. Intubation of the trachea, ligation of both carotid arteries, and cannulation of the right femoral vein were performed under ether anesthesia. The animals were then made decerebrate at the precollicular level. At least two hours were allowed for the animal to recover from ether before any recordings were taken.

A lumbosacral laminectomy was performed to expose the spinal cord from $L_5$ through $S_1$. Following mechanical immobilization by fixing the head of the animal in a stereotaxic apparatus, clamping the spinous processes of $L_3$ and $L_4$, and pinning the heads of both femurs to a rigid framework, the animals were routinely paralyzed with gallamine triethiodide (Flaxedil®, 2 mg/kg, i.v.) and artificially respired.

Extracellular recordings were made from single cells in the left laminae IV and V at the level of $L_6$ and $L_7$ using glass micropipettes filled with 2M NaCl, the impedance of which was 3 to 9 megohms. The microelectrodes were placed with a stepping hydraulic microdrive unit. The unit's activity was elicited by natural stimulation (pinch) to the left hind limb or electrical stimulation (rectangular pulses, 0.1 msec, 1/sec) to the left sural nerve exposed in the popliteal fossa. Potentials were amplified (bandwidth: 100 Hz to 1 kHz), displayed on a storage oscilloscope and recorded permanently on films. In some experiments, dot raster displays were used to study the cell

firing patterns.  Laminae IV and V type cells were identified according
to the electrophysiological properties cited by Wall *(1967)* and Hillman
and Wall *(1969)*.

Brain stimulations consisted of 100 msec trains of rectangular
pulses (0.1 msec, 100 Hz, 3/sec for 1 min, 5-10 V intensity).  Stimulus
trains were delivered via concentric bipolar electrodes placed stereo-
taxically to substantia nigra (SN, $A_4 L_4 H_{-2.5}$), periaqueductal gray
($A_1 L_1 H_0$) and raphe nucleus (R, $P_1 L_0 H_0$) in the midbrain.  Placements of
electrode tips were checked histologically following each experiment.
Modification of dorsal horn interneurons activity activated by peripheral stimuli were tested by stimulating the brain stem sites one
at a time.

After establishing a cell response to peripheral activation and
modifications by brain stem stimulations, one of a number of dopaminergic modifying drugs were given and the previous responses redetermined.  Drugs tested include dopamine receptor blockers, bulbocapnine
(20 mg/kg) and tetrabenazine (40 mg/kg), and dopamine stimulating
drugs, L-dopa (20 mg/kg) and apomorphine (20 mg/kg).  All drugs were
dissolved in 0.9% saline and given intravenously.

All exposed nervous tissues were bathed in warm mineral oil.
Rectal temperature was monitored and maintained at about $38^{\circ}$C.

## RESULTS

In the current experiments, cells were selected only from those
animals with correct brain stem electrode placements as verified from
histological examinations.  Other cells sampled from animals with
incorrect placements were not used in the present analysis.

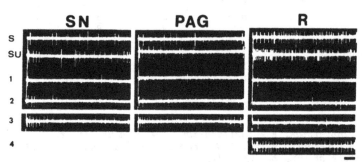

*Figure 1.   Effect of brain stem stimulations on spinal interneuron.
Stimulation intensity: 10 V.  S: spontaneous.  SU: sural-
evoked activity.  1: immediately after cessation of brain
stem site stimulation.  2: 1 minute after.  3: 5 minutes
after.  4: 10 minutes after brain stem stimulation.  Time
scale: 0.5 sec.  SN: substantia nigra.  PAG: periaqueductal
gray.  R: raphe nucleus.*

Spinal interneurons excited by peripheral stimuli were consistantly located at 1200 and 2000 microns below the surface of the lumbar cord. Their spontaneous firing rates were observed to differ from one cell to another and may even change over a period of time for the same cell (Figure 1). The duration of activation in response to sural nerve stimulation varied from a few spikes to long bursts of repetitive firing. Pinching invariably evoked a repetitive discharge which persisted as long as the stimulus was applied.

Throughout the course of the experiments, different types of responses including both inhibitory and facilitatory could be obtained following the cessation of the brain stem stimulation. These are summarized in Table 1. Of the 75 cells activated by sural nerve

TABLE 1.  MODIFICATION OF LAMINAE IV AND V CELL ACTIVITY BY MIDBRAIN STIMULATIONS.

| Peripheral stimuli | Effects | SN | PAG | R |
|---|---|---|---|---|
| Sural nerve | I | 20 | 16 | 17 |
|  | F | 16 | 13 | 10 |
|  | N | 39 | 36 | 32 |
|  |  | 75 | 65 | 59 |
| Pinch | I | 6 | 4 | 4 |
|  | F | 1 | 1 | 1 |
|  | N | 2 | 3 | 3 |
|  |  | 9 | 8 | 8 |
| Touch | I | 2 | 2 | 2 |
|  | F | 1 | 1 | 1 |
|  | N | 17 | 17 | 15 |
|  |  | 20 | 20 | 18 |

*I - Inhibition; F - facilitation; N - without effect.*
*SN - substantia nigra, PAG - periaqueductal gray, R - raphe nucleus*
*Numbers show number of cells sampled*

stimulation, 25% of cells sampled were inhibited, 20% facilitated and the remaining were uneffected following brain stem stimulations.

By using the pinch stimulus, neural inhibition was exhibited by the majority of cells following stimulation of SN, PAG or R separately. Only one out of nine cells was facilitated, the rest remained unchanged.

Touch sensitive cells were also encountered in the study. Brain stem stimulations were primarily without effect on the tactile units. However, 2 out of 17 cells were inhibited and 1 cell was facilitated from stimulating the three sites.

It should be noted that a fraction of the cells examined exhibited an overlap in the type of peripheral stimuli that could excite them. In this instance, brain stem stimulation was again found to modify the cell firing evoked by noxious stimuli but not when the activity was induced by the touch stimulus.

The inhibitory effect on laminae IV and V cells was further investigated in order to elucidate the antinociceptive nature of the brain stem evoked inhibition.

Figure 1 represents the typical inhibitory effect obtained from stimulating SN, PAG and R on the sural-evoked activity. The firing rates were markedly diminished immediately following cessation of stimulation to each of three sites. Inhibition from SN and PAG stimulations followed a similar time course and lasted for more than one but less than five minutes. R stimulation revealed the most powerful effect, the inhibitory action lasted beyond five minutes.

In some instances, pinching was used to introduce a natural noxious input to the laminae IV and V cells. Similar inhibition was observed from brain stem stimulations, however it was usually less prolonged, lasting about one minute. Hence, it appears that sural nerve stimulation resembles the natural noxious pinch stimulus in exciting the interneurons in Rexed's laminae IV and V regions.

Based on the notion that high intensity stimulation to the sural nerve activates all fibre groups within the cutaneous nerve, this accounts for the fast and slow responses observed in sural-evoked activity (Figure 2). The fast activity was observed to have an onset

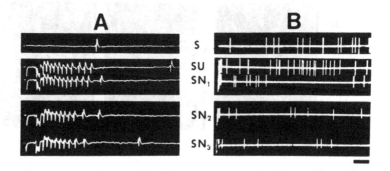

*Figure 2. Effect of substantia nigra (SN) stimulation on the fast and late responses evoked by sural nerve stimulation (SU) of a lamina V cell. S; spontaneous. $SN_1$: immediately post-stimulating SN. $SN_2$: 1 min. post-stimulation. $SN_3$: 2 min. post-stimulation. Time scale: 5 msec for A and 0.5 sec for B.*

of about 4 msec and to last no more than 30 msec following sural
nerve activation.  The late responses had a very long time course and
comprises the repetitive discharges.  SN stimulation was found to
inhibit the late activity without affecting the fast activity.  Corresponding selective inhibition upon the late activity of sural-evoked
units could be obtained from stimulating PAG and R as well.

It appears that brain stem stimulation produced inhibition acts
specifically on the late activity of sural response.  On reducing the
stimulation intensity to the sural nerve to a level just sufficient
to evoke a fast component, no effects were observed following SN, PAG
or R stimulations.  This substantiates the specific inhibition evoked
from brain stem stimulations acting on the late response.

Furthermore, measurement of conduction velocity revealed that
the late activity was transmitted at a rate of less than 2 m/sec
which is well within the range of conduction velocities for nociceptive fibres of the cutaneous nerve (*Gasser, 1943*).  Hence, the
antinociceptive role of midbrain stimulations on the spinal transmission of "painful" impulses was established.

The pharmacological nature of the descending inhibition could
be demonstrated by using dopamine antagonists, bulbocapinine and tetrabenazine, and dopamine stimulating drugs, L-dopa and apomorphine.

In Figure 3, brain stem evoked inhibitions on late sural response
were observed.  Marked inhibition from SN stimulation persisted
throughout the 32 sec testing period.  A relatively less marked

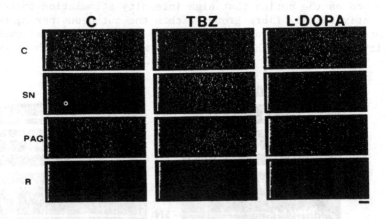

*Figure 3.  Effect of tetrabenazine (TBZ) and L-dopa on brain stem
stimulation induced inhibition of a lamina V cell.
C: predrug control.  Time scale: 0.1 sec.  Each picture
shows 32 sweeps running successively from the bottom
upwards.  SN: substantia nigra.  PAG: preiaqueductal
gray.  R: raphe nucleus.*

inhibitory effect was produced from PAG stimulation. R stimulation exhibited the most profound inhibitory effect among the three sites. In all cases, the fast sural-evoked activity remained relatively unchanged following brain stimulations.

Brain stimulations produced inhibitions were redetermined 10 minutes after TBZ administration. SN-evoked inhibition was abolished to the greatest extent, suggesting the previous descending inhibition may involve a dopaminergic mechanism. This was substantiated by the finding that subsequent treatment with L-dopa antagonized the dopaminergic blocking effect of TBZ and reestablished the marked inhibition on the late sural activity.

For PAG evoked inhibition, TBZ produced little effect. This may be due to the less powerful inhibition exhibited at predrug condition in this particular experiment. More marked inhibition was observed after L-dopa administration.

R-induced inhibition was only slightly diminished by TBZ. Subsequent injection of L-dopa reversed the TBZ effect, further prolonging the inhibition that was present before TBZ treatment.

Similar patterns of results could be produced by using bulbocapnine to antagonize the brain stem stimulation produced inhibitions. The bulbocapnine effect was again reversed by administering apomorphine. Injecting an equal volume of vehicle (0.9% saline) alone had no effect on brain stem stimulation induced inhibitory effect.

Different combinations of the dopaminergic modifying drugs were tested. Despite the variation in the duration of inhibition effect on the late sural activity, there appears to be a corresponding blocking effect of brain stem evoked inhibition by TBZ or bulbocapnine, which was consistently reversed by using L-dopa or apomorphine.

## DISCUSSION

Results of the present study indicate that brain stem stimulations evoke a descending inhibition on activation of laminae IV and V cells. The antinociceptive action outlasts the brain stimulations for 1 minute or more in many cases. The long duration of suppression effect correlates with that demonstrated in rats (*Mayer et al., 1971*).

Both inhibition and facilitation could be seen in the current experiments. This may account for the specific inhibition controlling the spinal transmission of noxious impulses. According to Melzack and Wall (*1965*), brain stimulations facilitate some interneurons which in turn exert a neural inhibition on those cells which carry the nociceptive messages.

It can be seen that a relatively high percentage of cells sampled were not affected by stimulating SN, PAG or R. This may be explained by the potent brain stem inhibition exerting on some dorsal horn cells upon decerebration (*Besson et al., 1975*).

Previous reports have demonstrated that reaction to noxious stimuli can be diminished or abolished by focal electrical stimulation

of various brain stem areas in the rat *(Liebeskind et al., 1973)* and
cat *(Mayer et al., 1971)*.  The present study shows that apparent
analgesic effect can be obtained from stimulating SN as well as PAG
or R, thus substantiating the behavioral studies on stimulation
produced analgesia.

In their study of monoamine systems with regard to stimulation
produced analgesia, Akil and Liebeskind *(1975)* suggested that dopamine should have a role in the modification of analgesia.  Pharmacological findings in the present study have demonstrated a possible
dopaminergic neurotransmission in the descending control of spinal
interneurons.  The fact that SN-evoked inhibition can be reversibly
modified by dopamine blocking and stimulating agents indicates that
the descending influence depends on the integrity of a dopaminergic
link between SN and lumbar cord *(Carlsson et al., 1964)*.

In comparison with SN, PAG-induced inhibition was less affected
by the dopamine modifying drugs.  Hence it is unlikely that the dopaminergic link occurs between SN and PAG.  Other monoamine systems
have been shown to participate in the PAG-evoked descending effect
*(Akil and Liebeskind, 1975)*.  That R induced effects were relatively
unaltered by dopamine modifying drugs would imply a SN-spinal cord
relay at this site *(Hopkins and Niessen, 1976)*.

In a previous study, Anden et al. *(1966)* demonstrated the presence of serotonergic neurons in R.  Besides, Akil and Mayer *(1972)*
showed that R-evoked analgesia involves a serotonergic mechanism.  In
the current study, R-induced inhibition may be attributed to this
serotonergic system.  This would explain the lack of blocking effect

It would appear that both SN and PAG are relayed to R to exert
their descending influences.  Upon stimulating SN or PAG, a part of
the triggering system of R is activated.  Direct stimulation of R,
which is the common final relay, produced the most potent inhibition
on laminae IV and V cells.

## ACKNOWLEDGEMENTS

This research was supported in part by a grant from the Tarbox
Parkinson's Disease Institute of Texas Tech University School of Medicine.
The authors wish to thank Mr. Robert Polzin and Mr. William L.
Adams for their excellent technical assistance.

## REFERENCES

Akil, H. and Liebeskind, J.C.  (1975).  Monoaminergic mechanisms of
    stimulation-produced analgesia. *Brain Res. 94*, 279-296.
Akil, H. and Mayer, D.J.  (1972).  Antagonism of stimulation-produced
    analgesia by p-CPA, a serotonin synthesis inhibitor. *Brain
    Res. 44*, 692-697.
Anden, N.E., Dahlstrom, A., Fuxe, R., Larsson, K., Olson, L. and

Ungerstedt, T.V. (1966). Ascending monoamine neurons to the telecephalon and diencephalon. *Acta physiol. scand. 67*, 313-326.

Besson, J.M., Conseiller, C., Hamann, K.F. and Maillard, M.C. (1972). Modification of dorsal horn cell activities in the spinal cord after intra-arterial injection of bradykinin. *J. Physiol. 221*, 189-205.

Besson, J.M., Guilbaud, G. and LeBars, D. (1975). Descending inhibitory influences exerted by the brain stem upon the activities of dorsal horn lamina V cells induced by intra-arterial injection of bradykinin into the limbs. *J. Physiol. 248*, 725-739.

Carlsson, A., Falck, B., Fuxe, K., and Hillarp, N.A. (1964). Cellular localization of monoamines in the spinal cord. *Acta physiol. scand. 60*, 112-119.

Gasser, H.S. (1943). Pain producing impulses in peripheral nerves. *Res. Publ. Ass. Nerv. Ment. Dis. 23*, 44-59.

Hillman, P. and Wall, P.D. (1969). Inhibitory and excitatory factors influencing the receptive fields of lamina V spinal cord cells. *Exp. Brain Res. 9*, 284-306.

Hopkins, D.A. and Neissen, L.W. (1976). Substantia nigra projections to the reticular formation, superior colliculus and central gray in the rat, cat and monkey. *Neurosci. Letters 2*, 253-259.

Liebeskind, J.C., Guilbaud, G., Besson, J.M. and Oliveras, J.L. (1973). Analgesia from electrical stimulation of the periaqueductal gray matter in the cat: behavioral observations and inhibitory effects on spinal cord interneurons. *Brain Res. 50*, 441-446.

Mayer, D.J. and Hayes, R.L. (1975). Stimulation-produced analgesia: development of tolerance and cross-tolerance to morphine. *Science 188*, 941-943.

Mayer, D.J., Wolfle, T.L., Akil, H., Carder, B. and Liebeskind, J.C. (1971). Analgesia from electrical stimulation in the brainstem of the rat. *Science 174*, 1351-1354.

Melzack, R. and Wall, P.D. (1965). Pain mechanisms: A new theory, *Science 150*, 971-979.

Minton, J.P. (1975). The response of breast cancer patients with bone pain to L-dopa. *Cancer 33*, 358-362.

Nixon, D.W. (1975). Use of L-dopa to relieve pain from bone metastasis. *N. Eng. J. Med. 292*, 647.

Pomeranz, B., Wall, P.D. and Weber, W.V. (1968). Cord cells responding to fine myelinated afferents from viscera, muscle and skin. *J. Physiol. 199*, 511-532.

Snider, S.R., Rahn, S., Cote, L.J. and Isgree, W.P. (1975). Pain, paresthesia and parkinsonism. *N. Eng. J. Med. 293*, 200.

Tolis, G.J. (1975). L-dopa for pain from bone metastasis. *N. Eng. J. Med. 292*, 1352-1353.

Verri, R.A., Graeff, F.G. and Corrando, A.P. (1967). Antagonism of mophine analgesia by reserpine and a-methyltyrosine and the role played by catecholamines in morphine analgesic action. *J. Pharm. Pharmac. 19*, 264-265.

Wagmann, I.H. and Price, D.D.  (1969).  Responses of dorsal horn cells
    of Macaca mulatta to cutaneous and sural nerve A and C fibre
    stimuli.  *J. Neurophysiol. 32*, 803-817.
Wall, P.D.  (1967).  The laminar organization of dorsal horn and effects
    of descending impulses.  *J. Physiol. 188*, 403-423.

# THE PARKINSONIAN SYNDROME AND ITS DOPAMINE CORRELATES

MARGARET M. HOEHN[1], THOMAS J. CROWLEY[2], AND CHARLES O. RUTLEDGE[3]

Departments of Neurology[1] and Psychiatry[2]
University of Colorado Medical Center
Denver, Colorado 80201
and
Department of Pharmacology and Toxicology [3]
University of Kansas School of Pharmacy
Lawrence, Kansas 66601

## ABSTRACT

The urinary excretion of free dopamine in 37 untreated parkinsonian patients correlated negatively with the severity of rigidity and akinesia ($p<0.025$) and with total neurologic deficit ($p<0.05$). In a parallel study of psychiatric patients, those with the lowest levels of urinary free dopamine before treatment were the most vulnerable to, and developed the most severe, secondary parkinsonian rigidity ($p<0.005$), akinesia ($p<0.05$), and total deficit ($p<0.01$) when they were subsequently treated for two weeks with trifluoperazine. In neither study was there a significant correlation between free urinary dopamine and tremor.

These studies directly associate the level of free dopamine in the urine with the severity of the parkinsonian syndrome. Therefore, although many peripheral sources contribute to urinary free dopamine, a small decrease in the level may actually reflect the severity of the disturbance of central dopamine metabolism and the known deficiency of dopamine in the neurons of the parkinsonian brain.

## INTRODUCTION

The motor abnormalities of Parkinson's disease are related to the degeneration of dopamine-containing neurons in the nigrostriatal pathway of the brain *(Carlsson, 1959; Ehringer and Hornykiewicz, 1960; Birkmayer and Hornykiewicz, 1961)*, and there is considerable

evidence that dopamine (DA) is excreted in reduced quantities in
patients with Parkinson's disease *(Barbeau et al., 1961a, 1961b;
Bischoff and Torres, 1962; Weil-Malherbe and Van Buren, 1969; Barbeau,
1969a; Kott et al., 1971)*. However, correlations between the severity of motor abnormalities and the degree of DA deficiency are less
well established. In the brain, deficiencies of DA and homovanillic
acid (HVA) in the nigrostriatal complex do correlate with the severity of akinesia *(Bernheimer et al., 1973; Hornykiewicz, 1974)*. With
regard to urinary levels of DA, Barbeau *et al.* (1961a, 1961b) found
that hospitalized parkinsonian patients had lower levels of urinary
DA than did outpatients; they suggested that this difference might
be due to the lesser mobility of the hospitalized patients. In a
later study, Barbeau *(1969a)* demonstrated that both the total group
of 60 parkinsonian patients he studied and a subgroup of 8 with "pure"
akinesia had low excretion of DA; however, in a subgroup of 6 patients
with "pure" tremor, DA excretion was normal.

   This study was undertaken to determine whether there is a relationship between the severity of parkinsonian signs and the amount of
free (unconjugated) DA in the urine. Although many peripheral sources
contribute more to urinary DA than does the central nervous system,
a small decrease in the level of free DA in the urine may reflect
the known deficiency of DA in the neurons of the parkinsonian brain
*(Hornykiewicz, 1974)*.

## METHODS

### SUBJECTS

   Twenty-eight patients with primary parkinsonism (Parkinson's
disease) and nine with secondary parkinsonism (not drug-induced)
were studied in hospital. The 18 men and 19 women were between 30
and 82 years old (mean, 65.7 ± SEM 10.8 years). Parkinsonism had
been present for 2 to 36 years (mean, 8.7 ± SEM 9.5 years). Patients had not been treated with antiparkinsonian medications for at
least one week before initial evaluation. All received diets free
of catecholamines for three days before evaluation.

   Two groups of psychiatric patients were studied. All were voluntary inpatients who had received no antipsychotic or antidepressant medications for at least 11 days before entering the study,
and who had no recent heavy use of alcohol or other drugs of abuse.
Group 1 consisted of 16 patients (8 men and 8 women) between 20 and
57 (mean, 31) years old; their diagnoses were schizophrenia (14),
psychotic organic brain syndrome (1), obsessive-compulsive personality disorder (1). The 10 women and 8 men in group 2 all had schizophrenia; the mean age was 28.2 years (range 20-50). None had overt
neurologic disease. Data from the two psychiatric groups were analyzed separately, but there actually was considerable overlap of
membership in the two groups.

NEUROLOGIC EVALUATIONS

Extrapyramidal signs were graded on a scale of increasing severity from 0 to 4 (*Yahr et al., 1969*). The maximal deficit score is 100; tremor contributes a possible 20; rigidity, 20; akinesia, 44; and other parkinsonian phenomena, 16. All patients were evaluated first in the drug-free state. Psychiatric patients were examined also during trifluoperazine administration about 3 times a week for 2 weeks or until unmistakable parkinsonian signs developed.

BIOCHEMICAL EVALUATIONS

All patients had at least one 24-hour urine collection when they were receiving no medications. Collections from psychiatric patients were repeated after they had been receiving trifluoperazine for 2 weeks or when the study was terminated because of the development of drug-induced parkinsonism. All voidings for 24 hours were added immediately to one bottle containing 2.0 gm sodium metabisulphite and stored at $4^{\circ}C$ until the end of the collection. Samples then were frozen and stored at $-5^{\circ}C$. Two or more assays were done of the free and of the total (free plus conjugated) forms of DA, 3,4-dihydroxyphenylacetic acid (DOPAC), and HVA by methods described previously (*Rutledge and Hoehn, 1973; Hoehn et al., 1976*). The means of the daily values were used to calculate each patient's excretion. All results were corrected for recovery, which was 70-80 percent for DA and HVA and 50-60 percent for DOPAC. The biochemical technicians and neurologic examiners were unaware of each other's results.

DRUG ADMINISTRATION

After completion of the initial evaluations, psychiatric patients received oral trifluoperazine HCl (Stelazine®) either by a low-dose schedule increasing by 4 mg/day (15 patients in group 1, 15 patients in group 2) or by a high-dose schedule increasing by 8 mg/day (1 patient in group 1, 3 patients in group 2). The schedules were determined independently by the patients' personal physicians, who were requested to stop increasing at a maximum of 40 mg/day, or when clinical improvement or side effects occurred. No antiparkinsonian drugs were administered during the study.

Correlations were analyzed by the Pearson product-moment method.

## RESULTS

PARKINSONIAN PATIENTS

The mean scores (± SEM) on the evaluation for extrapyramidal

dysfunction in these untreated parkinsonian patients were: tremor
5.1 ± 3.7; rigidity 9.4 ± 4.1; akinesia 24.9 ± 8.9; total neurologic
deficit 45.7 ± 14.9.

The urinary excretion of free and total DA, DOPAC, and HVA is
shown in Table 1. There were no significant differences between the

TABLE 1.   24 HOUR DA, DOPAC, AND HVA EXCRETION IN 37 UNTREATED
           PARKINSONIAN PATIENTS

|        | FREE       | TOTAL        | % CONJUGATED |
|--------|------------|--------------|--------------|
| DA     | 157 ± 34   | 937 ± 191    | 83           |
| DOPAC  | 478 ± 68   | 2299 ± 471   | 79           |
| HVA    | 2625 ± 633 | 3486 ± 780   | 25           |
| TOTAL  | 3260 ± 640 | 6722 ± 1344  | 52           |

Values are expressed as mean ± SEM µg/24-hour urine sample.  (Data
reprinted by permission of the Authors, the Editor, and the Journal
of Neurology, Neurosurgery, and Psychiatry, British Medical Association London, England.  See Reference: Hoehn et al., 1976).

patients with primary and secondary parkinsonism.  Eight-three percent of the DA was present as a conjugate; 79 percent of DOPAC, and
only 25 percent of HVA, was conjugated.

The excretion of free DA correlated negatively with the severity
of rigidity and akinesia ($p<0.025$) and with the total neurologic
deficit score ($p<0.05$) (Table 2).  There was no significant corre-

TABLE 2.   CORRELATIONS OF NEUROLOGIC DEFICIT AND URINARY DA, DOPAC,
           AND HVA IN 37 UNTREATED PARKINSONIAN PATIENTS

|                      | DA          || DOPAC        || HVA         ||
|----------------------|-------|-------|-------|-------|-------|-------|
|                      | FREE  | TOTAL | FREE  | TOTAL | FREE  | TOTAL |
| TREMOR               |       |       | +.307 |       |       |       |
| RIGIDITY             | -.327* |       |       |       |       |       |
| AKINESIA             | -.357* |       |       |       |       |       |
| TOTAL NEURO. DEFICIT | -.288 |       |       |       |       |       |

All, and only, values for which $p<0.05$ are shown.  *$p<0.025$ (Data
reprinted by permission of the Authors, the Editor, and the Journal
of Neurology, Neurosurgery, and Psychiatry, British Medical Association, London, England.  See Reference: Hoehn et al., 1976).

lation between free DA and the severity of tremor. Except for the positive relationship between free DOPAC and tremor, there were no other significant correlations between the severity of neurologic signs and the excretion of either individual or total metabolites.

PSYCHIATRIC PATIENTS

Figure 1 shows the mean daily dosages of trifluoperazine and

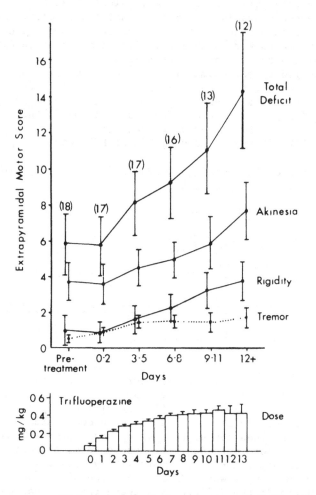

*Figure 1.* *Extrapyramidal motor deficit scores and daily dosage of trifluoperazine (mean ± SEM) for 18 schizophrenic patients. N available at each examination is in parentheses at top.*

mean neurologic deficit scores for patients in group 2 (the results
in group 1 were similar). From the pre-treatment evaluations to the
final evaluations, the mean scores increased as follows: akinesia,
from 3.8 to 7.9 ($p<0.01$; analysis of variance); rigidity, from 1.0
to 3.8 ($p<0.001$); tremor, from 0.6 to 1.7 ($p<0.01$); and total neurologic deficit, from 5.8 to 14.1 ($p<0.001$). The curves shown in
Figure 1 minimize the mean changes, because 4 patients discontinued
the study after 4, 5, 8, and 9 days because of the development of
distressing extrapyramidal symptoms. Since these high-scoring
patients were not available for the final examination, the last
points on the curves derive from the patients who changed the least.
Two other patients were unavailable for examination on day 12 for
non-medical reasons. Nine patients in group 2 and 5 in group 1
were considered by the examiners to develop unequivocal clinical
parkinsonism during the treatment period; in all of these the neurologic deficit scores changed by 9 to 29 points (mean 19.3 ± SEM 4.8).

The urinary excretion of free and total DA, DOPAC, and HVA is
shown in Table 3. Seventy-four percent of the DA was present as a
conjugate; 77% of DOPAC, and only 29% of HVA, was conjugated.

TABLE 3.  24-HOUR DA, DOPAC, AND HVA EXCRETION IN 18 UNTREATED
          SCHIZOPHRENIC PATIENTS

|         | FREE          | TOTAL          | % CONJUGATED |
|---------|---------------|----------------|--------------|
| DA      | 229 ± 29      | 887 ± 191      | 74           |
| DOPAC   | 2031 ± 502    | 8848 ± 1329    | 77           |
| HVA     | 3526 ± 513    | 4980 ± 662     | 29           |
| TOTAL   | 5786 ± 935    | 14715 ± 1713   | 61           |

*Values are expressed as mean ± SEM μg/24-hour urine sample.*

Table 4 lists the significant correlations between the patients'
pretreatment biochemical variables and their subsequent neurologic
change during treatment with trifluoperazine (group 2). Those patients who excreted relatively less free (unconjugated) DA, free DOPAC,
and total metabolites tended to develop more severe rigidity, akinesia, and total neurologic deficit. Conversely, patients with more
conjugation of DA or DOPAC were more likely to develop these signs.
The results in group 1 were similar, and one of the correlations is
shown in Figure 2: the difference between the pretreatment neurologic score and the highest (most pathologic) drug-period score for
each patient is plotted against the pre-drug excretion of free DA.
All 5 of the patients who developed obvious parkinsonism changed by

TABLE 4.   *CORRELATIONS OF PRETREATMENT URINARY DA, DOPAC, HVA, AND*
*EXTRAPYRAMIDAL CHANGES IN 18 SCHIZOPHRENIC PATIENTS DURING*
*TREATMENT WITH TRIFLUOPERAZINE*

| | TOTAL NEURO DEFICIT | AKINESIA | RIGIDITY | TREMOR |
|---|---|---|---|---|
| Free DA | -.52* | -.42 | -.62** | |
| Free DOPAC | -.42 | | | |
| Free DA+DOPAC+HVA | -.43 | | | |
| | | | | |
| Free+conjugated (total): | | | | |
|  DOPAC (77% conjugated) | | | | -.47 |
|  DA+DOPAC+HVA (61% conjugated) | -.41 | | | -.51 |
| | | | | |
| Conjugated DA | +.45 | | | |
| Conjugated DA+DOPAC+HVA | | | | -.47 |
| % Conjugated DA | +.68** | +.68** | +.47 | |
| % Conjugated DOPAC | +.55* | +.45 | +.46 | |

*All significant (p < 0.05) correlations between the biochemical vari-*
*ables listed in Table 3 and changes in neurologic score are listed.*
*\*p < 0.01; \*\*p < 0.005 (one-tailed)*

18 points or more.  The other 11 patients changed by less than 11
points; their extrapyramidal signs were transient, less severe, less
definite.  The median 24-hour free DA excretion was 190 µg.  The 5
patients in this group who developed parkinsonism were among the 8
patients who excreted less than 190 µg/24 hours.  None of the 8 patients who excreted more than that amount developed the syndrome.
This difference is significant ($p < 0.025$, Fisher's exact test).

The development of extrapyramidal signs did not correlate
significantly with age, sex, total dosage received during the study,
dosage of drug on the day of most severe extrapyramidal signs, highest daily dosage received by each patient, or a rough estimate of
post drug exposure.  Except for a decrease in the percentage of HVA
which was conjugated, there were no consistent or significant differences between pre- and post-drug biochemical variables.

## DISCUSSION

Although there is considerable evidence that free DA is excreted in reduced quantities in patients with Parkinson's disease,

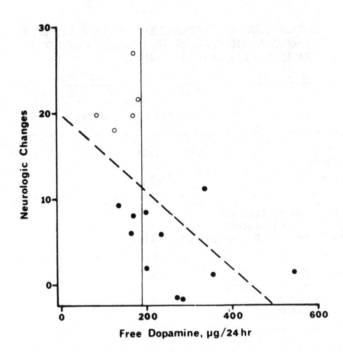

*Figure 2.  Pretreatment free dopamine excretion and neurologic change
with trifluoperazine therapy.  Higher neurologic scores
indicate the development of more marked extrapyramidal
signs.
○ Patients who developed clear-cut parkinsonism
• Patients who did not develop a parkinsonian syndrome
Regression: Y = a + b$_{xy}$ X.  (Figure in part reprinted
by permission of the American Journal of Psychiatry.
See Reference: Crowley et al., 1976).*

correlations between the severity of disease and the degree of DA
deficiency are less well extablished.  Among the parkinsonian patients in this study, the lower the level of free DA in the urine,
the more severe were rigidity, akinesia, and total neurologic deficit.  Similarly, among the psychiatric patients studied, the lower
the level of free DA in the urine before treatment, the more susceptible were the patients to the development of rigidity and akinesia when they were treated with the DA-receptor blocking agent trifluoperazine, and the more severe were their drug-induced rigidity,
akinesia, and total neurologic deficits.  In neither group of
patients did tremor correlate with low levels of free DA in the
urine.

The strength of these correlations is surprising, since animal
studies indicate that only a small proportion of urinary DA derives
from brain (Hoeldtke et al., 1974).  In the parkinsonian patients,

decreased motor activity might have resulted in decreased excretion
of free DA from peripheral sources, as has been suggested by Post
*et al.*, *(1973)*. However, in the psychiatric patients, the relative
deficiency of free DA antedated the drug-induced akinesia; and there
was no correlation between the pretreatment catatonic motor abnormalities of schizophrenia and any biochemical values. It seems more
likely that reduced nigrostriatal DA content is part of a generalized
central and peripheral disorder of DA metabolism, resulting in
reduced DA excretion. Thus the urinary excretion of free DA, although
it is primarily of peripheral origin, may accurately reflect a disturbance of central DA metabolism. The findings of this study are
an unexplained contradiction of earlier reports *(Bozzi et al., 1965;*
*Bruno and Allegranza, 1965)* of more urinary DA and HVA before treatment in patients who subsequently became parkinsonian than in those
who did not.

In neither parkinsonian nor psychiatric patients did tremor
correlate with free DA. There are clinical, therapeutic, pathologic,
and experimental reports that suggest that the tremor of Parkinson's
disease differs from the akinesia and rigidity *(Owen and Marsden,*
*1965; Stadlan et al., 1965; Yahr et al., 1967, 1969; Barbeau, 1969b;*
*Cotzias et al., 1969; Godwin-Austen et al., 1969; Abramsky et al.,*
*1971; Hornykiewicz, 1971; Chase et al., 1972; Strian et al., 1972;*
*Lloyd et al., 1973).* The present study suggests that the mechanism
of neuroleptic-induced tremor also differs in some way from that
of the rigidity and akinesia.

Neither age nor sex was correlated with drug-induced parkinsonism
in this study, although these factors appear to be important in older,
more chronic inpatient populations *(Crane, 1974; Klett and Caffey,*
*1972).* Nor was dosage of trifluoperazine correlated with the development of extrapyramidal signs; however, this protocol may not have
allowed great enough differences in dosages to systematically alter the
results; higher dosages might increase the incidence of parkinsonian
disorders, as has been reported by others *(Prien et al., 1969).*

Dopamine and HVA excretion have been reported to rise during
neuroleptic therapy *(Bozzi et al., 1965; Bruno and Allegranza, 1965).*
In this study, each patient's 24-hour excretion of DA and its metabolites remained reasonably constant during the days before treatment,
and trifluoperazine produced little mean change in excretion patterns.
However, these post-treatment values may be less reliable, since they
were derived from only one sample in most patients, and the excretion
of amine metabolites apparently varies more during, than before, neuroleptic therapy *(Bozzi et al., 1965; Bruno and Allegranza, 1965).*

The mean 24-hour excretion of free DA and of free and total
DOPAC and HVA was lower in the parkinsonian patients than in the
psychiatric patients. This suggests a hypothetical continuum: people who excrete very little free DA probably also have markedly
nigrostriatal DA and spontaneously show parkinsonian akinesia and
rigidity; neuroleptic drugs produce parkinsonian signs in people who
have only moderately deficient levels of DA, while those with the

highest urinary levels also have enough nigrostriatal DA to avoid
parkinsonian signs at the usual dosages of these drugs. We conclude from these studies that the urinary excretion of DA may
quantitatively reflect aspects of extrapyramidal DA metabolism which
are relevant to neuroleptic drug effects and to Parkinson's disease.

## ACKNOWLEDGEMENTS

This work was supported in part by U.S. Public Health Service -
National Institutes of Health Grant NS 09199 and Grant (RR-51) from
the General Clinical Research Program of the Division of Research
Resources, National Institutes of Health. The authors appreciate
the statistical advice of Donald Stilson, Ph.D.; the clinical assistance of Seymour Sundell and Mary Ann Stallings; the technical assistance of Amelia Marlowe, Robert Arnold, Diann Miller, and Marilyn
Hydinger; the secretarial help of Linda Greco-Sanders; the cooperation
of the staffs of the Clinical Research Center of the University of
Colorado Medical Center, the adult psychiatric unit of the Colorado
Psychiatric Hospital, and the Denver Veterans' Administration Hospital, where the patients were treated. Norman Weiner, M.D., offered
continuing encouragement for the work.

## REFERENCES

Abramsky, O., Carmon, A. and Lavy, S. (1971). Combined treatment
    with propranolol and levodopa. *J. Neurol. Sci. 14*, 491-494.
Barbeau, A. (1969a). Parkinson's disease as a systemic disorder.
    *In Third Symposium on Parkinson's Disease* (Gillingham, F.J.
    and Donaldson, I.M.L., Eds.) pp. 66-73. E.S. Livingstone Ltd.,
    Edinburgh and London.
Barbeau, A. (1969b). L-dopa therapy in Parkinson's disease: A crit-
    ical review of nine years' experience. *Can. Med. Assoc. J. 101*,
    791-800.
Barbeau, A., Murphy, G.F. and Sourkes, T.L. (1961a). Excretion of
    dopamine in diseases of the basal ganglia. *Science (Wash.)*
    *133*, 1706-1707.
Barbeau, A., Sourkes, T.L. and Murphy, G.F. (1961b). Les catéchol-
    amines dans la maladie de Parkinson. *In Monoamines et système*
    *Nerveux Central* (de Ajuriaguerra, J., Ed.) pp. 247-262. Georg
    + C$^{ie}$ S.A., Geneva.
Bernheimer, H. Birkmayer, O., Hornykiewicz, O., Jellinger, K. and
    Seitelberger, F. (1973). Brain dopamine and the syndromes
    of parkinsonism and Huntington's chorea. Clinical, morpholo-
    gical and neurochemical correlations. *J. Neurol. Sci. 20*,
    415-455.
Birkmayer, W. and Hornykiewicz, O. (1961). Der L-3,4-Dioxyphenyla-
    lanin (= Dopa) - Effekt bei der Parkinson - Akinese. *Weiner*
    *Klin. Wochenschr. 73*, 787-788.

Bischoff, F. and Torres, A. (1962). Determination of urine dopamine. *Clin. Chem. 8*, 370-377.

Bozzi, R., Bruno, A. and Allegranza, A. (1965). Urinary metabolites of some monoamines and clinical effects under reserpine and chlorpromazine. *Brit. J. Psychiat. 111*, 176-182.

Bruno, A. and Allegranza, A. (1965). The effect of haloperidol on the urinary excretion of dopamine, homovanillic and vanilmandelic acids in schizophrenics. *Psychopharmacologia (Berl.) 8*, 60-66.

Carlsson, A. (1959). The occurrence, distribution, and physiological role of catecholamines in the nervous system. *Pharm. Rev. 11*, 490-493.

Chase, T.N., Ng, L.K.Y. and Watanabe, A.M. (1972). Parkinson's disease: Modification by 5-hydroxytryptophan. *Neurology (Minneap.) 22*, 479-484.

Cotzias, G.C., Papavasiliou, P.S. and Gellene, R. (1969). Modification of parkinsonism - Chronic treatment with L-dopa. *New Eng. J. Med. 280*, 337-345.

Crane, G.E. (1974). Factors predisposing to drug-induced neurologic effects. *In The Phenothiazines and Structurally Related Drugs* (Forrest, I.S., Carr, C.J. and Usdin, E., Eds.) pp. 269-279. Raven Press, New York.

Crowley, T.J., Rutledge, C.O., Hoehn, M.M., Stallings, M.A. and Sundell, S. (1976). Low urinary dopamine and prediction of phenothiazine-induced parkinsonism: A preliminary report. *Am. J. Psychiat. 133*, 703-706.

Ehringer, H. and Hornykiewicz, O. (1960). Verteilung von Noradrenalin und Dopamin (3-Hydroxytyramin) im Gehirn des Menschen und ihr Verhalten bei Erkrankungen des extrapyramidalen Systems. *Klin. Wochenschr. 38*, 1236-1239.

Godwin-Austen, R.B., Tomlinson, E.B., Frears, C.C. and Kok, H.W.L. (1969). Effects of L-dopa in Parkinson's disease. *Lancet ii*, 165-168.

Hoehn, M.M., Crowley, T.J. and Rutledge, C.O. (1976). Dopamine correlates of neurologic and psychiatric status in untreated parkinsonism. *J. Neurol. Neurosurg. Psych. 39*, 941-951.

Hoeldtke, R., Rogawski, M. and Wurtman, R.J. (1974). Effect of selective destruction of central and peripheral catecholamine-containing neurones with 6-hydroxydopamine on catecholamine excretion in the rat. *Br. J. Pharm. 50*, 265-270.

Hornykiewicz, O. (1971). Histochemistry, biochemistry, and pharmacology of brain catecholamines in extrapyramidal syndromes in man. *In Monoamines Noyaux Gris Centraux et Syndrome de Parkinson* (de Ajuriaguerra, J. and Gauthier, G., Eds.) pp. 143-157. Georg + C$^{ie}$ S.A., Geneva.

Hornykiewicz, O. (1974). Metabolism of dopamine and L-dopa in human brain. *Biochem. Pharmacol. 23 (Suppl.)*, 917-923.

Klett, C.J. and Caffey, E. (1972). Evaluating the long-term need for antiparkinson drugs by schizophrenic patients. *Arch. Gen. Psychiat. 26*, 374-379.

Kott, E., Bornstein, B. and Eichhorn, F. (1971). Excretion of dopa metabolites. *New Eng. J. Med. 284*, 395.

Lloyd, K.G., Davidson, L. and Hornykiewicz, O. (1973). Metabolism of levodopa in the human brain. *In Advances in Neurology.* (Calne, D.B., Ed.) *3*, pp. 173-188. Raven Press, New York.

Owen, D.A.L. and Marsden, C.D. (1965). Effect of adrenergic β blockade on parkinsonian tremor. *Lancet ii*, 1259-1262.

Post, R.M., Kotin, J., Goodwin, F.K. and Gordon, E.K. (1973). Psychomotor activity and cerebrospinal fluid amine metabolites in affective illness. *Amer. J. Psychiat. 130*, 67-72.

Prien, R.F., Levin, J. and Cole, J.O. (1969). High dose trifluoperazine therapy in chronic schizophrenia. *Am. J. Psychiat. 126*, 305-313.

Rutledge, C.O. and Hoehn, M.M. (1973). Sulphate conjugation and L-dopa treatment of parkinsonian patients. *Nature 244*, 447-450.

Stadlan, E.M., Duvoisin, R. and Yahr, M.D. (1965). The pathology of parkinsonism. *In Proceedings of the Fifth International Congress of Neuropathology* (Lüthy, F. and Bischoff, A., Eds.) pp. 569-571. International Congress Series No. 100, Excerpta Medica, Amsterdam.

Strian, F., Micheler, E. and Benkert, O. (1972). Tremor inhibition in parkinson syndrome after apomorphine administration under L-dopa and decarboxylase inhibitor basic therapy. *Pharmakopsych. Neuro-Psychopharmakol. 5*, 198-205.

Weil-Malherbe, H. and Van Buren, J.M. (1969). The excretion of dopamine and metabolites in Parkinson's disease and the effect of diet thereon. *J. Lab. Clin. Med. 74*, 305-318.

Yahr, M.D., Duvoisin, R.C., Hoehn, M.M., Schear, M.J. and Barrett, R.E. (1968). L-dopa - its clinical effects in parkinsonism. *Trans. Amer. Neurol. Assoc. 93*, 56-63.

Yahr, M.D., Duvoisin, R.C., Schear, M.J., Barrett, R.E., and Hoehn, M.M. (1969). The treatment of parkinsonism with levodopa. *Arch. Neurol. 21*, 343-354.

# CNS COMPENSATION TO DOPAMINE NEURON LOSS IN PARKINSON'S DISEASE

KENNETH G. LLOYD

Departments of Psychiatry and Pharmacology
University of Toronto
and
Department of Psychopharmacology
Clarke Institute of Psychiatry
Toronto, Ontario, Canada

## ABSTRACT

Postmortem studies in brains from parkinsonian patients consistently reveal a minimum loss of 75% of the nigrostriatal dopamine neurons. This indicates that over a prolonged period, before Parkinson's disease is clinically evident, there is a physiological compensation for the slow loss of dopamine neurons (i.e. compensated stage of Parkinson's disease). Only when the dopamine neuron loss is sufficiently severe (greater than 75% of nigrostriatal dopamine neurons) does the disease become clinically evident (decompensated state). Postmortem examination of Parkinson's disease brains and study of animal models indicate that the following mechanisms may contribute to this CNS compensation:

1) A decrease in striatal cholinergic activity, in an attempt to maintain a critical DA:ACh balance; and 2) A decrease in activity of GABA neurons in the striatum and substantia nigra, resulting in an increased firing rate of nigral dopamine cells. These mechanisms allow the brain to readjust to the initial dopamine cell loss in Parkinson's disease.

## INTRODUCTION

It is well known that in patients with idiopathic or post-encephalitic Parkinson's disease there is a major loss of nigro-striatal dopamine (DA) neurons *(cf Hornykiewicz, 1966; Lloyd, Davidson and Hornykiewicz, 1975)*. Thus, melanin-containing cell bodies in the substantia nigra are specifically lost and this loss is associated with severe (80-95%) decreases in the striatum (caudate nucleus and putamen) of DA, its major metabolite homovanillic acid (HVA) and its synthetic enzyme L-dopa decarboxylase (DOPA-D) *(Lloyd, Davidson and Hornykiewicz, 1975; Bernheimer, Birkmayer, Hornykiewicz, Jellinger and Seitelberger, 1973)*. Alterations of a lesser magnitude are seen in other neuronal systems (e.g. serotonin, noradrenaline, choline-acetyltransferase, glutamic acid decarboxylase) *(Hornykiewicz, 1966; Bernheimer, Birkmayer and Hornykiewicz, 1961; Lloyd, Möhler, Heitz and Bartholini, 1975; Lloyd and Hornykiewicz, 1973; McGeer, McGeer and Fibiger, 1973; Rinne, Laaksonen, Riekkinen and Sonninen, 1974)*. That the loss of dopamine is of major clinical importance is seen by the ability of l-dopa to reverse the symptoms of Parkinson's disease, an effect which is dependent on the increase of DA levels in the striatum *(Lloyd, Davidson and Hornykiewicz, 1975)*.

## RESULTS AND DISCUSSION

One striking finding is that the degree of dopamine neuron loss, as indicated by levels of DA or DOPA-D in L-dopa treated cases *(Hockman, Lloyd, Farley and Hornykiewicz, 1971)* is at least 75-80% in all cases of clinically evident idiopathic or post-encephalitic Parkinson's disease *(Lloyd, 1972)*. This is illustrated in Table 1 which shows the DA, HVA and DOPA-D levels of non-L-DOPA treated parkinsonian patients with varying degrees of clinical severity. It is evident that in all cases there is a high degree of DA neuron loss, even in the less severe clinical stages of Parkinson's disease. This implies that before Parkinson's disease becomes clinically evident (or at least diagnosed, *cf R. Duvoisin, this volume*), there must be a very severe loss of DA neurons. Therefore, at a lesser degree of DA neuron loss it appears that there are homeostatic mechanisms by which the CNS can overcome this initial loss. From our present knowledge, two likely mechanisms are suggested: physiological alterations in the striatal DA:ACh balance and/or the nigral (and possible striatal) GABA:DA balance.

### (1) STRIATAL DA:ACh BALANCE

There is evidence that in the striatum, DA neurons normally inhibit the activity of striatal cholinergic neurons and that interference with DA neuron function increases striatal cholinergic activity. DA agonists reverse this increased cholinergic function. This control of ACh neurons by DA appears to be localized in the striatum and is not functional in other brain regions (e.g. accum-

TABLE 1.   CONCENTRATIONS OF DOPAMINE (DA), HOMOVANILLIC ACID (HVA)
           AND L-DOPA DECARBOXYLASE (DOPA D) IN THE PUTAMEN OF NON-
           L-DOPA TREATED PATIENTS WITH DIFFERENT CLINICAL STAGES OF
           PARKINSON'S DISEASE

| Patient | Clinical Stage | DA (µg/g) | HVA (µg/g) | DOPA D (nmol $CO_2$/100 mg Protein/30 min) |
|---------|----------------|-----------|------------|--------------------------------------------|
| 70-4 | III | ND | 1.45 | 28.5 |
| 70-16 | IV | ND | 0.49 | 24.6 |
| 69-1 | V | 0.40 | 0.35 | 84.6 |
| 71-26 | V | ND | 0.78 | 18.7 |
| 72-46 | V | ND | – | 17.1 |
| Controls | 0 | 5.06 | 4.29 | 431.9 |

ND = not detectable; Patient rating scale: 0 = non-Parkinsonian;
I = unilateral involvement; II = bilateral involvement; III = evidence of impaired balance and righting reflex; IV = fully developed
severe disease; V = confined to bed or wheelchair.
Data from Lloyd, 1972 and Lloyd, Davidson and Hornykiewicz, 1975.

bens, septum, hippocampus, cortex) (Agid, Guyenet, Glowinski, Beaujouan and Javoy, 1975; Bartholini, Stadler, Gadea-Ciria and Lloyd,
1975; Lloyd, Stadler and Bartholini, 1973; Sethy and Van Woert,
1974a and b; Trabucchi, Cheney, Racagni and Costa, 1974 and 1975).
The release of striatal cholinergic activity by neuroleptic drugs
(via blockade of DA receptors) is likely related to their catalep-
togenic activity (Lloyd, 1976).   Thus, at clinically equivalent
doses, haloperidol (and similar drugs) induces catalepsy and increases
striatal ACh release and turnover, whereas clozapine induces neither
catalepsy nor increased striatal ACh release (Bartholini, Stadler,
Gadea-Ciria and Lloyd, 1975).   An analogous situation is seen in man
where haloperidol produces a relatively high incidence of drug-induced
parkinsonism (Hornykiewicz, 1975) whereas the incidence of this side
effect to clozapine is extremely low (Simpson, 1974).
     It appears that there is a homeostatic mechanism which attenuates
a prolonged perturbation to this striatal DA:ACh balance.   Thus, upon
prolonged administration there is a tolerance to the haloperidol-
induced catalepsy in rats (Lloyd, Shibuya, Davidson and Hornykiewicz,
1976; Asper, Baggiolini, Burki, Lauerner, Ruch and Stille, 1973).
Acutely, haloperidol (5 mg/kg i.p., rats sacrificed 18 hours after
injection) produces a rise in striatal choline acetyltransferase
(ChAt) activity.   After 167 days of daily haloperidol administration
(5 mg/kg, i.p., rats sacrificed 18 hours after last injection) the
degree of catalepsy produced is greatly attenuated and the ChAt
activity is no longer elevated following haloperidol (Table 2).   Most

TABLE 2.   *CATALEPSY MEASUREMENTS AND STRIATAL CHOLINE ACETYLTRANS-*
*FERASE ACTIVITY IN RATS TREATED WITH HALOPERIDOL (5 mg/kg,*
*i.p.) ACUTELY (SINGLE INJECTION) OR CHRONICALLY (167 DAILY*
*INJECTIONS)* [1]

| Group | Duration of Catalepsy (Maximum 120 Sec) 60 Minutes After Haloperidol | Choline Acetyltransferase (nMol ACh/mg Protein/ 20 min) |
|---|---|---|
| Controls | 2 ± 1 (6) | 42.3 ± 1.9 (6) |
| Acute Haloperidol | 120 ± 0 (4)[3] | 48.7 ± 1.7 (4)[2] |
| Chronic Haloperidol | 36 ± 5 (9)[3,4] | 39.6 ± 2.3 (7)[5] |

[1]*Results expressed as Mean ± S.E.M.   Number of animals in parentheses.*
[2]*$p<0.05$ vs controls*
[3]*$p<0.001$ vs controls*
[4]*$p<0.001$ vs acute haloperidol*
[5]*$p<0.02$ vs acute haloperidol*
*Data from Lloyd, Shibuya, Davidson and Hornykiewicz, 1976.*

importantly when the data from individual acute and chronic animals
were examined there was a very high correlation ($r = 0.91$; $p<0.001$)
between the cataleptic effect of haloperidol and the degree of elevation of striatal ChAt activity.  This high correlation does not
exist between catelepsy and ChAt in other brain regions or between
catalepsy and glutamic acid decarboxylase (GAD) activity, DA, NA
or GABA levels in different brain areas (e.g. striatum, substantia
nigra, n.accumbens, septum).  In humans, a similar tolerance to the
neuroleptic-induced parkinsonism occurs, but not to the antipsychotic
effect of the drugs *(Hollister, 1972; Klett and Caffey, 1972)*.
     These findings show that the activity of the striatal choliner-
gic system is altered by acute changes in the activity of the nigro-
striatal DA path but that upon chronic blockade of this DA path (at
the DA receptor level) the response of the striatal cholinergic system is markedly attenuated.  It is likely that this or a similar
mechanism is operative in Parkinson's disease.  Thus, there is strong
evidence for a striatal DA:ACh imbalance in Parkinson's disease as (1)
anticholinergics mildly reduce symptoms *(Greenblatt and Shader, 1973)*
and cholinergic drugs exacerbate them *(Duvoisin, 1967)*; and (2) The
converse is true of drugs which affect DA neurons *(cf Lloyd and
Hornykiewicz, 1974)*.  This author suggests that in the initial
stages of Parkinson's disease, as DA neurons slowly drop out (due
to progressive cell loss in the pars compacta of the substantia

nigra) there is a homeostatic dampening of striatal cholinergic activity, which maintains a normal striatal DA:ACh balance.  Upon continued DA neuron loss this compensatory mechanism fails to maintain this
balance and a state of relative striatal cholinergic hyperactivity
exists.  Supportive evidence for this hypothesis is found in studies
on post-mortem brains.  Thus, in material from parkinsonian patients
who were not treated with L-DOPA, ChAt levels are lowered to the
greatest extent (30-50% of control) in those areas specifically
associated with Parkinson's disease (striatum, substantia nigra,
thalamus) *(Lloyd, Möhler, Heitz and Bartholini, 1975)*.  This lowering
of striatal ChAt activity is not subsequent to cell loss, as morphological changes are not reported in the striatum of parkinsonian patients.  Therefore these alterations in striatal ChAt activity are
likely part of a compensatory system to DA neuron loss, as outlined
in Figure 1.

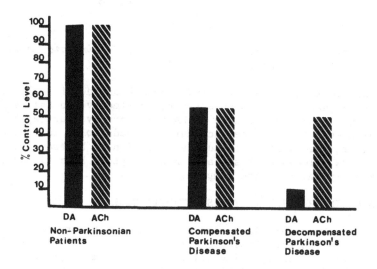

*Figure 1.  Striatal DA:ACh Balance in Parkinson's Disease*

This hypothesis explains a clinical observation which has been
one obstruction to the complete acceptance of the imbalance of DA:ACh
interregulation in Parkinson's disease.  The observation is that in
Parkinson's disease anticholinergic drugs only mildly reduce akinesia
and rigidity whereas in neuroleptic-induced parkinsonism (or catalepsy in rats) anticholinergics are very effective in reducing symptoms.  The situation is outlined in Figure 2.  The explanation according to the present hypothesis is that in idiopathic Parkinson's
disease the striatal cholinergic tone is already maximally dampened

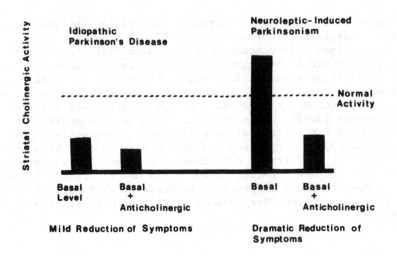

*Figure 2.   Hypothetical Response of Striatal Cholinergic Activity to Anticholinergic Medications*

by homeostatic mechanisms.  The additional blockade of cholinergic receptors by anticholinergics is rather ineffective in this situation. In contrast, the acute blockade of DA receptors by neuroleptics, which disinhibits striatal cholinergic neurons, leads to an increased striatal cholinergic activity.  In such a situation of hyperactive cholinergic neurons, blockade of striatal ACh receptors by anticholinergics drugs markedly reverses the symptoms.

## (2) GABA:DA INTERACTION IN THE SUBSTANTIA NIGRA

There is considerable evidence that an inhibitory neuronal path utilizing GABA projects from the striatum (or globus pallidus) to the substantia nigra.  Thus, stimulation of the striatum produces a monosynaptic inhibition of cells in the substantia nigra, an effect which is specifically mimicked by iontophoretic GABA administration and blocked by picrotoxin or bicuculline (*Crossman, Walker and Woodruff, 1973; Dray and Straughan, 1976; Precht and Yoshida, 1971; Feltz, 1971*).  That there is an interaction between these GABA neurons and nigral DA neurons is shown by:

(i) the disappearance of putative GABA receptors in the substantia nigra of parkinsonian patients (*Lloyd, Shemen and Hornykiewicz, 1976*) a condition in which only the DA cell bodies degenerate;

(ii) the acute lowering of nigral GABA levels by neuroleptic drugs and their elevation by DA agonists *(Kim and Hassler, 1975; McGeer, Grewaal and McGeer, 1976; Lloyd, Shibuya, Davidson and Hornykiewicz, 1976)*;

(iii) the decrease in GABA turnover brought about by apomorphine in regions of DA cell bodies *(Perez de la Mora, Fuxe, Hokfelt and Ljundahl, 1975)*;

(iv) the lowering of GAD activity in the striatum and substantia nigra of brain from non-L-DOPA treated parkinsonian patients *(Lloyd and Hornykiewicz, 1973; Lloyd, Möhler, Heitz and Bartholini, 1975; Rinne, Sonninen, Riekkinen and Laaksonen, 1974)*.

It is apparent that the decreased GAD activity in Parkinson's disease is not as a result of cell degeneration, but rather is due to a physiological process. Thus, upon prolonged L-DOPA therapy the striatal GAD levels in parkinsonian brain return to control levels in a manner dependent upon the duration of L-DOPA treatment *(Lloyd, Möhler, Bartholini and Hornykiewicz, 1976)*. Other evidence for a homeostatic regulation of this system is that upon chronic (167 day) haloperidol or L-DOPA treatment of rats, the changes in nigral GABA levels no longer occur *(Lloyd, Shibuya, Davidson and Hornykiewicz, 1976)*.

The proposed physiological alterations of nigral GABA terminal activity during the development of Parkinson's disease is presented in Table 3. Thus, as nigral DA cell bodies degenerate there is a compensatory homeostatic decrease in the inhibitory GABA input to the remaining DA cell bodies. This allows these cell bodies to fire at a more rapid (and eventually maximal) rate. There is evidence from post-mortem studies in parkinsonian brain that this occurs. Thus, the ratio

*TABLE 3. HYPOTHETICAL ACTIVITY OF GABA INPUT TO NIGRAL DA CELL BODIES IN PARKINSON'S DISEASE*

| Clinical Condition | Activity of GABA Input to Substantia Nigra | DA Cell Activity | DA Release in Striatum |
|---|---|---|---|
| Non-Parkinsonian (Control) | 100% | Tonically inhibitied | Normal DA release |
| Parkinson's Disease: Compensated | 30-50% | Firing maximally | Augmented - can maintain normal DA release |
| Decompensated | 20-40% | Firing maximally | Too few neurons to maintain Sufficient DA release |

of striatal HVA:DA is higher in parkinsonian than in control brains,
indicating an increased DA turnover in the surviving DA neurons.
Also, the decrease in striatal tyrosine hydroxylase activity (to 60-70
percent of control) in Parkinson's disease is much less than that for
DOPA D, or DA (to 20 percent or less of control) *Lloyd, Davidson and
Hornykiewicz, 1975).* It is significant that tyrosine hydroxylase
activity may be increased by enzyme induction *(Axelrod, 1971).* Further support for this hypothesis is found in the observation that
after partial lesion of the nigro-striatal neurons in the rat by
6-hydroxydopamine, the remaining DA neurons synthesize DA at an
increased rate *(Agid, Javoy and Glowinski, 1973).*
    The overall situation is summarized in Table 4.  Thus, in the

TABLE 4.  *SUMMARY OF COMPENSATORY MECHANISMS IN PARKINSON'S DISEASE*

---

*Normally* i.  DA neurons inhibit striatal ACh Neurons
          ii. GABA neurons inhibit DA cell bodies in substantia nigra.
*Parkinson's Disease:* loss of DA cell bodies in substantia nigra re-
                sults in decreased DA release in striatum
*Compensated State:* (i) striatal ACh neurons reduce synthesis and re-
                lease of ACh to maintain normal DA:ACh balance
                       (ii) GABA input to SN decreases synthesis and release
                of GABA, allowing maximal firing of remaining DA neurons
                       (i) + (ii) overcome DA deficit
*Decompensated Stage:* DA cell loss is too great for above compensation
                mechanisms.
                ACh preponderance in striatum leads to akinesia, rigid-
                ity (catalepsy in laboratory animals).

---

normal brain the nigro-striatal DA neurons inhibit striatal cholinergic interneurons.  Also, at the level of the substantia nigra, GABA
terminals control the firing rate of the DA cell bodies.  In the
initial stages of Parkinson's disease there is a slow loss of DA
neurons.  To compensate for this, the activity of the striatal cholinergic interneurons decreases, maintaining a normal striatal DA:ACh
balance.  Simultaneously there is a decrease in the activity of GABA
neurons terminating in the substantia nigra, allowing the still
intact DA neurons to fire at an increased rate.  These two mechanisms overcome the loss of the DA neurons and a state of compensated
Parkinson's disease exists (i.e. biochemically the disease is present but is not clinically evident).  As the DA neuron loss progresses these compensatory mechanisms are insufficient to overcome
the severe DA deficit and Parkinson's disease become clinically
evident.

## ACKNOWLEDGEMENTS

This work was supported by the Clarke Institute of Psychiatry and by the National Institute of Mental Health, U.S.A. (Grant No. MH20500-04).

## REFERENCES

Agid, Y., Javoy, F. and Glowinski, J. (1973). Hyperactivity of remaining dopaminergic neurons after partial destruction of the nigrostriatal dopaminergic system in the rat. *Nature, New Bio. 245*, 150-151.

Agid, Y., Guyenet, P., Glowinski, J. Beaujouan, J.C. and Javoy, F. (1975). Inhibitory influence of the nigrostriatal dopamine system on the striatal cholinergic neurons in the rat. *Brain Research 86*, 488-492.

Asper, H., Baggiolini, M., Burki, H.R., Lauener, H. Ruch, W. and Stille, G. (1973). Tolerance phenomena with neuroleptics catalepsy, apormophine stereotypies and striatal dopamine metabolism in the rat after single and repeated administration of loxapine and haloperidol. *Europ. J. Pharmacol. 22*, 287-294.

Axelrod, J. (1971). Noradrenaline: Fate and control of its biosynthesis. *Science 173*, 598-606.

Bartholini, G., Stadler, H., Gadea-Cirea, M. and Lloyd, K.G. (1975). The effect of antipsychotic drugs on the release of neurotransmitter in various brain areas. *In Antipsychotic Drugs - Pharmacodynamics and Pharmacokinetics* (Sedvall, G., Ed.) pp. 105-116. Pergamon Press, New York.

Bernheimer, H., Birkmayer, W. and Hornykiewicz, O. (1961). Verteilung des 5-Hydroxytryptamin (Serotonin) im Gehirn des Menschen und sein Verhalten bei Patienten mit Parkinson-Syndrom. *Klin. Wsch. 39*, 1056-1059.

Bernheimer, H., Birkmayer, W., Hornykiewicz, O., Jellinger, K. and Seitelberger, F. (1973). Brain dopamine and the syndromes of Parkinson and Huntington. *J. Neurol. Sci. 20*, 415-455.

Crossman, A.R., Walker, R.J. and Woodruff, G.N. (1973). Picrotoxin antagonism of γ-aminobutyric acid inhibitory responses and synaptic inhibition in the rat substantia nigra. *Brit. J. Pharmacol. 49*, 696-698.

Dray, A. and Straughan, D.W. (1976). Synaptic mechanisms in the substantia nigra. *J. Pharm. Pharmacol. 28*, 400-405.

Duvoisin, R.C. (1967). Cholinergic-Anticholinergic antagonism in parkinsonism. *Arch. Neurol. 17*, 124-136.

Feltz, P. (1971). γ-Aminobutyric acid and a caudate-nigral inhibition. *Can. J. Physiol. Pharmacol. 49*, 113-115.

Fonnum, F., Grofova, I., Rinvik, E., Storm-Mathisen, J. and Walberg, F. (1974). Origin and distribution of glutamate decarboxylase in substantia nigra of the cat. *Brain Research 71*, 77-92.

Greenblatt, D.J. and Shader, R.I. (1973). Anticholinergics. *New Engl. J. Med. 288*, 1215-1219.

Hattori, T., McGeer, P.L., Fibiger, H.C. and McGeer, E.G. (1973). On the source of GABA-containing terminals in the substantia nigra: Electron microscopic, autoradeographic and biochemical studies. *Brain Research 54*, 103-114.

Hockman, C.H., Lloyd, K.G., Farley, I.J. and Hornykiewicz, O. (1971). Experimental midbrain lesions: Neurochemical comparison between the animal model and Parkinson's Disease. *Brain Research 35*, 613-618.

Hollister, L.E. (1972). Mental disorders-antipsychotic and antimanic drugs. *New Engl. J. Med. 286*, 984-987.

Hornykiewicz, O. (1966). Dopamine (3-Hydroxytyramine) and brain function. *Pharmacol. Revs. 18*, 925-964.

Hornykiewicz, O. (1975). Parkinsonism induced by dopaminergic antagonists. *In Advances in Neurology, Vol. 9* (Calne, D.B. and Barbeau, A., Eds.) pp. 155-164, Raven Press, New York.

Kim, J.S. and Hassler, R. (1975). Effects of acute haloperidol on the gamma-aminobutyric acid system in rat striatum and substantia nigra. *Brain Research 88*, 150-153.

Kim. J.S., Bak, I.J., Hassler, R. and Okada, Y. (1971). Role of gamma-aminobutyric acid (GABA) in the extrapyramidal motor system. *Exp. Brain Research 14*, 95-104.

Klett, C.J. and Caffey, E. (1972). Evaluating the long-term need for antiparkinson drugs by chronic schizophenics. *Arch. Gen. Psychiat. 26*, 374-379.

Lloyd, K.G. (1972). Biogenic amines and related enzymes in the human and animal brain. Ph.D. Thesis, University of Toronto.

Lloyd, K.G. (1976). Observations concerning neurotransmitter interaction in schizophrenia. *In Cholinergic-monoaminergic interaction in the brain* (Butcher, L.L., Ed.) In Press, Academic Press, New York.

Lloyd, K.G. and Hornykiewicz, O. (1973). L-Glutamic acid Decarboxylase in Parkinson's disease: Effect of L-dopa therapy. *Nature 243*, 521-523.

Lloyd, K.G. and Hornykiewicz, O. (1974). Dopamine and Other monoamines in the basal ganglia: Relation to brain dysfunction. *In Frontiers in Neurology and Neuroscience Research, 1974.* (Seeman, P. and Brown, G.M., Eds.) pp. 26-35. University of Toronto Press, Toronto.

Lloyd, K.G., Davidson, L. and Hornykiewicz, O. (1975). The neurochemistry of Parkinson's disease: Effect of L-dopa therapy. *J. Pharmacol. Exp. Therap. 195*, 453-464.

Lloyd, K.G., Möhler, H., Bartholini, G. and Hornykiewicz, O. (1976). Pathological alterations in glutamic acid decarboxylase activity in Parkinson's disease. *In Fifth International Symposium on Parkinson's Disease* (Birkmayer, W. and Hornykiewicz, O., Eds.) In Press, Editiones Roche, Basel.

Lloyd, K.G., Möhler, H., Hertz, Ph. and Bartholini, G.  (1975).
    Distribution of choline acetyltransferase and glutamic acid
    decarboxylase within the substantia nigra and in other  brain
    regions from control and parkinsonian patients.  *J. Neurochem.*
    *25*, 789-795.
Lloyd, K.G., Shemen, L. and Hornykiewicz, O.  (1976).  Distribution
    of high affinity Sodium-independent $^3$H-gamma-aminobutyric acid
    ($^3$H-GABA Binding) in the human brain: Alterations in Parkinson's
    disease.  *Brain Research*.  In Press.
Lloyd, K.G., Shibuya, M., Davidson, L. and Hornykiewicz, O.  (1976).
    Chronic neuroleptic therapy: Tolerance and GABA Systems.  *In*
    *Symposium on Non-Striatal Dopamine* (Costa E. and Gessa, G.L.,
    Eds.)  In Press, Raven Press, New York.
Lloyd, K.G., Stadler, H. and Bartholini, G.  (1973).  Dopamine and
    acetylcholine neurons in striatal and limbic structures: Effect
    of neuroleptic drugs.  *In Frontiers in Catecholamine Research*
    (Usdin, E. and Snyder, S., Eds.) pp. 777-779.  Pergamon Press,
    Oxford.
McGeer, P.L., McGeer, E.G., Wada, J.A. and Jung, E.  (1971).  Effects
    of globus pallidus lesions and Parkinson's disease on brain
    glutamic acid decarboxylase.  *Brain Research 32*, 425-431.
McGeer, P.L., McGeer, E.G. and Fibiger, H.C.  (1973).  Glutamic-acid
    decarboxylase and choline acetylase in Huntington's Chorea and
    Parkinson's disease.  *Lancet ii*, 623-624.
McGeer, P.L., Grewaal, D.S. and McGeer, E.G.  (1976).  Effect on
    extrapyramidal GABA levels of drugs which influence dopamine
    and acetylcholine metabolism.  *In Fifth International Sympos-*
    *ium on Parkinson's Disease* (Birkmayer, W. and Hornykiewicz, O.,
    Eds.)  In Press, Editiones Roche, Basel.
Perez de la Mora, M., Fuxe, K. Hokfelt, T. and Ljungdahl, A.  (1975).
    Effect of apomorphine on the GABA Turnover in the dopamine
    cell group rich area of the mesencephalon: Evidence for the
    involvement of an inhibitory GABAergic feedback control of the
    ascending dopaminergic neurons.  *Neurosci. Letts. 1*, 109-114.
Precht, W. and Yoshida, M.  (1971).  Blockage of caudate-evoked
    inhibition of neurons in the substantia nigra by picratoxin.
    *Brain Research 32*, 229-233.
Sethy, V.H. and Van Woert, M.H.  (1974a).  Regulation of striatal
    acetylcholine concentrations by dopamine receptors.  *Nature*
    *251*, 529-530.
Sethy, V.H. and Van Woert, M.H.  (1974b).  Modification of striatal
    acetylcholine concentrations by dopamine receptor agonists
    and antagonists.  *Res. Comm. Chem. Pathol. Pharmacol. 8*, 13-28.
Simpson, G.M.  (1974).  Clozapine: A new antipsychotic drug.  *Curr.*
    *Therap. Research. 16*, 679-686.
Trabucchi, M. Cheney, D., Racagni, G. and Costa, E.  (1974).  Involve-
    ment of brain cholinergic mechanisms in the action of chlorpro-
    mazine.  *Nature 249*, 664-666.

Trabucchi, M., Cheney, D.L., Racagni, G. and Costa, E.   (1975).
    *In vivo* inhibition of striatal acetylcholine turnover by
    L-dopa, apomorphine and (+)-amphetamine.   *Brain Research 85*,
    130-134.

# BRAIN DOPAMINE TURNOVER AND THE RELIEF OF PARKINSONISM

U.K. RINNE, V. SONNINEN AND R. MARTTILA

Department of Neurology
University of Turku
Turku, Finland

## ABSTRACT

Levodopa alone or combined with a decarboxylase inhibitor elevated the concentration of homovanillic acid (HVA) in the cerebrospinal fluid (CSF). This increase correlated significantly with the
dose of the drug but not with the clinical improvement, although
some correlations with clinical side effects were evident. Nevertheless, the concentrations of HVA in the CSF during combined treatment were considerably lower than with therapeutically equivalent
doses of levodopa alone. Obviously, a part of the HVA found in the
CSF during levodopa treatment originates from the capillary walls.
Treatment with dopamine receptor agonists, Piribedil or Bromocriptine decreased significantly both the basal level and probenecid-
induced accumulations of HVA and CSF. But there were no changes in
concentrations of 5-hydroxyindoleacetic acid (5-HIAA). Correlation
analyses showed that patients who improved with both dopamine agonists used had significantly lower probenecid response of HVA in the
CSF and less severe disease than those without beneficial effect.
This relationship between dopamine receptor activation and improvement of parkinsonian disability suggests that the therapeutic efficacy of dopamine receptor agonists depends on the functional capacity
of brain dopaminergic mechanisms.

267

## INTRODUCTION

There is no doubt that clinical condition of parkinsonian patients can be improved by replacing the deficiency of brain dopamine
by levodopa.  Moreover, there is recent evidence that also dopamine
receptor agonists could be beneficial in the treatment of patients
with Parkinson's disease (Vakil et al., 1973; Calne et al., 1974: Chase
et al., 1974; Rinne et al., 1975).

In the present study we have investigated the possible relationship between dopamine receptor activation and the relief of parkinsonian clinical features.  Clinical responses and changes in the basal
levels and probenecid-induced accumulations of homovanillic acid (HVA)
and 5-hydroxyindoleacetic acid (5-HIAA) in the cerebrospinal fluid
(CSF) during treatment with levodopa or dopamine receptor agonists
were studied.

## RESULTS

LEVODOPA

Concentration of HVA in the CSF of parkinsonian patients was
significantly lower than those of controls both in the basal state
and after probenecid (Table 1).

TABLE 1.   CONCENTRATION (ng/ml) OF HVA IN THE CSF OF CONTROL AND
           PARKINSONIAN PATIENTS IN BASAL STATE AND AFTER ADMINISTRA-
           TION OF PROBENECID.  MEAN ± SEM.

| Group | HVA | |
|---|---|---|
| | Basal | Probenecid |
| Controls | 34.4 ± 1.9 | 104.6 ± 13.9 |
| | (64) | (28) |
| Parkinsonian patients | 15.8 ± 1.1 | 76.2 ± 6.3 |
| | (125) | (91) |
| P | <0.001 | <0.05 |

The basal concentration of HVA in the CSF of patients with
Parkinson's disease showed a significant ($P<0.05$) negative correlation with the severity of hypokinesia but not with other clinical
variables.  However, among the parkinsonian patients the HVA response to probenecid showed a significant negative correlation not
only with the degree of hypokinesia ($P<0.05$) but also with the
degree of rigidity and the severity of the disease as well as with

the disability of the patients ($P<0.05$ in all cases).   There was also
a tendency towards a positive correlation with tremor.
    Clinically, it is important to know whether the basal level of
HVA in the CSF or its response to probenecid can predict the clinical
responses to levodopa treatment.   Nevertheless, among many parkinsonian patients treated with levodopa alone or combined with a decarboxylase inhibitor we did not find any significant correlations.
    As can be seen in Table 2 the concentration of HVA in the CSF

TABLE 2.   *CONCENTRATION (ng/ml) OF HVA IN THE CSF OF CONTROL SUBJECTS
AND PARKINSONIAN PATIENTS IN BASAL STATE AND AFTER 3 MONTHS
OF TREATMENT WITH VARIOUS DOSE RATIOS OF LEVODOPA AND
BENSERAZIDE OR LEVODOPA ALONE.   MEAN ± SEM.*

| Group | Basal level | After 3 months' treatment |
|---|---|---|
| Controls | 34.4 ± 1.9 (64) | – |
| Parkinsonian patients | | |
| Levodopa and benserazide 4 x (200 mg + 50 mg) | 18.6 ± 2.2 (31) | 122.9 ± 15.3 (29) |
| 4 x (150 mg + 100 mg) | 21.8 ± 3.5 (28) | 64.8 ± 7.3 (38) |
| Levodopa 4 x 1,000 mg | 15.7 ± 1.5 (94) | 144.1 ± 14.4 (57) |

of parkinsonian patients increased significantly during long-term
treatment with levodopa alone or combined with a decarboxylase inhibitor.   This increase correlated significantly for levodopa ($P<0.05$)
and for levodopa and a decarboxylase inhibitor ($P<0.01$) with the dose.
Nevertheless, the concentrations of HVA in the CSF during combined
treatment were considerably lower than with therapeutically equivalent doses of levodopa alone (Table 2).   Moreover, with an increase
in the daily dose of decarboxylase inhibitor the concentration of
HVA significantly decreased ($P<0.001$).
    There was no correlation between the concentrations of HVA in
the CSF during treatment with levodopa alone or combined with a
decarboxylase inhibitor and clinical improvement, although some
correlations with clinical side effects were evident during treatment with levodopa alone (Table 3) and during combined treatment
with a decarboxylase inhibitor (Table 4).

TABLE 3.  *SIGNIFICANT CORRELATIONS BETWEEN CONCENTRATIONS OF HVA IN THE CSF AND VARIOUS CLINICAL SIDE EFFECTS DURING LONG-TERM TREATMENT WITH LEVODOPA.*

| Variable | Duration of treatment (months) | | |
|---|---|---|---|
| | 1 | 3 | 9 |
| Nausea | | $P<0.01$ | |
| Vomiting | | $P<0.01$ | |
| Anorexia | | | $P<0.05$ |
| Sweating | | | $P<0.05$ |
| Mood elevation | $P<0.05$ | | |
| Insomnia | $P<0.05$ | | |
| Involuntary movements | | | $P<0.01$ |

TABLE 4.  *SIGNIFICANT CORRELATIONS BETWEEN THE CONCENTRATIONS OF HVA IN THE CSF AND VARIOUS CLINICAL SIDE EFFECTS DURING LONG-TERM TREATMENT WITH LEVODOPA AND BENSERAZIDE.*

| Side effects | Duration of treatment (months) | | |
|---|---|---|---|
| | 1 | 3 | 9 |
| Mood elevation | $P<0.05$ | | |
| Psychotic behavior | | $P<0.05$ | |
| Postural hypotension | | | $P<0.01$ |

PIRIBEDIL

Table 5 shows that during long-term treatment a daily dose of 120 mg of Piribedil elicited a moderate, but significant ($P<0.001$) therapeutic response in parkinsonian patients.  The effect seemed to increase within the first two months.  But a significant ($P<0.01$) exacerbation of total disability took place when changed from Piribedil to placebo.  However, the beneficial effect of Piribedil seems to be significantly less to that of levodopa.

The basal concentration of HVA in the CSF of parkinsonian patients decreased during Piribedil treatment.  However, more significantly ($P<0.05$) Piribedil treatment led to a decrease in probenecid-induced accumulations of HVA after one month treatment with 120 mg of Piribedil daily (Table 6).  On the contrary, Piribedil treatment caused no significant changes either in the basal

TABLE 5.  *IMPROVEMENT OF MAJOR CLINICAL FEATURES OF PARKINSONIAN*
         *PATIENTS DURING PIRIBEDIL TREATMENT (120 MG/DAY).*
         *MEAN ± SEM.*

| Duration of treatment (weeks) | No. of patients | Mean improvement (% ± SEM) | | | |
|---|---|---|---|---|---|
| | | Total disability | Tremor | Rigidity | Hypo-kinesia |
| Piribedil | | | | | |
| 2 | 16 | 5 ± 1 | 8 ± 3 | 3 ± 1 | 3 ± 1 |
| 4 | 15 | 10 ± 2 | 19 ± 4 | 8 ± 3 | 8 ± 3 |
| 8 | 15 | 15 ± 3 | 20 ± 5 | 15 ± 4 | 10 ± 4 |
| 16 | 15 | 16 ± 3 | 22 ± 5 | 14 ± 5 | 12 ± 5 |
| Placebo | | | | | |
| 4 | 15 | 6 ± 2 | 7 ± 4 | 5 ± 4 | 6 ± 6 |

TABLE 6.  *EFFECT OF PIRIBEDIL TREATMENT ON PROBENECID-INDUCED ACCUMU-*
         *LATIONS (ng/ml) OF HVA AND 5-HIAA IN THE CSF OF 11 PARKIN-*
         *SONIAN PATIENTS.  MEAN ± SEM.*

| Piribedil | HVA | | 5-HIAA | |
|---|---|---|---|---|
| | Basal | Probenecid | Basal | Probenecid |
| Before | 17.1 ± 4.0 | 102.2 ± 12.1 | 32.6 ± 4.7 | 91.1 ± 12.1 |
| During | 13.7 ± 3.4 | 68.0 ± 10.0 | 33.1 ± 3.7 | 87.1 ± 13.5 |
| $P$ | >0.05 | <0.05 | >0.05 | >0.05 |

concentration of 5-HIAA or in its response to probenecid (Table 6).

Correlation analysis showed a significant ($P<0.05$) negative correlation between HVA accumulation in the CSF produced by probenecid and improvement of total disability during Piribedil treatment.  This can be seen in Table 7, showing that after one month treatment the probenecid-induced rise of HVA in the CSF is significantly ($P<0.05$) lower in patients with clear improvement, as compared to those without beneficial effect.  In the former patients there was also a clear tendency to have a higher rise in HVA when the probenecid test was carried out prior to treatment.  Moreover, there was significant correlation between these changes and the severity of the disease.  Patients showing more improvement and greater decrease in probenecid response of HVA had significantly less severe disease than others.

TABLE 7.   *CORRELATION OF PROBENECID-INDUCED ACCUMULATIONS (ng/ml)*
           *OF HVA IN THE CSF OF PARKINSONIAN PATIENTS WITH IMPROVE-*
           *MENT ON PIRIBEDIL.   MEAN ± SEM.*

| Improvement on Piribedil | Probenecid-induced accumulations of HVA | |
| --- | --- | --- |
| | Before | During |
| >10% | 124.6 ± 33.7 | 35.2 ± 14.3 |
| (20 ± 2) | (5) | (5) |
| <10% | 81.8 ± 16.6 | 95.3 ± 14.3 |
| (3 ± 1) | (6) | (6) |
| P | >0.05 | <0.05 |

BROMOCRIPTINE

Table 8 shows that the daily dose of 30 mg of Bromocriptine
elicited a significant long-term improvement of parkinsonian patients.
The improvement in total disability seems to be better than with Piribedil but less than with levodopa.  The effect increased within the
first 3 months of treatment while the dose was gradually increased.

TABLE 8.   *IMPROVEMENT (%) OF PARKINSONIAN PATIENTS DURING BROMOCRIP-*
           *TINE TREATMENT (30 MG/DAY).   MEAN ± SEM.*

| Duration of treatment (months) | No. of patients | Mean improvement (% ± SEM) | | | | |
| --- | --- | --- | --- | --- | --- | --- |
| | | Total disability | Tremor | Rigi-dity | Hypo-kinesia | Perfor-mance |
| Bromocriptine | | | | | | |
| 1 | 24 | 9 ± 2 | 21 ± 4 | 11 ± 3 | 5 ± 2 | 5 ± 2 |
| 2 | 24 | 17 ± 3 | 35 ± 5 | 16 ± 3 | 13 ± 3 | 18 ± 4 |
| 3 | 24 | 22 ± 4 | 37 ± 5 | 24 ± 4 | 18 ± 4 | 17 ± 4 |
| 4 | 23 | 26 ± 4 | 43 ± 5 | 30 ± 5 | 21 ± 4 | 22 ± 5 |
| 5 | 23 | 31 ± 4 | 46 ± 6 | 34 ± 5 | 23 ± 4 | 26 ± 5 |

Bromocriptine induced changes in dopamine turnover, which were
similar to those obtained with Piribedil.  Both the basal level of
HVA in the CSF and its response to probenecid decreased significantly during Bromocriptine treatment.  But there were no changes in
concentrations of 5-HIAA (Table 9).  As in the case with Piribedil

correlation analyses showed that patients who improved with Bromo-
criptine had significantly lower probenecid response of HVA in the
CSF and less severe disease than those without beneficial effect
(Table 10).

TABLE 9.   BASAL CONCENTRATIONS (ng/ml) AND PROBENECID-INDUCED
           ACCUMULATIONS OF HVA AND 5-HIAA IN THE CSF OF PARKINSONIAN
           PATIENTS.   EFFECT OF BROMOCRIPTINE TREATMENT.   MEAN ± SEM.

| Bromo-criptine treatment | No. of patients | HVA | | 5-HIAA | |
|---|---|---|---|---|---|
| | | Basal | Probenecid | Basal | Probenecid |
| Before | 12 | 20.8 ± 2.2 | 145.0 ± 17.2 | 20.0 ± 3.3 | 46.5 ± 7.4 |
| During | 10 | 10.3 ± 2.3 | 92.6 ± 15.3 | 18.4 ± 2.3 | 62.2 ± 8.6 |
| P | | <0.05 | <0.01 | >0.05 | >0.05 |

TABLE 10.  CORRELATION OF PROBENECID-INDUCED ACCUMULATIONS (ng/ml) OF
           HVA IN THE CSF OF PARKINSONIAN PATIENTS WITH IMPROVEMENT ON
           BROMOCRIPTINE.   MEAN ± SEM.

| Improvement on Bromocriptine | Probenecid-induced accumulations of HVA | |
|---|---|---|
| | Before | During |
| >25% | 140.5 ± 23.5 | 68.7 ± 17.5 |
| (47 ± 8) | (6) | (6) |
| <25% | 149.5 ± 27.3 | 128.1 ± 17.1 |
| (14 ± 4) | (6) | (4) |
| P | >0.05 | <0.05 |

## DISCUSSION

The results obtained showed that levodopa increased the concentration of HVA in the CSF, indicating increased metabolism.  Nevertheless, the difference between the concentration of HVA in patients
treated with levodopa alone and in those treated with levodopa combined with a decarboxylase inhibitor showed that at least part of
the HVA found in the CSF during levodopa treatment originates from
the capillary walls, as has also been suggested as a result of
experimental studies (Bartholini et al., 1971).  It is thus under-

standable that the concentration of HVA in the CSF during long-term
treatment with levodopa showed no significant correlation with the
therapeutic response.

The results showed that dopamine receptor agonists such as
Piribedil *(Vakil et al., 1913; Chase et al., 1974; Rinne et al., 1975)*
and Bromocriptine *(Calne et al., 1974)* have a beneficial effect in
the treatment of patients with Parkinson's disease. However, the
efficacy seems to be significantly less than that of levodopa.

Biochemical determinations of acid monoamine metabolites in the
CSF indicated that dopaminergic agonists have significant neuropharmacological effects. Changes in the basal level and especially
in probenecid-induced accumulations of HVA in the CSF suggest that
these drugs reduce the turnover of endogenous dopamine in the brain.
According to experimental studies *(Andén et al., 1967)* the pharmacological mechanism for these changes in dopamine turnover may be
stimulation of the dopaminergic receptors.

Both dopaminergic agonists used in the present study induced
not only corresponding changes in dopamine metabolism in the brain
but also had similar clinical correlations. There was a significant
relationship between dopamine receptor activation and improvement of
parkinsonian disability suggesting that the therapeutic efficacy of
dopamine receptor agonists depends on the functional capacity of brain
dopaminergic mechanisms.

The results suggest that dopamine receptor agonists may help us
to understand the relationship between brain dopaminergic mechanisms
and improvement of parkinsonian symptoms.

## ACKNOWLEDGMENTS

This study was supported by a grant from the Signe and Ane
Gyllenberg Foundation.

## REFERENCES

Anden, N.-E., Rubensson, A., Fuxe, K., Hökfelt, T. (1967). Evi-
    dence for dopamine receptor stimulation by apomorphine. *J.
    Pharm. Pharmacol. 19,* 627–629.

Bartholini, G., Tissot, R., Pletscher, A. (1971). Brain capillaries
    as a source of homovanillic acid in cerebrospinal fluid. *Brain
    Res. 27,* 163–168.

Calne, D.B., Teychenne, P.F., Claveria, L.E., Eastman, R., Greenacre,
    J.K., Petrie, A. (1974). Bromocriptine in Parkinsonism.
    *British Medical Journal 4,* 442–444.

Chase, T.N., Woods, A.C., Glaubiger, G.A. (1974). Parkinson disease
    treated with a suspected dopamine receptor agonist. *Arch. Neu-
    rol. 30,* 383–386.

Rinne, U.K., Sonninen, V., Marttila, R. (1975). Dopaminergic Agonist
    Effects on Parkinsonian Clinical Features and Brain Monoamine

Metabolism. *In Advances in Neurology* (Ed. by Calne, D.B.,
Chase, T.N., and Barbeau, A.) *9*, pp. 383-392. Raven Press,
New York.

Vakil, S.D., Calne, D.B., Reid, J.L. Seymour, C.A. (1973).
Pyrimidyl-piperonyl-piperazine (ET 495) in parkinsonism.
*In Advances in Neurology* (Ed. Calne, D.B.) *3*, pp. 121-125.
Raven Press, New York.

# EVALUATION OF AN EXPERIMENTAL ANTICHOLINERGIC DRUG, ELANTRINE, IN TREATING THE TREMOR OF PARKINSONISM

ALVIN RIX

Department of Neurological Surgery
University of Oklahoma School of Medicine
Oklahoma City, Oklahoma 73190

## ABSTRACT

An experimental anticholinergic drug, elantrine, had shown significant improvement in tremor of parkinsonism in 89 patients not taking L-dopa. A double-blind study of 22 parkinsonian patients stabilized on L-dopa showed marked improvement in tremor and moderate improvement in rigidity and bradykinesia when elantrine was added to their treatment program. Nine of 15 patients taking L-dopa (or Sinemet®) and elantrine had cessation of all tremor and have continued free of tremor to date, over two years.

## INTRODUCTION

A morphanthridine derivative originally developed by Lakeside Laboratories (now part of Merrill-National Laboratories) has been assigned an USAN name, elantrine. The drug (Fig. 1) was originally synthesized as a possible anti-depressant but laboratory studies indicated it has anti-tremor and anticholinergic properties. Clinical studies in treatment of depression showed no benefits. For clinical evaluation of this drug in the treatment of parkinsonism, a double-blind study was carried out comparing elantrine to trihyxyphenidyl (Artane®). A total of 89 patients studied in five clinics of five different medical schools gave statistically significant results

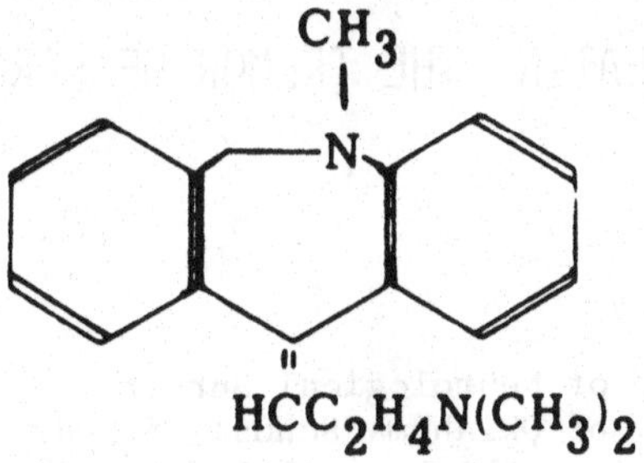

*Figure 1.   Elantrine*

in that 73 of 89 (82%) patients showed significant improvement in
total signs and symptoms while taking elantrine as compared to the
pre-treatment period.  Of the 89 patients, improvement of tremor
was greater with elantrine than with trihexyphenidyl in 43%; there
was no difference in tremor control in the two groups in 43%, and 14%
of the patients were noted to have less tremor while taking trihexyphenidyl.  Of the 51 patients in the two groups with difference in
tremor scores, elantrine was superior to trihexyphenidyl in 75%.
Common anticholinergic side-effects were noted but no serious complications resulted.  *(Rix and Fisher, 1972; Blonsky et al., 1974).*

## METHODS

A double-blind study designed for 40 patients was then devised.
During the time interval alloted only 22 patients qualified for this
double-blind study.  These were patients who had been stabilized on
L-dopa for three months or more and this dose maintained during the
study.  These patients had not been taking, and did not take during
the study, any antidepressant drugs, tranquilizers, reserpine, α-
methyl dopa (Aldomet®), or guanethidine (Ismelin®).  Patients with
glaucoma, stage V parkinsonism, renal disease, hepatic disease, cardiovascular disease, pulmonary disease or blood dyscrasia, patients
under 18, and pregnant patients were excluded.  Hoehn and Yahr *(1967)*
ratings of degree of disability due to parkinsonism, Stages I-V, were
utilized.  A rating scale was devised and individual patient's signs
and symptoms were noted weekly for four weeks for baseline period of
observation.  Then each patient was started on a capsule once daily,
according to the double-blind schedule, either placebo or elantrine,
the first week, increased to two capsules daily the second week and

increased to three capsules daily the third week. The patient was
then maintained on that dosage with his usual amount of L-dopa for
the next nine weeks. After this time all patients were knowingly
placed on elantrine.

## RESULTS

At the end of the study it was found that of the ten patients
taking placebo and L-dopa, only one of the ten showed any significant
improvement during the 16 week period. Whereas eleven of the twelve
patients taking elantrine and L-dopa showed significant improvement
during this same period. After the "placebo patients" had been placed
on elantrine, ten of ten showed striking improvement, and the one patient who had improved on placebo became free of tremor while taking
elantrine. Five of the ten in the placebo group were tremor-free in
six months.

Tremor scores were comparable for the two groups during the
baseline period (Fig. 2). Those on placebo at the end of 16 weeks

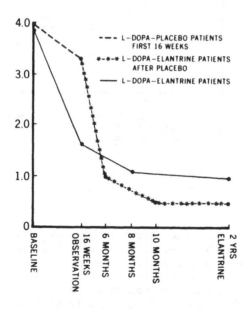

Figure 2.  Tremor scores from 22 patients in L-dopa - elantrine -
placebo double blind study.

showed very slight improvement whereas the patients taking elantrine
showed a 50% improvement in tremor the first two months they took the
drug.  The placebo group showed a slightly better response to elantrine
in reducing their tremor score in their first two months on this drug.
Both groups showed further gains and additional improvement in tremor
the first six months of taking elantrine, then stayed essentially the
same between six months and two years.  Nine of the 15 patients taking
elantrine over two years are currently free of tremor.

Combining the scores for rigidity and bradykinesia the placebo
patients started with slightly lower baseline scores and showed only
a trace of improvement during the 16 week observation period (Fig. 3).

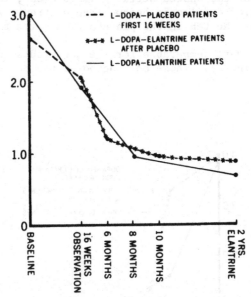

*Figure 3.   Rigidity and bradykinesia scores from 22 patients in
L-dopa - elantrine - placebo double blind study.*

The group taking elantrine showed 33% improvement the first two months
of drug therapy.  After the placebo group had been on elantrine for
two months, there was almost fifty percent (50%) reduction in their
scores.  Slight gains were noted after six months of elantrine, with
very minimal change over the course of the following 18 months.

There were no significant changes in blood pressure, pulse,
weight, electrocardiogram, tonometry, complete blood count, urine
analysis, and blood chemistry.

## DISCUSSION

This observer has used this experimental drug with 95 patients. Four patients with essential tremor and one with multiple sclerosis and tremor were not helped. Of the 90 patients with parkinsonism, 14 could not be properly evaluated. Of the remaining 76 patients, 72 improved significantly and four were not helped by the drug. It may require two months or longer to establish dosage and achieve maximum benefit with elantrine.

About half of these patients have been taking L-dopa five years or longer and only one has developed "on and off" syndrome while taking elantrine. One other patient, when being changed from L-dopa to Sinemet® stopped his elantrine and developed "on and off" syndrome which entirely subsided when he resumed elantrine.

For most Stage III parkinsonism patients, use of L-dopa or Sinemet® is quite basic, but the addition of a suitable anticholinergic drug may have striking benefits, particularly insofar as control of tremor is concerned. Study to date has indicated that elantrine has less peripheral effect and more central effect than some other anticholinergic drugs, and this could be helpful in the treatment of parkinsonism.

## REFERENCES

Rix, A., and Fisher, R.G. (1972) Comparison of trihexyphenidyl and dihydromorphanthridine derivative in control of tremor of parkinsonism. *South. Med. Journal 65*, 1385-1389.

Blonsky, E.R., Ericsson, A.D., McKinney, A.S., Rix, A., Wang, R.I.H., and Rimm, A.A. (1974) Phase II multiclinic study of elantrine in parkinsonism. *Clinical Pharmacology and Therapeutics 15*, 46-50.

Hoehn, M.M. and Yahr, M.D. (1967) Parkinsonism: onset, progression and mortality. *Neurology 17*, 427-442.

# MATERNALLY DETERMINED SUSCEPTIBILITY TO D-AMPHETAMINE-INDUCED STEREOTYPY IN RATS

ROBERT W. BELL AND HENRY L. SCHREIBER, III

Department of Psychology
Texas Tech University
Lubbock, Texas 79409

## ABSTRACT

During the first week after parturition, rat pups were removed
and returned to a mother-present nest, were removed and returned to
a mother-absent nest, were separated from their mothers by removal
of the mothers, or were undisturbed.  In adulthood, when repeatedly
injected with a dose of D-amphetamine which induces progressively
higher levels of stereotypy (2.5 mg/kg), only subjects which had
been removed and returned to a mother-present nest in infancy showed
a retarded rate of increase in stereotypy.

## INTRODUCTION

Many of the preceeding papers have re-affirmed the well-established involvement of dopamine (DA) in Parkinson's disease.  Perhaps
equally well-established is DA's involvement in other severe disturbances of central nervous system function, for example, schizophrenia
(*Davis, 1975*).  However, despite DA's importance in proper mental
function, few studies have investigated the non-genetic, early
experiential factors which might influence DA synthesis and metabolism in the adult animal or might influence neurochemical systems
affecting DA.  D-Amphetamine-induced stereotypy in rats purportedly
depends on DA or a neurotransmitter in balance or conjunction with
DA (*Randrup, Munkvad, Fog and Ayhan, 1975*).  The antagonism of D-

amphetamine-induced stereotypy in rats is frequently used as a
screening device to test new neuroleptic agents (Iversen and Iversen,
1975). Therefore, the present study was undertaken to investigate
a complex, non-genetic, early experiential factor which might influence D-amphetamine-induced stereotypy in adulthood--maternal behavior
elicited by handling rat pups.

In rats, the preweaning period is one of rapid developmental
change in aminergic neurotransmitter systems; during this period DA,
norepinephrine and serotonin, their precursors, metabolites and
associated enzymes show various profound ontogenetic changes (Bennett
and Giarman, 1965; Loizou, 1972). Behavioral manipulations might be
expected to have their greatest inductive impact during or just prior
to such a period of rapid developmental change. Since early handling
must occur during the preweaning period in order to exert its effects
on the adult animal, being particularly potent during the first week
following parturition (Levine and Lewis, 1959), early handling might
directly influence the rat pup's developing neurochemistry. Although
early handling produces a range of physiological effects on the adult
animal, its primary underlying mechanism of action traditionally has
been thought to be the adrenal stress response (Denenberg and Zarrow,
1971; Levine and Mullins, 1968). Since responsiveness to chronic
stress is known to affect the biosynthesis of brain catecholamines
(Stone, 1975), early handling conceivably could influence brain
catecholamines indirectly through an altered adrenal stress response
in addition to any direct inductive effect on neurochemistry.

Early handling consists of removing all pups from the nest,
placing them individually in shavings-filled containers for a period
of time (usually three minutes), and then returning them to the
mother-present nest. This procedure induces ultrasonic vocalizations
by the rat pups, which, in turn, induce maternal behavior (Bell,
Nitschke, Bell and Zachman, 1974; Smotherman, Bell, Starzec, Elias
and Zachman, 1974). In fact, early handling of the first litter
determines the rat mother's maternal behavior toward subsequent un-
handled litters (Villescas and Bell, unpublished observations).
Therefore, the present study investigated not only the direct effects
of handling on the pups themselves, but also the indirect effects of
maternal behavior elicited by early handling.

## METHOD

### EARLY HANDLING AND MATERNAL SEPARATION

Sixteen litters of Sprague-Dawley rats were reduced to eight pups
per litter on their first day after parturition. Litters and mothers
were housed in 45.0 x 22.5 x 22.0 cm opaque plastic maternity cages,
with cedar shavings as bedding and nest material, in a colony room
with controlled temperature and lighting (12 hr lighted). Litters

were randomly assigned to the following four treatments for the second to the sixth day after parturition: (1) handled, mother-present
litters were removed for three minutes and returned to the mother-
present nest; (2) the handled, mother-absent litters were removed
for 3 min and when returned to the nest, the mother rats were separated from them for one hour by a solid or perforated hardboard
partition.  The hour long period of separation for the handled, mother-
absent group would allow handled pups to return to nest temperature,
cease ultrasonic vocalizations or otherwise return to "normal"; (3)
as a control for the hour long period of separation, mother-absent
litters were undisturbed, but the mother rat was separated from the
pups by a solid or perforated hardboard partition for one hour; and
(4) other control litters were undisturbed.

## MATERNAL BEHAVIOR AND OPEN-FIELD TESTING

Following reunion of mothers with pups, observations of maternal
behavior, classified as described by Bell, Nitschke, Bell and Zachman
(1974), were recorded at 15 sec intervals for 20 min.  Since mere
observation may disturb rat mothers, the undisturbed controls were
not incorporated in the observations of maternal behavior.  Litters
were weaned at 21 days and housed individually in standard laboratory
cages (25 x 18 x 17.5 cm).  At 55 days of age the offspring, both
males and females, received 4 daily 4 min tests in an open-field
measuring 182.5 x 182.5 cm with walls 31.25 cm high.  Behaviors
observed were Response Latency, Number of Rearings, Number of Squares
Entered, and Defecation (number of fecal boli).  To reduce the effects
of interdependence of observed behaviors, maternal and offspring
observations were subjected to arcsin transformations.  The measure
of litter defecation in the open-field was transformed with a square
root transformation $(X + .5)^{\frac{1}{2}}$ because of the large number of zeroes.
At 60 days of age, the offspring were observed during a single 10 min
trial in an exploratory maze with 4 arms providing differing amounts
of tactile stimulation.

## AMPHETAMINE INJECTION PERIOD

At 75 ± 5 days of age, 12 male subjects were randomly selected
from each group and randomly assigned to one of 3 treatments, 0.0
mg/kg, 2.5 mg/kg, or 10.0 mg/kg (comparable volume of saline vehicle,
s.c.), thus N=4 per cell.  Female subjects were used in other experiments (Schreiber, Bell, Kufner and Villescas, in press).  Subjects
were injected 30 ± 5 minutes prior to testing in one of 2 dark gray
Y-mazes with 30 cm high x 13 cm wide x 45 cm long arms.  Two observers
independently recorded rearings, entries, and stereotypy for 3 min
trials for 8 days.  "Entries" and "Rearings" were combined to form a
Locomotion score.  A "Rearing" was defined as the subject standing

on its hind limbs with neither forepaw touching the Y-maze floor; the
rearing was terminated when a single forepaw touched the floor.  An
"Entry" occurred when the base of the subject's tail passed beyond
the red line marking the entrance to the arm of the Y-maze.  "Stereotypy" was defined as repetitive head bobbing, licking, biting, and
sniffing.  Testing was arranged such that each observer saw half of
the subjects per cell on one day and the other half on the following
day.  Food and water were available continuously in home cages.
Subjects were weighed on odd-numbered days.  Data was summed over
two-day blocks to reduce day-to-day variation and to equate any
possible observer effects.  In order to meet the homogeneity of
variance requirements of analyses of variance, data was transformed
with a square root transformation $(X + 1)^{\frac{1}{2}}$.  Locomotor activity and
stereotypy were separately analyzed using split plot factorial analyses of variance for the 8 day test period, 3 (DOSE) x 2 (EARLY HAND-
LING) x 2 (MATERIAL SEPARATION) x 4 (TWO-DAY BLOCKS), according to
Kirk *(1968)*.  All results reported here were significant at $p < .05$
or better.

## RESULTS

### MATERNAL BEHAVIOR AND OPEN FIELD TEST

No significant differences in maternal behavior were observed
between groups when data reflecting type of partition was collapsed.
(Mothers separated from their pups with a solid partition were more
active when reunited with their pups than mothers separated with a
perforated partition, indicating that pup stimulus characteristics
were changed by handling.)  Handled pups (from both the handled,
mother-present group and the handled mother-absent group) had a
shorter response latency in the open-field than non-handled pups
(mother-absent group and undisturbed control group).  Moreover,
handling produced differences in rearings in the open-field that
interacted with the day of testing.  Handled pups exhibited a higher
frequency of rearings in the open-field on days 1-3 of testing, with
day 4 indicating no difference between handled and non-handled pups.
Handled, mother-absent males exhibited less defecation across days
than males simply maternally separated (mother absent group).  No
significant differences among groups were found in the exploratory-
maze results.  The changes in maternal behavior and the changes in
the male and female offsprings' open-field activity are reported more
fully elsewhere *(Villescas, Bell, Wright and Kufner, in press)*.

### AMPHETAMINE INJECTION PERIOD

As may be seen in Figure 1. the dose of amphetamine significantly
influenced the amount of stereotypy observed over the test period:

(a) The saline groups showed virtually no stereotypy; (b) the 2.5 mg/kg groups showed an increasing pattern of stereotypy; (c) the 10.0 mg/kg groups showed virtually the maximum amount of stereotypy. The following pattern of stereotypy arose for the handled, mother-present group: (a) Handled, mother-present group subjects were not significantly different from the other groups on the first two-day block.  (b) The handled, mother-present group was significantly lower than the other groups on the second two-day block.  (c) Handled, mother-present subjects were significantly lower on the third two-

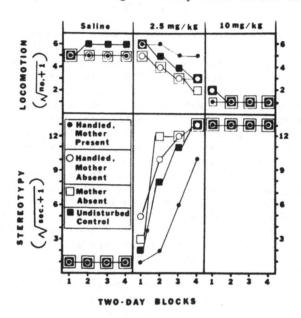

TWO-DAY BLOCKS

*Figure 1.    Mean locomotion and stereotypy scores for handled/mother-present group, handled/mother-absent group, mother-absent group and undisturbed control group (N for each X̄=4) during the 8 day injection period. (For clarity, each mean graphed was rounded to the nearest whole number.)*

day block also.  (d) However, by the fourth two-day block, the handled, mother-present group did not significantly differ from the other groups. As may be seen in Figure 1, the dose of amphetamine also significantly influenced the amount of locomotor activity observed over the test period: (a) A high level of locomotor activity was exhibited by the saline groups. (b) A declining pattern of locomotion was exhibited by the 2.5 mg/kg groups. (c) Virtually no locomotor activity was exhibited by the 10.0 mg/kg groups.  Subjects which had experienced maternal separation (the mother-absent group and the handled, mother-absent

group) locomoted less than the other two groups. At 2.5 mg/kg, subjects which had not received early handling (the undisturbed control
and the mother-absent group) showed a greater rate of decline in locomotion than groups which had received early handling (the handled,
mother-present group and the handled, mother-absent group). Locomotor
activity is to be reported in greater detail elsewhere (Schreiber,
Bell, Wood, Carlson, Kufner, Wright and Villescas, unpublished observations).

## DISCUSSION

In general, the results conformed with previous findings concerning amphetamine-induced stereotypy. At higher doses of D-amphetamine (e.g., 10 mg/kg), the absence of locomotor activity has been used
to define drug-induced stereotypy (Schiørring, 1971). At lower doses of
repeatedly administered D-amphetamine (e.g., 2.5 mg/kg), progressively
lower levels of locomotor activity reciprocate progressively higher
levels of stereotypy at about 30 minutes post injection (Schreiber,
Bell, Conely, Kufner, Palet and Wright, in press; Segal and Mandell,
1974). However, in the present study, only the subjects which had
received early handling with rat mothers present had a slower rate
of increase in drug-induced stereotypy. These results indicate that
the effect of the maternal behavior elicited by early handling on the
handled pup, rather than the act of early handling alone or the changes
in maternal behavior produced by the act of maternal separation alone,
retarded the usual increase in stereotypy seen with repeated injections
of D-amphetamine. Since there were no apparent differences between
handled and non-handled groups in the measures of maternal behavior
taken at mother/litter reunion, the effect on the handled, mother present offspring probably operated through the mother/infant dyad rather
than upon maternal behavior in general. Apparently, similar maternal
behavior has differing consequences on stressed pups returned to the
mother-present nest in comparison with pups recovered from stress when
reunited with the mother rat. However, separating the pups from the
rat mother did have long-term consequences on the pups. Both groups
of maternally separated subjects (the mother-absent group and the
handled, mother-absent group) were significantly heavier than the two
groups of non-maternally separated subjects. Also, maternally separated subjects showed less locomotion overall during the amphetamine
injection period. Groups which had received early handling in infancy
showed differences in the open-field test of emotionality, a finding
of long standing (Denenberg, 1964). This seems to indicate a more-or-
less direct effect of early handling on emotionality. Although
changes in emotionality may have contributed to the present results,
these changes were not sufficient to explain the present results.
Whereas the handled, mother-absent subjects were similar to the handled, mother-present subjects in open-field activity, they differed

in response to D-amphetamine, suggesting that the effect on amphetamine-induced stereotypy was not a consequence of a general change in emotionality.  Moreover, the handled, mother-present group did not differ significantly from the other groups in the amount of stereotypy initially exhibited at 2.5 mg/kg or 10.0 mg/kg of D-amphetamine on the first two-day block of testing.  Thus, the effect on drug-induced stereotypy was not prepotent, but required repeated injections of D-amphetamine in order to be manifested.  Since Segal and Mandell *(1974)* have shown that repeatedly-administered low doses of D-amphetamine may produce changes in catecholamine biosynthetic capacity, early handling with return to a mother-present nest conceivably may influence those changes in catecholamine biosynthesis.  Although the present results must be substantiated by future neurochemical assays to specify the nature of the effect, the fact that altered mother-infant dyads produced a retarded rate of increase in amphetamine-induced stereotypy, and the fact that DA is involved in Parkinson's disease suggest that the onset of Parkinson's disease may be linked, in part, with early social-developmental events.

## ACKNOWLEDGEMENTS

This study was funded by a Texas Tech University Arts and Science Institute of Research grant.  The authors thank Dr. Richard H. Carlson for obtaining the D-amphetamine and Connie P. Schreiber for typing the manuscript.

## REFERENCES

Bell, R.W., Nitschke, W., Bell, N.J. and Zackman, T.A.  (1974).  Early experience, ultrasonic vocalization, and maternal responsiveness in rats. *Dev. Psychobiol. 7*, 235-243.

Bennett, D.S. and Giarman, N.J.  (1965).  Schedule of appearance of 5-hydroxytryptamine (serotonin) and associated enzymes in the developing rat brain. *J. Neurochem. 12*, 911-918.

Davis, J.M.  Catecholamines and psychosis. *In Catecholamines and Behavior* (Friedhoff, A.J., Ed.) pp. 135-154.  Plemun Press, New York.

Denenberg, V.H.  (1964).  Critical periods, stimulus input and emotional reactivity: A theory of infantile stimulation. *Psychol. Rev. 71*, 335-351.

Denenberg, V.H. and Zarrow, M.S.  (1971).  Effects of handling in infancy upon adult behavior and adrenocortical activity: Suggestions for a neuroendocrine mechanism. *In The Developmental of Self-Regulatory Mechanisms* (Walcher, D.N. and Peters, D.L., Eds.) pp. 40-74.  Academic Press, New York.

Iversen, S.D. and Iversen, L.L.  (1975). *Behavioral Pharmacology* pp. 269-292.  Oxford University Press, New York and Oxford.

Kirk, R.E.   (1968).   Experimental Design: Procedures for the Behavioral
    Sciences.   Brooks/Cole Publishing Co., Belmont.
Levine, S. and Mullins, R.   (1968).   Hormones in infancy.   *In Early
    Experience and Behavior* (Newton, G. and Levine, S., Eds.) pp.
    168-197.   Thomas, Springfield.
Loizou, L.A.   (1972).   The postnatal ontogeny of monoamine-containing
    neurones in the central nervous system of the albino rat.
    *Brain Res. 40*, 395-418.
Randrup, A., Munkvad, K., Fog, R. and Ayhan, I.H.   (1975).   Catechola-
    mines in activation, stereotypy and level of mood.   *In Catechol-
    amines and Behavior* (Friedhoff, A.J., Ed.) pp. 89-107.   Plenum
    Press, New York.
Schiørring, E.   (1971).   Amphetamine induced selective stimulation of
    certain behaviour items with concurrent inhibition of others in
    an open-field test with rats.   *Behavior 34*, 1-17.
Schreiber, H., Bell, R., Conely, L., Kufner, M., Palet, J. and Wright,
    L. (in press).   Diminished reaction to a novel stimulus during
    amphetamine withdrawal in rats.   *Pharmac. Biochem. Behav.*
Schreiber, H.L., Bell, R.W., Kufner, M. and Villescas, R. (in press).
    Maternal behavior: A determinant of amphetamine toxicity in rats.
    *Psychopharmacology.*
Segal, D.S. and Mandell, A.J.   (1974).   Long-term administration of
    d-amphetamine: Progressive augmentation of motor activity and
    stereotypy.   *Pharmac. Biochem. Behav. 2*, 249-255.
Smotherman, W.P., Bell, R.W., Starzec, J., Elias, J. and Zachman,
    T.A.   (1974).   Maternal response to infant vocalizations and
    olfactory cues in rats and mice.   *Behav. Biol. 12*, 55-66.
Stone, E.A.   (1975).   Stress and Catecholamines.   *In Catecholamines
    and Behavior v. 2*, (Friedhoff, A.J., Ed.) pp. 31-72.   Plenum
    Press, New York.
Villescas, R., Bell, R.W., Wright, L. and Kufner, M. (in press).
    Effect of handling on maternal behavior following return of
    pups to the nest.   *Dev. Psychobiol.*

# POSTMENOPAUSAL PARKINSONISM: BRAIN IRON OVERLOAD?

CHARLES N. STILL

William S. Hall Psychiatric Institute, and the
Department of Neuropsychiatry and Behavioral Science
The University of South Carolina School of Medicine
Columbia, South Carolina 29202

## ABSTRACT

Records of 11 postmenopausal parkinsonism patients were evaluated
in comparison with those of 11 postmenopausal depression patients.
None had a history of encephalitis, stroke, drug-induced or toxic
extrapyramidal disorders, or active bleeding within six months before
admission. There was no significant differences between the two groups
with regard to time interval from menopause to onset of symptoms,
height, weight, or age at first admission. Both groups showed normal
height, hemoglobin, hematocrit, and erythrocyte counts. Parkinsonism
patients were underweight and had a shorter interval from menopause to
onset of symptoms ($12.4 \pm 1.9$ vs. $16.8 \pm 2.5$ yr.). These findings are
compatible with the hypothesis that in parkinsonism, hereditary predisposition to positive body iron balance may be associated with
alteration of the blood-brain barrier in parkinsonism.

## INTRODUCTION

In classic style, James Parkinson defined the shaking palsy
(paralysis agitans) as follows: "Involuntary tremulous motion, with
lessened muscular power, in parts not in action and even when supported; with a propensity to bend the trunk forwards, and to pass
from a walking to a running pace: the senses and intellects being
uninjured." Anticipating therapeutic advances of the future, he

291

admonished, "Until we are better informed respecting the nature of the disease, the employment of internal medicines is scarcely warrantable; unless analogy should point out some remedy the trial of which rational hope might authorize... It is indeed much to be regretted that this malady is generally regarded by the sufferers... (as) so discouraging to the employment of remedial means... Seldom occurring before the age of fifty, and frequently yielding but little inconvenience for several months, it is generally considered as the irremediable diminution of the nervous influence, naturally resulting from declining life; and remedies are therefore seldom sought for" *(Parkinson, 1817)*. He gives no account of *bona fide* paralysis agitans in women, though Gowers *(1888)* later recorded a series of 42 females with average age of onset at 51 years, two years earlier than in 73 males. This male preponderance in parkinsonism has since been confirmed repeatedly, though not always approaching the ratio of two males to one female.

## METHODS

Retrospective review of the inpatient medical records of 22 postmenopausal women born between 1896 and 1922, and admitted to the William S. Hall Psychiatric Institute during 1969-1976, identified one group of 11 patients with manifestations of parkinsonism, and another group of 11 patients with manifestations of depression without parkinsonism. None had a documented history of encephalitis, stroke, drug-related or toxic extrapyramidal syndromes resembling parkinsonism, or a history of blood loss within six months preceding admission. Records were evaluated for age at menopause, onset of symptoms, and admission height, weight, erythrocyte count, hematocrit, and hemoglobin. The control group of depressed patients was selected for height and weight based on tables compiled from data provided by insured persons residing in the United States *(Diem and Lentner, 1970)*. Hematologic data from both groups were evaluated in comparison with postmenopausal women from the general population of Wales and from populations selected for income by poverty index ratios of one to four in the Comprehensive Nutritional Health Survey conducted in South Carolina from November 1969 to April 1970   *(Elwood, 1971; Dantzler, 1972)*. Progressively later ages of onset in parkinsonism occurring since 1920 led Poskanzer and Schwab *(1963)* to propose the hypothesis of a single etiology related to subclinical infection during the outbreaks of pandemic encephalitis from 1918 to 1926, with prediction of a precipitous decline in the number of cases of parkinsonism before 1980. As yet, no such trend has emerged. Moreover, genetic studies of parkinsonism in Minnesota and in Sweden show an estimated heritability of 79 to 91% with multifactorial causation, supporting the concept of abiotrophy introduced by Gowers *(Kondo, Kurland, and Schull, 1973)*. Findings of a seven-year gap in male (64 years) and female (71 years) ages of onset for parkinsonism in Minnesota during 1960-1964 (*Kurland et al., 1969*) suggest that hereditary predisposition to positive body iron balance may be the most crucial of many factors in the pathogenesis of parkinsonism (*Still, 1974*).

## RESULTS AND DISCUSSION

As summarized in Tables 1 and 2, there were no significant differences between the two groups.

*TABLE 1. PARKINSONISM VS. DEPRESSION IN POSTMENOPAUSAL WOMEN*

| CHRONOLOGY (MEAN AGE IN YEARS) | PARKINSONISM | DEPRESSION |
|---|---|---|
| ADMISSION | 63.5 ± 1.9 | 60.7 ± 1.5 |
| ONSET | 58.2 ± 1.7 | 60.5 ± 1.5 |
| MENOPAUSE | 45.8 ± 1.0 | 43.7 ± 1.9 |
| MENOPAUSE/ONSET | 12.4 ± 1.9 | 16.8 ± 2.5 |
| NUMBER IN GROUP | 11 | 11 |

*TABLE 2. PARKINSONISM VS. DEPRESSION IN POSTMENOPAUSAL WOMEN*

| | N | HEIGHT (CM) | WEIGHT (kg) |
|---|---|---|---|
| PARKINSONISM | 11 | 161.4 ± 1.9 | 60.7 ± 4.1 |
| DEPRESSION | 11 | 162.8 ± 1.9 | 70.7 ± 3.0 |
| TABLE * | - | 162.6 | 65.8 |

* (*Diem and Lentner, 1970*)

In Table 3, normal hemoglobin, hematocrit, and erythrocyte counts exclude iron deficiency anemia suggesting an inverse relationship between iron lack and parkinsonism, as demonstrated by threefold control levels of urinary iron excretion following a single intramuscular administration of the iron-chelating agent deferoxamine to 16 patients with parkinsonism. This Montreal series of patients showed no differ-

ences from controls with regard to hemograms, transferrin, serum iron,
or total iron-binding capacity *(Barbeau and Boileau, 1969)*.  Comparison
of postmenopausal patients from both parkinsonism and depressed groups
with groups of similar age in Wales or in South Carolina suggests that
geographic and economic factors do affect hemoglobin and hematocrit
levels.  Yet it is also clear that iron deficiency anemia associated

TABLE 3.   *PARKINSONISM VS. DEPRESSION IN POSTMENOPAUSAL WOMEN*

| GROUP | N | HEMOGLOBIN | HEMATOCRIT | RBC |
|---|---|---|---|---|
| PARKINSONISM | 11 | 14.3 ± 0.19 | 43.5 ± 0.51 | 4.74 ± 0.11 |
| DEPRESSION | 11 | 14.5 ± 0.38 | 43.8 ± 0.26 | 4.70 ± 0.13 |
| ELWOOD (1970) | 88 | 13.5 ± 0.11 | 41.9 ± 0.3 | |
| DANTZLER (1972) | | | | |
| PI-4 ** | | 13.6 | 41.9 | |
| PI-1 * | | 12.6 | 39.5 | |

* PI-1    *(family income equals upper limit of poverty level)*
** PI-4    *(family income equals 4 X upper limits of poverty level)*

with menstrual iron loss usually resolves itself by increased retention of body iron, in the decade following menopause, so that the
incidence of iron deficiency does not increase appreciably in the
elderly *(Elwood, 1971; Elwood, Rees, and Thomas, 1968)*.
     What is the evidence for brain iron overload in parkinsonism?
Earle *(1968)* studied 11 formalin-fixed brain specimens from 105
histologically verified cases of Parkinson's disease by means of
X-ray fluorescent spectroscopy.  Iron was "consistently increased
by a factor of two or more above normal, and the potassium was consistently decreased."  The potassium shift was thought to represent
an artefact of formalin fixation, but the generalized shift of iron
suggested severe alteration of the blood-brain barrier to permit
generalized iron storage in parkinsonian brain, i.e. brain iron
overload.  Recent studies of the blood-brain barrier by electron
microscopy show that mitochondria constitute 10-11% of capillary
cell cytoplasm in cerebral and cerebellar cortex, whereas the mitochondrial contribution to lung capillary cell cytoplasm is under
3%, suggesting that the excess work capacity of the blood-brain
barrier maintains ionic concentration gradients between brain extracellular fluid and plasma *(Oldendorf, Cornford, and Brown, 1976)*.
Evidence of mitochondrial involvement in parkinsonism has been reported
by Rojas *et al. (1965)*, who described iron impregnation of mitochondria

in biopsy specimens from the ventrolateral nucleus of the thalamus.
Mitochondria provide the structural matrix for the four complexes of
the electron transfer chain which governs energy coupling processes
required for cell survival (Green and Goldberger, 1967). Figure 1
shows that iron atoms form integral components of each complex, so
that iron overload must disrupt electron transfer within mitochondria.

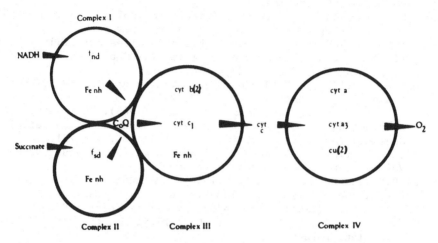

Figure 1.   Electron Transfer Chain Complexes of Mitochondria;
            CoQ = coenzyme $Q_{10}$; cu = copper; cyt = cytochrome;
            Fe nh = nonheme iron; $f_{nd}$ = NADH dehydrogenase;
            $f_{sd}$ = succinate dehydrogenase; NADH = nicotinamide
            adenine dinucleotide (reduced form); $O_2$ = oxygen.
            Adapted from Green and Goldberger (1967).

Mitochondrial dysfunction then cumulatively impairs blood-brain
barrier efficiency, setting up a vicious cycle of progressive iron
accumulation in the brain.  Focal iron storage affects areas of highest iron content, as follows: 1) globus pallidus 2) red nucleus 3)
substantia nigra 4) putaman 5) dentate nucleus 6) caudate nucleus 7)
motor cortex 8) thalamus 9) occipital cortex 10) frontal white matter
(Hallgren and Sourander, 1958).  As Greenfield (1955) noted, these
are areas of predilection in parkinsonism.  In recognizing that
hereditary predisposition to positive body iron balance may lead to
brain iron overload due to severe alteration of the blood-brain
barrier, we have come full circle back to James Parkinson (1817):
"In such a case then, at whatever period of the disease it might be
proposed to attempt the cure, blood should first be taken from the
upper part of the neck, unless contraindicated by any particular
circumstance".

# REFERENCES

Barbeau, A. and Boileau, J.L. (1969). Mobilizable iron in Parkin-
    son's disease. *Neurology 19, 314.*

Dantzler, M.U. (1972). Final Comprehensive Report. Comprehensive
    Nutritional Health Survey. p. 6. State Board of Health, Col-
    umbia, South Carolina.

Diem, K. and Lentner, C. (1970). Scientific Tables. Seventh Edition.
    p. 711, Geigy Pharmaceuticals, Ardsley, New York.

Earle, K.M. (1968). Studies on Parkinson's disease including X-ray
    fluorescent spectroscopy of formalin fixed brain tissue. *J.
    Neuropath. Exp. Neurol. 27, 1-14.*

Elwood, P.C. (1971). Epidemiological aspects of iron deficiency in
    the elderly. *Gerontol. Clin. 13, 2-11.*

Elwood, P.C., Rees, G., and Thomas, J.D.R. (1968). Community study
    of menstrual iron loss and its association with iron deficiency
    anemia. *In the Brit. J. Prev. Soc. Med. 22, 127-131.*

Gowers, W.R. (1888). A Manual of Diseases of the Nervous System.
    Volume 2, p. 588, Churchill, London.

Green, D.E. and Golberger, R.F. (1967). Molecular Insights into
    the Living Process. pp. 183-212, Academic Press, New York.

Greenfield, J.G. (1955). The Pathology of Parkinson's Disease. *In
    James Parkinson (1755-1824),* (Critchley, M., Ed.) pp. 219-243.
    Macmillan, London.

Hallgren, B. and Sourander, P. (1958). The effect of age on the
    non-haemin iron in the human brain. *J. Neurochem. 3, 41-51.*

Kondo, K. Kurland, L.T. and Schull, W.J. (1973). Parkinson's
    disease: genetic analysis and evidence of a multifactorial
    etiology. *Mayo Clin. Proceedings 48, 465-475.*

Kurland, L.T., Hauser, W.A., Okazaki, H., and Nobrega, F.T. (1969).
    Epidemiologic studies of parkinsonism with special reference to
    the cohort hypothesis. *In Third Symposium of Parkinson's
    Disease.* pp. 12-16, Livingstone, Edinburgh.

Oldendorf, W.H., Cornford, M., and Brown, W.J. (1976). The large
    apparent metabolic work capacity of the blood-brain barrier.
    *Arch. Neurol. (Chicago) 33, 390.*

Parkinson, J. (1817). An Essay on the Shaking Palsy. pp. 1-66.
    Sherwood, Neely, and Jones, London.

Poskanzer, D.C. and Schwab, R.S. (1963). Cohort analysis of Parkin-
    son's syndrome: evidence for a single etiology related to sub-
    clinical infection about 1920. *J. Chron. Dis. 16, 961-973.*

Rojas, G., Asenjo, A., Chiorino, R., Aranda, L., Rocamora, R. and
    Donoso, P. (19650. Cellular and subcellular structure of the
    ventrolateral nucleus of the thalamus in Parkinson disease.
    Deposits of iron. *Confin. Neurol. 26, 362-376.*

Still, C.N. (1974). Blood, bread, iron and the aging brain. *J.
    South Carolina Med. Assoc. 70, 279-284.*

# FAILURE OF L-DOPA TO RELIEVE ACTIVATED RIGIDITY IN PARKINSON'S DISEASE

DAVID D. WEBSTER* AND JAMES A. MORTIMER**

Neurology Service and Surgery Service
Veterans Administration Hospital
University of Minnesota
Minneapolis, Minnesota 55801

## ABSTRACT

Rigidity in Parkinson patients can be easily quantitated by determining net work required to passively flex and extend the forearm through an arc of $100^{\circ}$. Rigidity thus measured can be subdivided into two very distinct types, resting and activated. Resting rigidity, measured while the patient is relaxed, responds to all effective therapeutic agents and correlates closely to degree of clinical improvement. Activated rigidity, measured during voluntary activity, is not relieved by any presently available medical treatment. It remains unchanged at pre-therapy levels even in patients who may temporarily appear to have dramatic improvement in clinical symptomatology. Longitudinal measurements made in hundreds of parkinson patients over intervals ranging from 5 to 15 years show continuing high levels of activated rigidity through the entire period of study.

In marked contrast to our wide experience with parkinson patients is a single, well documented case of Wilson's disease who appears to have recovered completely both by clinical examination and by all of our machine measurements. This patient had high levels of extrapyramidal deficit, repeatedly measured over a period of four months when penicillamine therapy was being investigated. He then suddenly reverted to normal and returned to full time employment. High values of resting rigidity, activated rigidity, akinesia and resting tremor all reverted to normal and have

---

*Chief, Neurology Service
**Neurophysiologist, Stereotaxic Unit

remained normal for the past 6 years.

The implication of this study is that L-dopa and related treatments only mask the symptomatology of Parkinson's disease and are
not retarding the underlying pathological process.  Penicillamine,
on the other hand, probably does relieve the destructive process in
Wilson's disease and may, in early cases, permanently relieve the
extrapyramidal dysfunction.

## INTRODUCTION

It is a common clinical finding in parkinsonism that upper limb
rigidity can be revealed or considerably enhanced by having the
patient carry out a voluntary task with the arm contralateral to
that being examined.  The magnitude of this rigidity, which we have
termed "activated rigidity", has proven to be a reliable indicator
of the severity of the disease, permitting its advance over years
to be accurately assessed (Webster, 1972).  Paradoxically, despite
substantial improvement in the functional state of patients treated
with L-dopa, quantitative measures of activated rigidity have been
found to change very little with this therapy.  Its dramatic reduction by thalamotomy and by the use of penicillamine in Wilson's
disease, however, indicates that activated rigidity is related to
the basic disease process underlying extrapyramidal dysfunction.
In this paper, we review some of the major findings concerning the
efficacy of specific therapies for the improvement of function in
Parkinson's disease and for reduction of tremor and rigidity.  The
possible origin of activated rigidity is discussed.

Our interest in Parkinson's disease dates from the early 1960's
when we first designed a battery of automated tests to quantitate
rigidity, tremor, bradykinesia and shuffling gait.  After a great
deal of experimentation we standardized on five measurements of
right and left arm dysfunction and one of gait.  To date, these
standardized measurements have been carried out in over 500 parkinsonian patients, some of whom have been tested in our clinic for as
long as 16 years.  These measurements have permitted us to study
both the natural history of the advancing disease as well as the
effects of thalamotomy and various drug therapies.

## METHODS

Description of the electromechanical devices used to evaluate
extrapyramidal dysfunction in our laboratory have been given elsewhere (Webster, 1959, 1966), and will only be briefly summarized
here.

RIGIDITY

Rigidity can be felt clinically as resistance to slow, passive motion.  It has been classified as a waxy or plastic resistance, because it is characteristically non-elastic, changing direction as limb movement is reversed.  Rigidity can therefore be thought of as a torque opposing passive motion, and may be quantitated by integrating this torque over a complete cycle of flexion and extension to obtain a work value.  In our measurements the patients' forearms are pulled through a $100^o$ arc of passive motion at $20^o$ per second by a servo-controlled device, and the net work expended by the machine is printed out at the end of each cycle.  Ten or more cycles are averaged for a single test value.

Early in our work we found rigidity values varied considerably with degree of alertness and mental set.  To reduce variability we elected to measure rigidity with the patient relaxed but awake (resting rigidity) and while performing a series of voluntary movements with the opposite extremity (activated rigidity).  The voluntary movements were elicited by having the subject pursue a spot of light on a television tube.  The spot jumps to a new location each time the patient catches it with his hand.  Patients are encouraged to perform the task as rapidly as possible and are scored on the number of hits obtained in 50 seconds.  This *pursuit score* along with a supination/pronation score (described below), provide measures of motor function.

In normal controls activated rigidity is generally positive, but rarely exceeds 20 inch-pounds per hundred degree cycle.  Higher values are common in early Parkinson's disease and these continue to increase with advancing disease.  Resting rigidity is curiously negative in normal controls who average close to approximately minus 10 inch-pounds.  This indicates that normal subjects unitentionally push the machine along, thereby producing negative instead of positive work as seen by the machine.  We term this *negative rigidity*.  Early Parkinson patients usually have a degree of negative resting rigidity, but these values steadily advance in a positive direction with progressive untreated disease and frequently reach as high as +60 inch-pounds in advanced Parkinsonism.

TREMOR

Arm tremor is measured as the peak-to-peak envelope of the alternating torque about the elbow joint averaged over a 100 second period.  Since tremor is sensitive to mental stress, a standard activation procedure is followed where patients are instructed to count backwards by twos during the test.  Normal subjects range below 4 grams on this measure, whereas parkinsonian patients may have as much as 4,000 grams of tremor in extreme cases.  (Tremor measurements are given in grams, which is the force measured at a distance of 30 centimeters from the axis of rotation.)

SUPINATION-PRONATION

Failure of rapid alternating wrist movement, dysdiadochokinesia, is a cardinal sign of Parkinson's disease. We test this function by having the patient twist a doorknob mounted on an angular displacement transducer. The instrument counts the total number of degrees of wrist rotation both clockwise and counterclockwise during ten seconds of maximum supination-pronation effort. Normals average about 7,500 degrees per ten seconds. Patients with severe hand bradykinesia will score less than 100 degrees on this test.

WALK INDEX

This test is designed to produce high values for the so-called shuffling gait of Parkinson's disease (Webster, 1968). The patient is penalized for hesistancy, short steps and slow movement. The walk index is the product of the number of seconds required to negotiate a thirty foot obstacle course multiplied by the number of steps taken by the right foot. Normals average 60 step seconds. Parkinson patients are unable to ambulate alone as this index approaches 6,000 step seconds.

DATA REDUCTION

Since all of the above tests except the walk index produce data for both right and left sides, the entire test battery contains 11 separate items. Also, since each test is repeated three to ten times the machine is programmed to average all sub-tests, identify and print the final averaged test scores on paper tape. The entire battery requires 45 minutes to administer.

DISEASE EVALUATION BY THE PARKINSONIAN TEST BATTERY

Over the past 15 years, a variety of drug and surgical therapies were evaluated with our test battery. In the early 1960's, patients entered our clinic on combinations of anticholinergic, antihistaminergic, tranquilizing, antidepressive, and CNS-stimulating drugs. Because of the large number and variety of drugs and the necessity of maintaining patients on the best available therapy, it was not possible to carefully evaluate all of these older therapeutic agents. The relative merits of several of these agents, however, were assessed by cautious rotation and combination of various medications.

During the 1960's we also had the opportunity to measure the acute results of stereotaxic surgery in 85 patients, 14 of whom are still being followed in longitudinal measurements. In this paper, we will report the long term findings of one of these cases.

The advent of the era of amantadine hydrochloride and L-dopa in the late 1960's afforded an opportunity to look at the relative

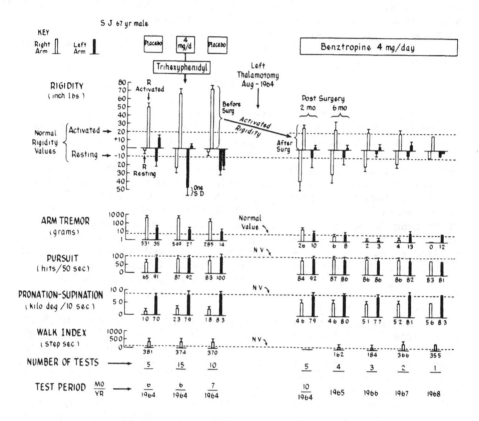

*Figure 1. Relative response to drug and thalamotomy therapies in unilateral Parkinson's disease. Each group of rigidity tests appears as two sets of adjacent bar graphs. Right sided data is coded open, left side as closed bars. The first bar in each set indicates resting rigidity and the second bar, activated rigidity. The normal value shown for activated rigidity is the upper limit of normal. Note the profound and lasting decrease of activated rigidity following thalamotomy.*

merits of these new agents.  More recently, it has become possible
to multiply the effects of L-dopa with methyldopa and finally with
carbidopa.  We will show the longitudinal course of one patient,
who remains in excellent control after initial anticholinergic therapy, followed by L-dopa, L-dopa combined with methyldopa, and finally
supplemented by amantadine.  We will also show average L-dopa
responses of a large group of parkinsonian patients and compare
those with machine measurements of penicillamine therapy in Wilson's
disease.

## RESULTS

Figure 1 shows the results of a four year study following a
thalamotomy done in 1964.  This is an especially interesting case
because this patient was afflicted with parkinsonism only on his
right side.  As frequently happens in unilateral Parkinson's disease,
this case progressed slowly and therefore was an ideal one for
thalamotomy.  The cause of this patient's disease was uncertain.
There was, however, a history of high fever and confusion diagnosed
as pneumonia early in World War II followed shortly by loss of
right hand dexterity.  Resting tremor first appeared in his right
hand ten years later and continued to increase until he was first
studied by us in 1964.  Examination then showed marked bradykinesia
of the right hand and severe resting tremor involving both the
arm and leg only on that side.  For several years he had been
totally dependent on his left hand for all self care activities
including handwriting.

The first data column of Figure 1 shows the averages of five
test batteries administered early in June.  By comparing the right-
sided (open bar) data in this column to the left-sided (solid bar)
data, one is able to observe how clearly the machine tests indicate
the presence of Parkinson's disease, since in this man all of the
right-sided values are markedly abnormal whereas the left-sided
values are not.  Starting with activated rigidity we see approximately
+50 inch-pounds on the right compared to +12 on the left.  Resting
rigidity is considerably more negative on the normal left side (-10).
Arm tremor plotted against a logarithmic scale is much larger on the
right (531 gm.) than on the left (35 gm.).  The relatively small
tremor shown on the left may actually originate from the very intense
right-sided tremor being mechanically transmitted in a diminished
amount through the bony structures of the patient's trunk and shoulder girdle into the left arm.  The pursuit score indicating upper
arm function is essentially normal on the left side but is substantially reduced on the right.  Inspection of the supination-pronation
data indicates normal left hand function compared to right hand
values measuring less than 1/7th normal.  The lowermost graph shows
the patient's walk index.  The abnormally high values here are due
primarily to the fact that he walked with a prosthesis after suffer-

ing an above-the-knee traumatic amputation of his right leg in 1949. Since thalamotomy often impairs balance, the principal significance of this data is that he did walk well after surgery despite this handicap.

Note in column 2 how dramatically the right resting rigidity is driven negative with the administration of trihexyphenidyl. Even the normal left side is driven considerably further negative. This sign of effective drug therapy is common to a wide variety of agents (Webster, 1966). It can also be seen that even though resting rigidity is significantly decreased, activated rigidity is not. Actually, it increases on the afflicted right side. Considering the other tests briefly, we see arm tremor unchanged, the pursuit score on the right significantly elevated towards normal and the supination-pronation rate doubled but still far from normal value. The 3rd column shows ten days of testing accomplished after trihexy-phenidyl was withdrawn from the placebo capsules unknown to the patient. Note that resting rigidity on the right side has returned to the previous no medication value. The functional tests of pursuit and supination-pronation have decreased but not to their initial low values.

In August of 1964 a left thalamotomy was performed. When the patient returned to our service for additional measurements several weeks later, he had already been re-started on an effective anti-cholinergic drug, this time benztrophine mesylate 4 mg. per day, and, because of the overall excellent results, we did not choose to further manipulate his drug therapy, even though the before and after comparisons are somewhat unsatisfactory. Note that the single most striking consequence of placing a small 6 mm. lesion within the left ventro-lateral nucleus is the reduction of activated rigidity to approximately normal limits. While it is possible that the initiation of benztrophine therapy could have influenced the level of activated rigidity, in our experience we have never seen a decrease in this variable with anticholinergic medication. We would expect that this drug would produce changes similar to the earlier trial with trihexyphenidyl. Following surgery there is also the striking reduction of arm tremor by a factor of approximately 50 to within normal limits and a concomitant gain in right hand function which now has increased to approximately two-thirds of normal. The remaining four columns show averages of multiple tests accomplished in the years 1965, 1966, 1967 and 1968. All of these figures indicate that this patient was substantially and permanently helped by his thalamotomy, and there is no evidence in this four year followup of any tendency towards a recurrence of parkinson symptoms. Clinically this patient remained free of all signs of tremor for as long as he was followed. He recovered all self-care activities fully, including right-sided handwriting. For the next four years he maintained his own home and walked 12 blocks daily without assistance. In 1969 this patient developed diabetic retinopathy secondary to diabetes

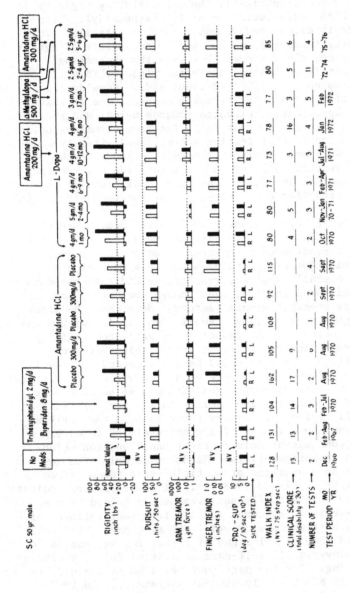

*Figure 2. Relative effectiveness of different therapeutic agents on slowly progressing Parkinson's disease. The relative effectiveness of each therapeutic manipulation is indicated by the downward movement of resting rigidity and the upward movement of the pursuit and pronation-supination scores compared to data in the time period immediately preceding each change of medication. Activated rigidity indicated by the uppermost set of bars is comparatively unresponsive to any therapy. See text for details.*

mellitus which he had had since 1959. This led to a rapid loss of
eyesight. He is now 79 years old and confined to a nursing home.
He is oriented to person and place and is clinically free of tremor
and rigidity. No antiparkinson medications have been given for the
past three years.

Figure 2 shows a ten year longitudinal case study of Parkinson's
disease in which a wide variety of therapeutic agents were conservatively manipulated to successfully maintain function despite a
constantly progressing illness. Before examining this complicated
plot in detail, let us first point out that this moderately advanced
case was initially controlled with anticholinergic therapy for three
years. As that therapy failed, amantadine hydrochloride was tried
with little improvement. When L-dopa was started a very significant
response occurred four to 12 months later. However, 16 months after
initiation of L-dopa therapy, function again began to deteriorate.
At this point methyldopa was added to multiply the L-dopa effect as
well as to decrease the daily L-dopa requirement. From that time on
in 1972, the patient showed evidence of having reached maximum
L-dopa tolerance. We judged this by the appearance some time in
the late morning or mid-afternoon of minimal dystonic movements of
face, tongue, head or limbs. We consider these adventitious movements to be damaging to our patients and we therefore cut back L-dopa
levels whenever they appear. For this reason when L-dopa again began
to fail in late 1972, amantadine was added producing further minimal
benefits which have continued through 1976.

A detailed inspection of the graph will show that this patient
is functioning far above the levels measured 10 years earlier even
though his Parkinson's disease now is markedly advanced. Activated
rigidity, which was slightly above the upper limits of normal in
1966, increased slowly over the first four years, reaching a moderately high level which has been maintained throughout therapy. The
apparent lack of a significant response to the variety of different
drugs administered is striking. By contrast, resting rigidity
decreased, albeit transiently, following the addition of each new
drug. The initial decrease in resting rigidity with anticholinergic
therapy in 1967 was reversed by 1970 due to a substantial further
progression of the underlying disease. The actual progression rate
can be estimated by averaging the right and left pursuit scores
recorded in 1966 before any treatment was started and comparing
this figure to the average pursuit scores measured in 1970 when the
patient was again not on any medication (seven tests done during
three rotations onto placebo amantadine). The pursuit score deterioration rate thus measured shows a yearly decline of 4.2 per cent from
the normal scale value of 100 hits per 50 seconds. At first inspection the two trials on amantadine 300 mg./day in 1970 look insignifi-
cant. However, by averaging the right and left pursuit scores for

each trial on amantadine, we get an average value of 42.5 hits/50 seconds on placebo compared 53.0 on amantadine, a gain of 10.5 per cent. When the same is done for supination-pronation, our figures show 1500 degrees per 10 seconds off-drug compared to 2700 degrees on amantadine, a gain of 17.5 per cent on a normalized scale. These are respectable gains for a very disabled patient who changed from 17 to 9 on our clinical evaluation score (Webster, 1968). The graphic plots of function in Figure 2 still were far from normal values and for this reason amantadine was stopped and L-dopa started in October of 1970. This resulted in very substantial improvement in all aspects of the testing measurements for the next nine months (October, 1970 through April, 1971). Both pursuit and the supination-pronation measurements responded at one month, whereas arm tremor was minimal at four months while resting rigidity reached maximum negativity at nine months. Activated rigidity also declined somewhat during this period but not in proportion to changes in all of the other measurements. At 10-12 months of therapy, many of the L-dopa gains can be seen to start declining and despite the addition of methyldopa and amantadine, this decline persists into 1976. Before leaving Figure 2, comments on the rate of functional decline on L-dopa should be made. By averaging the actual right and left pursuit scores over the initial nine month period of maximum benefit and comparing this figure to the 1975-76 average of four tests, our calculations show an initial pursuit score of 74.0 hits/50 seconds and a final score of 54.5. The time base, measuring from the mid point of the two test periods, is 4.75 years, and this works out to an average rate of decline on L-dopa of 4.1 per cent/year. This is identical to the original rate of decline and strongly suggests that L-dopa is effectively helping an injured neuronal mass to function but is in no way slowing the rate of deterioration of the underlying pathological process. We shall conclude with a brief reference to the clinical status of the patient.

This patient was a 50 year old dairy farmer first examined by us in 1966. He complained of increasing difficulty with his hands and fingers for the previous two years. His handwriting was severely impaired, he required help in dressing, and could no longer mount and operate his farm tractor. Resting tremor and cogwheel rigidity were present in the right arm. Clinically, he was 13/30th totally disabled. On biperiden therapy he recovered enough function to continue his farm work until three years later when the disease again advanced to the point of threatening his livelihood. After changing to L-dopa in 1970, he got along very well until January 1972, when he again felt he might have to sell his farm and retire. With the addition of methyldopa and eventually amantadine, this patient has continued to maintain all self care activities and to operate his farm successfully. Clinical examination shows that he is more than twice as functional as he was prior to any therapy 10 years earlier.

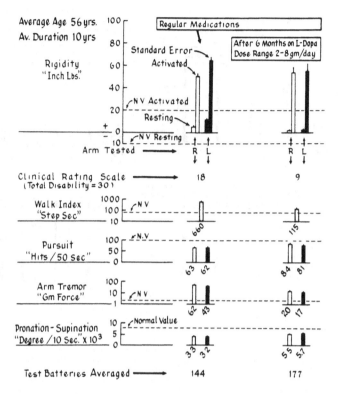

*Figure 3. Relative response of 30 parkinson's patients to L-dopa therapy. Means and standard errors are shown for each test. Normal values for each group are labeled N.V. Note that L-dopa causes significant changes toward normal values in all measures except activated rigidity and right arm tremor.*

Figure 3 shows the averaged results of maximized L-dopa therapy given to 30 parkinsonian patients. A total of 144 test batteries were administered prior to the addition of L-dopa to their regular medications. These results are compared to 177 test batteries given to the same patients after they had been on L-dopa for at least six months and had achieved the highest gains possible short of producing drug toxicity. The entire series of initial measurements improved remarkably except for activated rigidity, which remained essentially unchanged. Paired t-tests on the pre-therapy and post-therapy data indicate that significant ($p < .05$) improvements occurred in all measurements except activated rigidity bilaterally ($p < .2$) and arm tremor on the right side ($p < .1$). Despite the statistical signi-ficance of these changes, it is important to point out that even

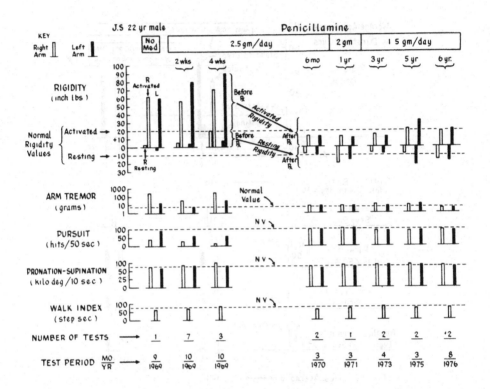

*Figure 4. Extrapyramidal dysfunction in Wilson's disease. Note the very high activated rigidity value, the positive value of resting rigidity, the high right arm tremor, and the very low value of right pursuit testing before penicillamine becomes effective. Six months after starting treatment, all tests became normal and have remained there.*

though major improvements were recorded, none of the averaged measurements returned to normal values.

Figure 4 shows a seven year study of a case of Wilson's disease. This 22 year old utility worker was referred to our clinic in September 1969 because of disabling right arm tremor which had started only two months earlier. On examination he looked very much like a parkinson patient except that he was mentally dull, euphoric, and had a facies unlike that of early parkinsonism. This consisted of a silly grin, forced mouth opening and copious drooling. A well developed Kayser-Fleischer ring was present in both corneas, and ceruloplasm levels were exceedingly low. A diagnosis of Wilson's disease was made and penicillamine therapy was started along with a restrictive copper diet. Inspection of Figure 4 shows only one test battery administered prior to starting penicillamine. These data, however, are relatively unchanged from seven tests administered the

first two weeks of therapy and an additional three tests obtained
after four weeks of therapy.  Actually, we obtained all of these
tests anticipating that penicillamine therapy would have an immediate
effect on the disease.  In retrospect, it can be recognized that no
beneficial improvements occurred within the first month of therapy
and therefore all of the tests given in that period have been
grouped as belonging to the pre-response stage of treatment.  When
we examine these test values we see that activated rigidity, which
initially was very high on both sides, actually increased during the
initial treatments.  This indicated that the disease continued to
evolve even though therapy had been started.  The same is true of
the initial high values of resting rigidity which proceeded to
become more positive in the first month of therapy.  Arm tremor
scores likewise show a progressive deterioration through the first
month starting at values unusually high for Parkinson's disease.
Strangely, the supination-pronation function was not abnormal, but
probably would have deteriorated in time since we have seen such
impairment in other cases of Wilson's disease.  The absence of hand
bradykinesia here is surprising even though the case is an early
one.  We have never seen this degree of extrapyramidal dysfunction
signaled by high levels of activated rigidity, resting rigidity
and arm tremor in parkinson patients without substantial reductions
of supination-pronation.  The patient's walk index likewise was
within normal limits.  This is not at all unusual even in Parkinson's
disease, especially in a younger patient.  The walk index is usually
one of the last functions to begin to deteriorate in Parkinson's
disease.

Now let us turn our attention to the after therapy data in
Figure 4.  The first column shows averages of two tests taken six
months after starting penicillamine therapy.  The profound changes
shown here exceed anything we have previously seen in the L-dopa
treatment of extrapyramidal disease.  Activated rigidity fell below
its upper normal limit (20 inch pounds) bilaterally, and continued
to remain normal until five years later when it minimally exceeded
this limit.  One year later, however, it again was within normal
limits.  Resting rigidity improved from positive values before therapy to significantly negative values after therapy.  These have
continued to be negative throughout the seven year course on penicillamine.  Note how the arm tremor and pursuit score have now
returned to essentially normal limits and remain there.  The supination-pronation data were not abnormal before therapy and have not
become abnormal since therapy.  The same is true of the walk index.

Clinically, this young man was profoundly disabled as indicated
by the introductory remarks.  He continued unchanged until discharged
from the hospital some four weeks after his penicillamine therapy had
been started.  He was then referred to an outpatient clinic for
continuing care; however, he did not return to our laboratory until
six months later.  At that time his clinical examination showed no
signs of Wilson's disease.  The patient's tremor had disappeared.

He was alert and his facial expression was normal.  All drooling
had ceased.  The patient had returned to his utility job of lineman
and was functioning adequately.  Two years after the onset of penicillamine therapy, the Kayser-Fleischer rings cleared and have not
returned.  He continues to perfrom well at this job even today.
Overall, we believe this represents a well documented case of
incipient Wilson's disease which now is completely controlled by the
daily administration of penicillamine.  This in itself is not unusual.
Similar cases have been reported and followed for even longer periods
(*Sternlieb and Scheinberg, 1968*).  What is unusual here is that we
did obtain important extrapyramidal deficit measurements at the
height of the disease process, and that all of these measurements
returned to normal as excessive copper deposits in the putamen were
gradually lowered by penicillamine.

## DISCUSSION

Although the patients in our study made substantial gains on
L-dopa therapy in the alleviation of resting rigidity, tremor and
bradykinesia, they failed to show comparable reductions in activated
rigidity.  This finding contrasts sharply with the lasting reduction
in activated rigidity achieved by penicillamine treatment of Wilson's
disease and by thalamotomy in parkinsonism.  Although we have no
clear explanation for these divergent findings, we believe they
indicate a fundamental limitation in the control of Parkinson's
disease by L-dopa therapy alone.  The failure of this therapy to
appreciably reduce activated rigidity suggests that the underlying
pathological process common to most forms of Parkinson's disease
may not be entirely controllable by this medication.

What is the cause of resting and activated rigidity?  It has been
known for some time that the plastic resistance to passive movement
is related to the presence of electromyographic activity (EMG) that
shifts from flexor to extensor muscles as passive motion changes
from extension to flexion (*Denny-Brown, 1960; Rushworth, 1961;
Andrews et al., 1972*).  We have confirmed this finding in several
patients by recording from the biceps and triceps brachii during
tests for rigidity.  Positive rigidity, both resting and activated,
was associated in all cases with a discharge occurring in either
the biceps or triceps or both muscles during those portions of the
cycles in which these muscles were stretched.  Negative rigidity
in both normal subjects and patients was found to be associated with
the opposite pattern, i.e., activation during the shortening phase
of passive movement.  These data do not permit us to state whether
the discharge of these muscles is reflex-mediated.  However, large
stretch reflexes, apparently conducted by long-loop pathways (*Tatton
and Lee, 1975*) and involuntary shortening reactions (*Denny-Brown,
1960; Rushworth, 1961; Andrews et al., 1972*) have been recorded in
rigid parkinsonians.  Similar shortening reactions have been described in normal subjects (*Landau et al., 1966; Andrews et al., 1972*),

consistent with the present findings that normals exhibit negative resting rigidity. The possibility of a common basis for activated and resting rigidity may explain why both forms of rigidity are simultaneously alleviated by thalamotomy. The finding that L-dopa affects resting rigidity to a greater extent than activated rigidity would therefore suggest that its action may be one of modification of the threshold for the release of an exaggerated EMG response to stretch, rather than of modification of the basic circuit involved in its generation.

The long-term success of thalamotomy shown in Figure 1 illustrates the potential benefit of surgery for certain well-selected cases. As stated earlier, this case was in all respects an ideal one, the symptoms being unilateral and slowly progressive (*Cooper et al., 1968; Van Buren et al., 1973*). The finding that resting and activated rigidity as well as bradykinesia were reduced to normal levels by surgery implies that these parkinsonism symptoms likely resulted from excessive or disordered discharge in pathways interrupted by the procedure. In support of this view, when we compared the outcome of 75 parkinsonian operations to 10 thalamotomies done for intention tremor in multiple sclerosis, the acute results in Parkinsonians were similar to the data presented in Figure 1, while the patients with multiple sclerosis generally had *decreased* motor function and less reduction of rigidity following the operation.

A comparison of the data for L-dopa therapy presented in Figures 2 and 3 with the thalamotomy data in Figure 1 illustrates the essential differences in these two forms of therapy. While both therapies produced reductions in resting rigidity, tremor and bradykinesia, only thalamotomy alleviated activated rigidity as well. Although the generality of this finding has been confirmed in 75 thalamotomy patients (*Webster, 1969*) and in over 100 patients whom we have followed on L-dopa (unpublished observations), two exceptions have been observed. In certain patients with mild forms of Parkinson's disease, L-dopa in therapeutic doses is also capable of reducing activated rigidity. In more advanced cases, patients receiving near toxic doses of L-dopa have also occasionally shown some reduction in this measure. (*One of these unusually sensitive cases is discussed by Webster, 1972*).

The complete reversibility of extrapyramidal symptoms in Wilson's disease illustrated in Figure 4 suggests that the pathological process underlying these symptoms is also reversible. We have never seen this kind of result in the treatment of Parkinson's disease with presently available drugs. Although L-dopa remains the single most effective medication for parkinsonism, we believe that it does not fundamentally reverse the underlying pathological process which continues to progress slowly, as illustrated in Figure 2. Rather this drug seems to mask over most of the symptoms of the still progressing disease process. A notable exception to this masking is the presence of activated rigidity, which appears to be little affected by L-dopa at appropriate therapeutic doses in most cases.

# REFERENCES

Webster, D.D. (1972). Clinical aspects of rigidity. *In* Parkinson's
    Disease: Rigidity, Akinesia, Behavior (Siegfried, J., Ed.)
    pp. 66-92, Hans Huber, Bern, Stuttgart, Vienna.
Webster, D.D. (1959). A method of measuring the dynamic characteris-
    tics of muscle rigidity, strength, and tremor in the upper
    extremity. *IRE Trans. on Medical Electronics 6*, 159-164.
Webster, D.D. (1966). Rigidity in extrapyramidal disease. The
    Second Symposium on Parkinson's Disease. *J. Neurosurg., Suppl.*
    Part II. 299-307.
Webster, D.D. (1968). A critical analysis of disability in Parkin-
    son's Disease. *Mod. Treat. 5*, 257-282.
Sternlieb, I. and Scheinberg, I.H. (1968). Birth Defects Original
    Article Series, *4* (No. 2), 122-125.
Denny-Brown, D. (1960). Diseases of the basal ganglia. Their rela-
    tion to disorders of movement. *Lancet ii*, 1099-1105, 1155-1162.
Rushworth, G. (1961). The gamma system in Parkinsonism. *Int. J.*
    *Neurol. 2*, 34-50.
Andrews, C.J., Burke, D. and Lance, J.W. (1972). The response to
    muscle stretch and shortening in Parkinsonian rigidity. *Brain*
    *95*, 795-812.
Tatton, W.G. and Lee, R.G. (1975). Evidence for abnormal long-loop
    reflexes in rigid Parkinsonian patients. *Brain Res. 100*, 671-
    676.
Landau, W.M., Struppler, A., and Mehls, O. (1966). A comparative elec-
    tromyographic study of the reactions to passive movement in
    Parkinsonism and in normal subjects. *Neurology (Minneap.) 16*,
    34-48.
Cooper, I.S., Riklan, M., Stellar, S., Waltz, J.M., Levita, E.,
    Ribera, V.A., and Zimmerman, J. (1968). A multidisciplinary
    investigation of neurosurgical rehabilitation in bilateral
    parkinsonism. *J. Amer. Geriat. Soc. 16*, 1177-1306.
Van Buren, J.M., Li, C.L., Shapiro, D.Y., Henderson, W.G., and
    Sadowsky, D.A. (1973). A qualitative and quantitative evalua-
    tion of Parkinsonians three to six years following thalamotomy.
    *Confin. neurol. 35*, 202-235.
Webster, D.D. (1959). A method of measuring the dynamic characteris-
    tics of muscle rigidity, strength, and tremor in the upper
    extremity. *IRE Trans. on Medical Electronics 6*, 159-164.
Webster, D.D. (1966). Rigidity in extrapyramidal disease. The
    Second Symposium on Parkinson's Disease. *J. Neurosurg., Suppl.*
    Part II. 299-307.

Webster, D.D. (1968).  A critical analysis of disability in Parkin-
    son's Disease.  *Mod. Treat. 5*, 257-282.
Webster, D.D. (1969).  Dynamic evaluation of thalamotomy in Parkinson's
    Disease: Analysis of 75 consecutive cases.  *In* Third Symposium
    on Parkinson's Disease (Gillingham, F.J. and Donaldson, I.M.L.,
    Eds) pp. 266-271.  E. & S. Livingstone, Ltd., Edinburgh and
    London.
Webster, D.D. (1972).  Clinical aspects of rigidity.  *In* Parkinson's
    Disease: Rigidity, Akinesia, Behavior (Siegfried, J., Ed.)
    pp. 66-92, Hans Huber, Bern, Stuttgart, Vienna.

# SUBJECT INDEX

Acetylcholine, 14, 256
Adenylate cyclase, 184
d-Amphetamine, 32, 39, 41,
      209, 212, 287
L-Amphetamine, 210
Apomorphine, 42, 59
Athetosis, 11

Bradykinesia, 47, 65, 111
Brain stem stimulation, 235
Bromocriptine, 28, 51, 59,
      60, 273

Caudate stimulation, 73
Cerebellocorticospinal pro-
  jection system, 69, 77
Cerebrospinal fluid, 23, 268
Chlordiazepoxide, 46, 47
Chlorpromazine, 31, 32, 226
Chorea, 161
Clozapine, 194

Dibenzoxazepine, 186
Dilantin®, 103, 106
Dopa decarboxylase, 256
Dopa decarboxylase inhibitors
      carbidopa, 39, 42,
      50, 53, 158
      benserazide, 50,
      223, 269
Dopamine, 184, 185, 246, 249,
      256, 257

Dopamine β-hydroxylase, 168,
    174
Dyskinesias
  L-dopa-induced, 28, 29, 50
  tardive dyskinesia, 30, 40,
     163, 169, 170
  choreiform dyskinesia, 44,
    47
  amphetamine-induced, 215
Dystonia, 159, 160, 169

Ethyl alcohol, 160
Epilepsy, 63
Essential tremor, 160

GABA, 14, 161, 261
Gilles de la Tourette syn-
    drome, 198
Globus pallidus, 73

Haloperidol, 32, 186, 200,
    204
Hemiballism, 111, 113, 162
Homovanillic acid, 23, 248,
    249, 257, 271,273
Huntington's disease
  deanol, 172
  akinetic form, 25
  GABA, 161
  levodopa, 204
  lithium carbonate, 172
6-Hydroxydopa, 14
6-Hydroxydopamine, 14

Printed in the United States
by Baker & Taylor Publisher Services